The Practical *Guide to*

Candida

Including the UK directory of complementary
practitioners who treat candida albicans holistically

Jane McWhirter MA (Hons) MC MMCA

All Hallows House Foundation

First published in 1995
by ALL HALLOWS HOUSE FOUNDATION
All Hallows House Centre for Natural Health and Counselling
Idol Lane, London EC3R 5DD

The author and publisher of this book and directory cannot be held liable for any errors and omissions, or actions that may be taken as a consequence of using it, nor actions taken or recommendations made by any practitioners or doctors listed. No health claims for specific products are made or intended, and nothing in this book should be used as substitutes for medical advice.

Cover design by PHD and James Fraser
Typesetting by Per Kaasen and Dr John Miller
Printed and bound by Fisher Print Services

British Library Cataloguing - in Publication Data:
A catalogue record or this book is
available from the British Library

ISBN: 0 952 6286 0 0

FOR FURTHER COPIES OF THIS BOOK PLEASE SEND £4.50 plus £1.25 p&p to:
Green Library, 9 Rickett Street, London SW6 1RU

ALL PROCEEDS FROM THE SALE OF THIS BOOK WILL GO TOWARDS RESEARCH ON THE HOLISTIC AND CLINICAL TREATMENT OF CANDIDIASIS

This book is printed on environmentally friendly paper.

The Practical Guide to Candida

including the UK directory of complementary practitioners who treat candida albicans holistically

Jane McWhirter was born in London in 1959. She was educated at the North London Collegiate School, Marlborough College and the University of St Andrews where she got an honours degree in Fine Arts. It was not until she put her back out in 1984 and received treatment from a McTimoney chiropractor that she knew she wanted a career in complementary medicine. She trained to be a McTimoney chiropractor in Oxford, qualified in 1989 and now has a busy and fulfilling practice. In 1990 she opened a multi-disciplinary complementary clinic, All Hallows House in the City of London. Here 16 like-minded practitioners, including two doctors, work as a team using an integrated approach to health and preventative care, for individuals and City companies.

Jane's interest in candidiasis and gut dysbiosis began in 1992 when such a high proportion of their clients were presenting with the symptom patterns of it and responding so well to holistic treatment. The scale of the problem and the fact that GPs do not generally recognise it became quite clear in October 1994, when a tiny mention of their Candida Support Group in the Daily Mail produced 700 enquiries from all over the UK within a fortnight. They were all asking where they could get treatment and advice.

She is married to David Lorimer, the Director of the Scientific and Medical Network and they are expecting their first baby in October 1995.

CONTENTS

II

ACKNOWLEDGEMENTS

There are so many people to thank for their practical and moral support in putting this guide and directory together. For the constant love and inspiration from the wonderful team of practitioners at All Hallows House, but especially Gillian Hamer, our nutritionist, who first alerted me to how debilitating a condition candidiasis can be, and how dramatically people can improve with the right advice and treatment. She has encouraged and advised me all the way. But equally to the sufferers who have come here for treatment, or written to us, and especially to Anya Harris whose idea it was to start the Candida Support Group and the other regulars who came to the Group for the first year. We have learnt at least as much about candidiasis and treating it from our remarkable sufferers as we have from books and doctors. Stephen Mossbacher and Angela Holden from Wild Oats gave us enthusiastic help with the Group and introduced us to the feast of foods one can have on the diet. Thanks also to Hazel Courtney whose mention of the Group in the Daily Mail triggered the massive response that confirmed our hunch that candidiasis is indeed the silent epidemic of the nineties.

We all owe a huge debt to Leon Chaitow for his excellent book which first gave sufferers and practitioners in the UK clues and answers back in 1985. I spoke to him before starting the directory and he has given it his whole-hearted encouragement. This was echoed by numerous practitioners, both medically qualified and otherwise, who sent messages of thanks and encouragement. Once their entries started to come in for the directory, Per Kaasen, our wizard on the database, simply took over. It would not have happened at all without him. He also helped turn the guide into the shape you now see, with some invaluable advice from Dr John Miller. James Fraser and Barry Hurd designed the cover in All Hallows' colours.

I learnt a great deal about candida from Dr John Stirling, Dr Nigel Plummer and Dr Ilyias, Rhaya Jordan, Dr Anthony Fox, Dr Alan Hibberd and Dr Ole van Hauen Drucker, all of whom have found in their clinical experience that the holistic, integrated approach to health is what works in the long run. Also thanks to Rohit Meta whose knowledge of the products is as good as the invaluable mail order service he offers at the Nutricentre. Gill Jacobs was been a tower of strength in the final (and most difficult) stages and her encouragement led to the setting up of the national network of support groups. Thank you also to Sarah Stacey for her unerring quality of advice and for her contacts in the media, and to Green Library for handling the distribution. Martin and Yvonne Arber have very kindly let me use their wonderful cartoons from InterAction, the Journal for Action for

M.E. Martin has suffered with M.E and candida himself for several years, which is why he hits the target every time! You'll agree it makes all the difference to be able to have a laugh about things when the going gets tough. Details are in Appendix 1 if you would like a copy of the whole book. (All proceeds go to local M.E. support groups).

In publishing this ourselves, I have to thank the trustees of the All Hallows House Foundation. It means at least £2 from every guide and directory sold will be able to go straight to research where it is so badly needed, but it also means I have not had the back up of professional editors and proof readers. So I am very grateful to friends and colleagues who have helped, particularly Chris Thomson. Last and most of all, my late mother Carole, for breast feeding me and bringing me up to love cooking and "real" food, and David Lorimer, my darling husband and eagle-eyed proof reader.

INTRODUCTION

It sounds funny to say how glad I am to "meet" you through a book, but I have met so many wonderful friends, both sufferers and practitioners through our work with candida, that I feel I'm meeting you too. The thought that I will be meeting thousands of you through this guide is a real joy, but also a huge responsibility. I have heard too many horror stories from people who have been given poor or conflicting advice, to underestimate the need for clear, simple and accurate advice. It really needs six months to begin to do justice to this subject, but I have done my best in the little time I have. I see clients for about 30 hours a week, run a natural health clinic and I am expecting our first baby in October. Strictly speaking, I am not qualified to write about candida, being a humble McTimoney chiropractor rather than a nutritionist or naturopath. But since I suspect most practitioners learn far more about candida from sufferers than from any formal training, perhaps I am better qualified than many. In any event, if you find anything in the guide or directory that you feel is wrong or misleading, or missing, please do tell me. We want this book to be a living thing and we need your help to make it grow. We have therefore decided to print fewer copies of this first edition so that it can be updated and reprinted in the near future, probably in the spring of 1996.

Let us begin at the beginning and tell you how this guide happened. In March 1990, I opened a Natural Health clinic in a wonderful Wren spire in the City of London. It had two main aims. The first was that the practitioners should work as a team, exchanging knowledge and experience freely for our own professional development, but above all for the good of our clients. The second was to make the benefits of natural therapies available to key influencers and decision makers (which is why we are in the City). In the first aim, I think we have succeeded, and this has been crucial in our success in treating chronic, multi-symptom syndromes like candida. The second aim is unfolding slowly but surely with major City companies waking up to the power of natural therapies in combating and preventing stress.

From the start, Gillian Hamer, our marvellous nutritionist, was diagnosing quite a few people with candidiasis and treating them successfully. Later, I found that some of my chronic back pain sufferers who had also seen her were miraculously out of pain for the first time in years. So I started to look into it. Then after a particularly stressful time, Gillian suspected that I too had candida. I was most indignant! Like all the practitioners at All Hallows who believe in practising what we preach, I thought my diet and lifestyle were exemplary. My tendency to work 12 hours a day plus might bear some improvement perhaps - but I have always done that. The key fact about the anti-candida diet is that it cannot do anyone any harm, and it seems to do most people a lot of good. So I thought "physician heal thyself - you'd better get on with it!" It was only when I started feeling much better a week later that I realised how lousy I had been feeling before. Mercifully, I was able to get things back in order after a couple of months, though I still find I am happier without wheat or cows' milk. In retrospect, I am sure that it was candida and food intolerance that blighted my existence in my early twenties at university when, like many of my friends, I was simply unable to keep my weight where I wanted it, and my rollercoaster eating habits (craving sugar and bread which I didn't even like) were preoccupying me on a pretty permanent basis and completely eroding my self-esteem. This may sound familiar to you.

In March last year (1994) Anya Harris, one of Gillian's clients, said we must start a support group for candida sufferers. We certainly had plenty by that time, and the numbers were on the increase. But would people suffering with exhaustion - most of whom were just about managing to hold down very demanding jobs by their fingernails - ever give up their precious time and come to such a group? Of course, Anya was right. Within a couple of weeks we had a full meeting room of 15 candida sufferers every third Thursday sharing their experiences, swapping tips, learning more about the problem, and feasting on sugar and yeast-free goodies together. By 11pm, Gillian and I were dropping but these people who were supposed to be suffering from chronic fatigue did not want to go home! You would not believe how 15 people, all supposed to be suffering from the same thing, could have such totally different stories to tell. Anya's illustrates the sort of trouble sufferers have with their GPs and employers. She had been struggling to keep going for two years when she read Leon Chaitow's book *Could Yeast be Your Problem?* It was quite clear to her that this was why she had been feeling so terrible, while at the same time being told there was nothing wrong with her. So she went her GP and told him about this. "Oh candida" he said, "It's a figment of the imagination of the upwardly mobile." Most women in this all too common situation burst into tears as soon as they get out of the surgery, but not Anya. She slammed Leon's book down on the GP's desk and said "Read that. I'm coming back to see you on Monday morning." She had been wearing shorts and a tee-shirt, but next time she went back in her City suit, fully made up, high heels (she is five foot nothing) and shoulder pads. To give him his due, her GP had read the book, and he admitted "You're right. It does sound as if you have candidiasis, but I'm afraid there's not a lot I can do to help you - but let me know if I can." He was actually very helpful in her battle with her employers, who were rather less sympathetic.

Then in October, Hazel Courtney, whose column "Alternatives" in the Daily Mail is so popular, got to hear about the Group. She wrote a three line mention and within a week we had received about 700 letters from desperate people all over the UK, all asking for more information and where they could get proper help locally. We seemed to have an epidemic on our hands. Since then, other journalists have rung. There have been other mentions of the group and we have sent basic information to over 4000 enquirers. Many journalists wanted to do major features on candida, but I pleaded with them not to do so just yet, as it would unleash such frustration on an even greater scale.

Whether you have two symptoms or twenty-two, candida is something which you should not treat by yourself. So the obvious answer was to compile a directory, for the whole of the UK, of complementary practitioners experienced in treating it. The other problem was how to get GPs to recognise the existence of candida. Since there is no definitive black and white test to indicate whether or not someone has it (mainly because it is present in all of us) and because there has been virtually no research done in this country, you cannot blame them for thinking it is a trendy fad. Having set up the directory, we would then organise some research and audits, but where would we get the money to pay for them? It is very unusual to get funding for medical research unless someone else has already done some in the same area and got it published, so we would have to raise the money ourselves. Why not publish the directory through our registered charity and put the funds into research and further training for practitioners? Simple! That is exactly what we are going to do. For every book sold, about £3 will go straight into the research kitty. In fact, subject to ethical approval, we have also won an award from the Research Council for Complementary Medicine to do a pilot study.

New books on candidiasis are coming out all the time. The second edition of Gill Jacobs' lovely book came out last December; Angela Kilmartin of cystitis fame has just written one, while Leon Chaitow, the UK pioneer in this field, is bringing out his second edition soon, which I am very much looking forward to seeing. They each have very different approaches and I hope you will look at them all. But all the books in the world are not going to get round the fact that you need a good practitioner to help you as well. Having heard hundreds of people's bitter experience, I firmly believe that this is essential in all but a few exceptional cases. The trouble with candida is that it is such a tenacious and opportunistic little so-and-so that you have to address all fronts simultaneously. Getting three quarters of the treatment right means you probably will not crack it completely and it will just come back. We have seen so many people who had spent months or years of their lives and literally hundreds of pounds on supplements (and some on treatment too) before getting the right help. And others who have spent years seeking and failing to find a diagnosis. How many times have we heard "Oh I *wish* I'd come and seen you years ago".

But a practitioner cannot do it all for you. If you are aiming for a full and permanent recovery, then there are no quick fixes - unless you want to take an anti-fungal drug (e.g. Nystatin) indefinitely, as people find that the symptoms come back (sometimes even worse) as soon as they stop taking it. If there is one thing that I hope this guide helps you to realise, it is that you have to take responsibility for your own health. We each have a little "ecosystem" in our gut that is nothing short of miraculous - when it is in balance. Yours, probably through no fault of your own, has got out of sync, but ultimately you are the only one that can make it strong and resilient again, and for some of you this may take some time.

You will need to ask for help. Many candida sufferers are the self-reliant types who find this very difficult. But you will find there is plenty of help around. You will experience the tremendous power of natural therapies, some of them using wisdom that is thousands of years old, to help your body heal and re-balance itself. And hopefully your practitioner will become a wise and trusted guide and teacher on your journey, with your family, friends, health food shop manager and fellow sufferers in your support group if you join one, all playing key roles.

The second thing that I hope you understand from this guide is that this game has common patterns, but no fixed rules. You are a totally unique individual and what is true for one person may not be so for you, so you simply have to learn what suits you. The quickest and easiest way to do that is to learn, or re-learn, how to listen to what your body is telling you all the time - but to do this, you have to clear your communication channels first.

How quickly and easily your particular journey passes and where it takes you, will depend on your attitude. As you will see in chapters 1 and 9, a positive attitude will have a measurable, physical effect on your body's ability to fight the candida. We practitioners reckon we can spot the ones who will be bouncing back into the clinic within a few months, glowing with their new found energy, thanking us for changing their lives (we always remind them that *they* did it). They are usually the ones who are so absolutely fed up with life passing them by, they say "I'll do *anything*" and they just go for it. Mary, for instance, is a lovely Irish lady of 46 who runs her own highly successful management consultancy and has a four-year-old little girl. She had been getting migraines lasting four days at a time, and heavy drugs were not really helping but just making her feel like a zombie the rest of the time. I discussed what would fit into her schedule and what she was prepared to do (*"anything!"*) so we agreed on the combination of the candida programme and McTimoney chiropractic, as (like so many migraine sufferers) the bones in her neck and upper back were in a real pickle. For someone as busy as she is, it was amazing how she went for it. She never looked back for an instant. One of most difficult times is usually at parties, but not for Mary. If any of her friends started the "Poor you" routine, "I don't know how you can bear to give up bread/chocolate/wine...." they were firmly shut up with "Oh stop whinging! If you only knew how much *better* I'm feeling - it is not a penance or a deprivation in the least. It is a complete joy! You'd think I had to give them up for ever the way you are going on - it'll only be for a few months." So if ever you feel sorry for yourself, or if your friends start up with the "poor you" bit, remember Mary!

No one is pretending this will be easy, but I hope this guide will make it much less difficult. So many ex-sufferers, once they are completely better - usually better than they have been for years - say afterwards that they are almost glad they had candida since they have changed for the better or learnt so much about themselves on the way, and that life is somehow richer. But whatever happens, remember you are not alone. Thousands have beaten candida before you and tens of thousands will be tackling it with you.

So Good Luck and Good Health!

Jane McWhirter

Jane McWhirter

A NOTE TO PRACTITIONERS

This guide has been written for sufferers, but even if it only saves you some of the considerable time needed to explain everything to individual clients and to give them constant encouragement, I hope it will help you too. We hope that the major supplement suppliers will stock copies so you can have one sent to your new patients with their first batch of supplements.

As you know, there is quite a bit of conflicting information out there on gut dysbiosis and how best to treat it. I have relied on advice and personal clinical experience rather than academic theories, so if your clinical experience differs, do please let me know. I have also emphasised that every practitioner has their individual style and experience, so I hope you do not get anyone complaining "oh but that's not what the book said."

What next?
New material, research, and products are coming out every week and we want this guide and directory to be a "living thing" that grows with feedback and new ideas and information. We are therefore printing fewer copies so that an updated edition of both the directory and guide can come out sooner. We are aiming for the spring of 1996. In the meantime, Gill Jacobs and I will be editing a newsletter for practitioners. Please send us any material, ideas, research, product news and feedback you have for the newsletter and so the next edition of this guide can be improved. Please also encourage all of your colleagues who you respect to send for an application form for the directory.

This little venture has highlighted a host of other needs of candida sufferers and the medical world and, with help, we are going to try to meet them, including a practitioners' newsletter, clinical audits, grants for research - your research if you will do it.

If you are not in this directory and would like to be, please send a C5 s.a.e. to Candida Directory, All Hallows House, Idol Lane, London EC3R 5DD for an application form. Depending on the number of new entries, supplements to the directory will be printed every two months until another edition needs to be printed. You will also receive the information mentioned at the back of the guide.

A NOTE TO GPs

The first man to publish substantially on the overgrowth of candida albicans, Dr Orion Truss, called his book "the Missing Diagnosis". That was in 1979, but as long as medicine is pathology-driven, candidiasis (or gut dysbiosis as it should more properly be referred to) and other underlying syndromes will continue to be missed. More seriously, when it is misdiagnosed, the treatment that is given for the presenting symptom can make the underlying condition even worse and more difficult to clear. Many GPs have told me that candidiasis is a 'trendy fad' that will pass like all the others. However its predisposing factors include the overuse of antibiotics, a junk diet and others that are typical of our modern industrialised lifestyles, so the timing of this syndrome makes sense. We have a hunch that it is no exaggeration to call candidiasis "the silent epidemic of the nineties" - and hope to start to show this in our research and audits. In the meantime, we believe that a great deal of misery on the patients' part and 'heartsink' (and money) on yours could be spared if you will for the moment at least suspend your disbelief, keep an open mind and read on.

We appreciate that it can be difficult to be presented with a syndrome with such diverse symptoms, and for which there is no definitive test. We are also aware that until more research is done in the UK, you can be forgiven for dismissing candida. This is precisely why this guide is being published through a registered charity, so that all the proceeds can go straight back into research. We are delighted that, subject to ethical approval, we have also been given a First Rung Award to do a pilot study by the Research Council for Complementary Medicine. We are also doing a trial in a fund holding practice working with the partners there to diagnose and treat cases of candidiasis. The statistical analysis will compare cost and number of GP visits and SF36 (quality of life) before and after treatment and should be ready for publication by the middle of 1996.

In the meantime, we hope that this directory provides a means of contacting well qualified practitioners who are experienced in treating gut dysbiosis, and that you will refer a patient or two and see how they get on. We also hope that you will consider getting involved in our research, audits and cost comparisons. (Please contact All Hallows House for details.)

I am not making a penny out of this and would not have made the effort unless I was convinced that there are thousands more people out there who can regain their health and quality of life like the hundreds we have seen. Patients cannot all be imagining it when they say that their waist grows by 4" and they put on 3lb after one piece of toast and Marmite, or that they wake up exhausted and aching all over after 9 hours sleep, and then find that they have all their energy back after less than a month on the programme. We have heard many stories about what doctors have said to their patients. A 5'6" woman who had put on 5 stone in the 6 months after being prescribed the Pill for period pains was told "but girls often put on weight at your age". A nurse who had given up hope of having children had a hysterectomy when she was 38 to cure her Endometriosis and found that her pain, bloating and fatigue became even worse after the operation. She was told "it's all part of being a woman. You'll have to learn to live with it."

Some of the most likely presenting symptoms are:

- Recurrent thrush or cystitis, PMS, Endometriosis, prostatitis

- IBS

- headaches

- depression, anxiety,

- asthma

- fungal and allergic skin complaints

- chronic back / neck pain with no obvious physical cause

- unable to lose weight

- hypoglycaemia

- in children - recurrent ENT infections and hyperactivity

The most common indicators that candidiasis / gut dysbiosis may be an underlying factor are:

- grey, dull quality to skin, often with dark rings under the eyes - generally toxic-looking

- abdominal pain, bloating, flatulence and/or heart burn. IBS-type symptoms, a noticeable change in type of stool and frequency of motion

- some patients look puffy and overweight

- waking up tired even after 9+ hours sleep, constant lethargy or energy dips

- chronic aches and stiffness, often feeling "ill all over"

- food cravings, particularly sugar, bread, alcohol and chocolate

- fuzzy-headedness, memory lapses, poor concentration

- allergies, sensitivities to fumes and food intolerances

HOW TO USE THIS BOOK.

Every one of you picking up this guide will have done so at a different stage in your journey towards being free from candida or gut dysbiosis. Probably only two thirds of it or less will be appropriate to you - but which two thirds will vary.

1. Put yourself in a calm frame of mind when reading, so you can "listen" to what is right for your body and you as an individual. Remember you are doing this for yourself and nobody else.

2. Be selective and discerning, and remember that this is going to take some time and that you can only take one step at a time.

3. Have a pencil or highlighter as you read. Tick the bits that feel like priorities for you and mark any queries.

4. If negative feelings come up or you find yourself making excuses, make a note of them. Just leave them there and review them later.

5. Scan the list of contents and mark your key chapters. You do not have to read the whole thing, or in the order written.

7. Record and score your symptoms now and date them (See chapter 2). You will be surprised how much you have improved when you look back at them.

8. *The baseline treatment in Chapter 5 is for everyone,* but it is not always necessarily the thing to start with. Don't rush in, be prepared before you start.

9. Please let us know how we can improve the directory and guide.

CHAPTER 1.

WHAT IS CANDIDA AND HOW CAN IT AFFECT US?

Candida is short for **Candida albicans,** one of the most common of the many types of yeasts and parasites which live on the lining *(mucosa)* of the gut *(gastro intestinal tract)*. As long as your gut is healthy, the candida is harmless. Over the last 30 years, a combination of factors such as the over-use of antibiotics, our diet, stress and pollution, has changed the environment in the guts of many people in the industrialised world into one in which yeasts can flourish. The toxins they produce and the damage done to the gut lining can cause a devastating list of apparently unrelated symptoms that commonly includes fatigue, abdominal bloating and pain, food sensitivities and cravings, but can also range from athlete's foot to depression, irritable bowel diseases to recurrent thrush and cystitis, and a damaged immune system. (See Chapter 2 for a full list.) The important thing to understand is that *candidiasis* (overgrowth of *candida albicans)* is symptomatic of and part of a general imbalance in the gut (known as *gut dysbiosis)*.

When the whole digestive system and gut wall is out of balance and damaged, the hormonal, immune and nervous systems are also affected - in fact the whole body-mind. Some doctors are moving towards the conviction that gut dysbiosis and the subsequent suppression of the immune system, is involved in many of the 'mystery' diseases that have become so much more common over the last 30-40 years. These include the irritable bowel diseases, rheumatoid arthritis and chronic fatigue syndrome (M.E.). Also the recurrent infections such as middle-ear infection in children and cystitis and thrush in women. Some are now agreeing with doctors working back in the 30's and 40's such as Josef Issels and Max Gerson and think that in some cases, fungal infections are a precursor to cancer.

The silent epidemic of the nineties'?

At a much lower level, and thanks to our modern industrialised diet and lifestyles, and the inappropriate use of antibiotics, candidiasis has become alarmingly common, particularly among women, who make up about 60% of all sufferers, with men and children making up the other 20% each. Dr Trowbridge, working in the States, wrote in 1986 that it affects at least one-third of the population, that is over half of all women in the urban areas of industrialised countries. (Trowbridge 1986)

Geoffrey Cannon, in his excellent new study of the pros and cons of antibiotics, *SUPERBUG, Nature's Revenge, Why Antibiotics Can Breed Disease* documents examples of clear links between the increasing use of antibiotics from the sixties onwards, and drastically increased incidence of certain diseases - all of which we observe are closely associated with candidiasis.

"The second most common use of antibiotics in the UK is for urinary tract and bladder infections, notably cystitis...The urinary tract should be sterile, but nowadays, around two and a half million women in the UK suffer from cystitis in any one year, and about half of all women are sufferers at some time in their lives. Of these, around 100,000 are estimated to be 'problem patients', with symptoms recurring four or more times a year. In the USA it is reckoned that the cost of treating cystitis is around $2 billion a year.

"Irritable bowel syndrome is at some time now suffered by up to one third of the British people, and by twice a many women as men. Commonly the disease starts early in life and never clears up.....The number of British children under the age of sixteen suffering from Crohn's disease tripled between the 1960s and the 1980s.

Rheumatoid arthritis (affecting mostly women) and ankylosing spondilitis (severe stiffness and degeneration in the lower spine affecting mostly men from their twenties) now afflict up to two million people in Britain. They were very rare before the War.

"Middle-ear inflammation is now very common, afflicting around on in five British children under the age of four every year...this is one of a number of childhood diseases, such as asthma, childhood diabetes and eczema, mow much more common in the UK that they were in the early twentieth century."

Geoffrey Cannon also cites a study done by Dr Hunter at Adenbrokes Hospital in Cambridge in 1985, involving 113 women who had hysterectomies (removal of the womb). 74 were given antibiotics (metronidazole) as routine prophpylaxis ('just in case', to prevent other infections) and 39 were not. Within 6 weeks, 12 of the 74 had developed irritable bowels; whereas only one of the 39 had similar symptoms.

Most of the diseases mentioned above are classified as 'functional', which is medical code for 'We can't find anything physically wrong.' As Geoffrey Cannon says, "Candidiasis is a controversial disease. Doctors don't understand it."

But in 1986, the *Journal of American Medical Association* carried a signed leading article entitled *"Is there an epidemic of chronic candidiasis in our midst?"* It began:

There is a growing underground of public controversy surrounding the reputed presence of a 'new epidemic'. This epidemic involves chronic candidiasis, a condition in which there is an overgrowth of and systemic invasion by the yeast organism *Candida albicans*. The proponents indicate that non-specific symptoms such as fatigue, intestinal gas, depression, muscle aches, constipation, diarrhoea, loss of sexual desire and pre-menstrual syndrome are but a few of the signals that one may have chronic candidiasis.

So why do doctors not recognise candidiasis?
Fungal infections have been recognised in very ill people since Hippocrates if not before. Today, the medical profession generally accepts that candidiasis is common in AIDS patients and others whose immune systems have been very badly damaged, and in those who are on immuno-suppressant drugs (transplant patients for instance). But most doctors do not recognise it as being at the root of a host of other more everyday symptoms *outside* the gut, vagina or throat. This is partly because two areas that have been comparatively little studied and therefore barely taught in the medical schools are nutrition, and the human intestinal flora and the *beneficial* roles these bacteria play in the health of our whole body-mind.

One of the main problems is that the symptoms are so diverse and vary so much between individuals that patterns are not obvious. Many women suffer from candidiasis miserably for years without ever having thrush or cystitis, so their GPs do not recognise any link. Because it is not generally considered serious nor that common, no statistics on a mass scale have yet been collated. Only a very little research has been done in the UK - partly because it is a syndrome that is so difficult to define clearly and simply, so it does not lend itself to elegantly designed trails.

So how does candida overgrow?

Candida can live happily on any mucosal surface in the body, in your throat and nose and in the vagina and on the skin, but for the moment let us concentrate on the gut where it usually seems to start and can act as a 'reservoir'.

If your gut and digestive system are healthy, there will be an intricate balance *(biosis)* kept by the literally billions of friendly bugs which make up our gut *flora* (e.g. *lactobacilli and bifido bacteria*). There are 400-500 different species of bacteria known to live in our guts at various times and the hundred, thousand billion of them outnumber all the cells in our bodies. Different types inhabit different parts of the intestine and each have specific roles to play (see the diagram below, kindly supplied by BioCare). The friendly bugs help to ensure both the efficient digestion and absorption of our food and the destruction of any potentially harmful bugs before they can do any damage. A strong and healthy gut in balance is like a mini ecosystem in which potentially harmful yeasts are controlled such that they remain dormant and harmless. However, if the balance gets upset *(dys-biosis)* and the numbers of friendly inhabitants are reduced, it is not just our digestion and absorption that is affected.

Typical Microbial Flora of the Gastro-intestinal Tract of Man

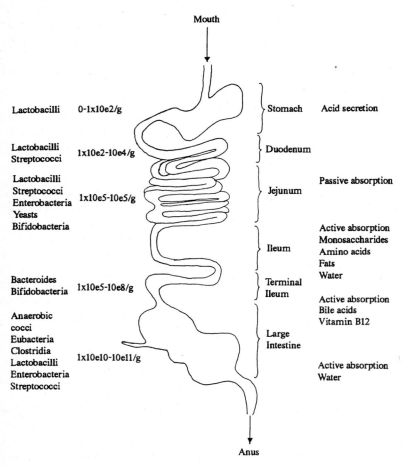

Candida is a very versatile and opportunistic organism and, given half a chance, it will waste no time in multiplying and claiming the territory on the lining of our gut, previously held by our friendly bugs. This is when it can change in form from a yeast to a fungus, described as going from its commensal (i.e. living together happily) to its invasive or *mycelial* form, growing microscopic whiskers *(hyphae)* rather like mould on bread. At this stage it can produce lots of gases and waste products including some alcohol, but the real problems begin when the candida puts down roots through the gut lining and into the tissues, causing what is known as a **"leaky gut"**.

This means that the yeasts' poisonous waste products and our incompletely digested food can escape along the hyphae and get into our bloodstream. Then they may be recognised by the body's immune system as "invaders" and trigger an inappropriate immune reaction causing inflammation and a host of other associated symptoms, from unexplained fatigue to pre-menstrual syndrome, headaches, allergies and arthritis.

As you can see, the right balance in your gut ecosystem is crucial for your health. There is no point in killing off the candida without rebalancing its environment, i.e. your gut, and making sure it is completely healed, or the yeasts will simply come back again. (See chapter 5 for the treatment programme).

Of course, in an unhealthy environment, the candida might not be the only parasite having a field day. There are 70 other types of candida for a start, as well as other parasites such as *Giardia, Helicobacter pyloris, Cryptosporidium and Blastocystis hominis,* to name just a few. The bacteria from outside the body such as those which cause food poisoning such as *salmonella* will also have an easy way in. Equally, parasites and infections found in the vagina are also more likely to get a hold in someone whose endocrine and immune systems are below par. What is more, it is now recognised that drugs, whether antibiotics or anti-fungals cause the bugs to build up a stronger resistance to them and become even more virulent and persistent.

The Law of Symbiosis

As you know, a symbiotic relationship between two or more people is one that is mutually beneficial to all of them. It is exactly the same between organisms living in the same environment, whether they are yeasts or other types of parasites, viruses or bacteria. If there are a few bugs established in an area, they make it much easier for other bugs of similar types to move in too. So if your gut is in a bad way, it is likely to get even worse. However, it works in our favour too. When things are in a healthy balance, they will stay that way to a remarkable degree. One sees examples of this again and again. This is true of the multitude of factors affecting the health of the gut and the immune system as a whole, and also in the brain and the liver, the joints and so on. So if you feel you have reached a plateau in your process of betting better, hang on, think of the law of symbiosis and you'll take a leap forward.

How do I get candidiasis? Or rather, how does the candida get me?

The following factors are the most likely to upset the balance in the gut and / or, to affect the immune system, giving the yeast the opportunity to change and take over.

Taking antibiotics, especially the broad spectrum ones taken orally at a low dosage over long periods for ear, nose and throat infections, or recurring infections. These kill the bad bugs, but the friendly ones are knocked out indiscriminately along with them. Many women in the UK see-saw from cystitis to thrush because the antibiotics given for the cystitis cause the thrush and the cystitis comes back again because the whole balance has not been restored, resulting in a dependency on antibiotics that can be difficult to break. Interestingly, in France, many GP s will give probiotics automatically to women who know from past experience that antibiotics will give them thrush.

The effects on the friendly gut flora vary between different types of antibiotic: Tetracyclines and Erythromycins are the worst, Ampicillin moderate and Penicillin has only a slight effect. Antibiotics also have also been shown to have an immuno-suppressant effect themselves.

Taking corticosteroidal medication, again usually over a long period, for example for asthma, eczema and rheumatoid arthritis. These have a general depressive effect on the immune system.

The Pill and HRT (hormone replacement therapy) behave as female sex hormones in the body. Statistics show that the Pill increases the risk of candidiasis. A slight depression of the immune system among Pill-takers has been shown, but the more likely explanation is its effect on the delicate balance and cycles of oestrogen and progesterone which have a very clear correlation with candidiasis. (Our changing hormone levels is one of the main reasons why 60% of candidiasis sufferers are women.) Thrush is most common the week before one's period and during pregnancy when progesterone levels are high - the Pill has a similar effect. Again paradoxically, the Pill and HRT are often prescribed for the very menstrual problems we suspect were resulting from candidiasis and gut dysbiosis in the first place.

NSAIDs (Non-steroidal anti-inflammatory drugs)   This is a whole class of drugs, often used as painkillers, which can cause inflammation in the gut lining, making life much easier for the microbes that cause a leaky gut. They also interfere with the production of prostaglandins which coat the mucous lining of our guts, protecting them from our digestive acids and enzymes. NSAIDs are given for many of the very things we believe can result from gut dysbiosis, such as chronic back pain, arthritis, migraine, gout and menstrual problems

Poor diet. A diet that is high in refined sugars and carbohydrates, processed and preserved foods will put a strain on the digestive and hormone systems. The gut lining will become inflamed and unhealthy and the flow of food through the small intestine will be too fast - making perfect conditions for the candida to take hold.

A diet that is low in fresh, whole foods will mean that you will be deficient the essential nutrients your gut needs to repair itself to stay strong and healthy. This diet will also be *low in fibre*, so your food will rush through the small intestine too fast for the friendly bugs to maintain a footing.

High meat, dairy and sugar diets. If you eat lots of meat and/or dairy products, you will be favouring the establishment of the *coliforms and streptococci* respectively. Resistant bacteria are also most likely to reach us through the food chain from the livestock industry (see below). Sugars favour yeasts. On the other hand, plenty of fresh fruit and vegetables promote the growth of our *friendly lactobacilli and bifidobacteria.*

Stimulants and depressants. Any substance which artificially boosts or depresses our energy levels or moods, when used regularly over time, will weaken our hormone and immune systems. The very cup of coffee or cigarette that you have to pick you up, though it gives you a temporary lift, only puts a strain on the system; it exhausts your adrenal glands and causes stored sugars to spurt out into the blood stream which then have to be brought back into balance again by the pancreas. In the meantime, the candida has had a feast.

Alcohol not only plays havoc by feeding candida with food in its pre-digested form, but also drains our vitamin and mineral reserves, dehydrates us, and in the long term strains our liver so that it cannot cope with any extra waste products.

With diabetes, thrush is known to be more common in the mouth and the vagina because there is more sugar in the blood and urine.

Stress or trauma of any sort, whether prolonged or during a crisis, is now recognised as one of the main contributory preconditions to candidiasis. It is known that stress causes actual physical changes to occur in our guts. These include decreased acid production in the stomach and small intestines, leading to a higher pH (more alkaline environment) in which the yeasts can thrive. The rate of flow through our intestines also increases and this favours the bad bugs, especially the *streptococci* family, which grow twice as fast as our friendly bugs. Stress also suppresses the immunoglobulins which form the first line of defence in our gut's immune system.

Lack of good quality sleep. Stimulants taken during the day may affect those periods of your sleep known as REM (rapid eye movement) sleep, the time that is especially important for your body's general rest and repair. Candida sufferers often need a lot of sleep and still wake up feeling tired and unrefreshed because of this, plus the extra load of toxins their systems have to cope with.

If you were not breast fed for the first 6 months, or had a diet high in sugar in your early years, the gut flora and immune system would not have been able to get themselves so well established. This will make you more susceptible to recurrent infections in childhood (which are usually treated with antibiotics, getting you on the drug 'treadmill' at an early age) and candidiasis later in life.

In old age as the gut lining and immune system become more fragile, one becomes more vulnerable generally.

Vaccinations and immunisations? Not enough research has been published on this area to say anything categorically, but it is a common pattern that people with candidiasis, ME(CFS), MS and so on, have a higher than usual history of vaccinations and/or travel jabs - whether just before the onset of problems or in the past.

The five stages of candida overgrowth.

One of the clearest analyses of the steps by which candida overgrowth and its toxins invades the body that I have seen is defined by Dr. Ole van Hauen-Drucker, who pioneered holistic medicine and cancer treatment in Denmark and Dr. Howard Hagglund, allergy specialist at the University of Oklahoma. They identify five stages of overgrowth as follows:

1. Commensal - present in everyone's gut, only causing problems (quite temporary in all healthy individuals) if the 'host' overindulges in alcohol or the pudding trolley, for example.

2. Invasive - the yeast changes to its fungal form resulting in abdominal/bowel symptoms, damage to gut lining so that toxins and undigested nutrients leak into the blood stream. Toxins are carried to the liver (our main organ for detoxification) via the hepatic portal vein.

3. Liver overload - as toxins and antigens begin to build up, sporadic flare-ups of allergies and sensitivities to foods and chemical fumes are likely. Muscle and joint aches and pains are common.

4. Liver breakdown - toxins circulating freely and yeast buds are likely to be found anywhere in the blood. Depending on the state of the host's immune system, fungal infection outside the gut is possible.

5. Crosses the blood-brain barrier - the concentration of toxins outside the brain reaches a steep enough gradient for them to pass through. Fungal infection possible in the brain.

If I am getting mental symptoms, does that mean I am at stage 5?
Absolutely not! People who are at level 5 are really very ill, with severe M.E. or AIDS for example. Remember that once the gradient is steep enough, many other neurotoxins (i.e. substances that affect our brains) such as alcohol and methyl mercury (from mercury fillings), can cross the blood-brain barrier. So symptoms such as "foggy brain", poor memory or concentration, headaches, depression or anxiety, and hormonal disturbances can all be present in people at only stage 3.

Why does candida go to certain parts of the body and not others and what can I do?

It is widely recognised that problems such as pain and stiffness in joints, for example, focus in certain areas and not others - and that they move around (though this tends to baffle many doctors). Whether one has candidiasis or not, this is often the site of an old injury or is referred due to nerve interference from spinal misalignment (i.e. pains in the elbow or wrist can be stemming from an old neck injury). But where there is no physical explanation, alternative practitioners explain that it may be on an energy meridian (see under acupuncture in chapter 11) that is blocked or over stimulated. The underlying cause of this may be a lowered organ function, or emotional, but usually both. Either way, this can interfere with the regulatory systems and result in a *local* reduction in blood, nerve, lymph or energy flow and a drop in immunity. Improving the circulation of energy and body fluids at the troublesome sites, whether by seeing an acupuncturist, reflexologist, chiropractor/osteopath, rubbing or dry-skin brushing them yourself, taking exercise, or visualisation, will help in the short term. Taking any unnecessary strain off your structure by checking your posture and chairs (see chapter 4) will also be very worthwhile. However, it goes without saying that you also have to solve the underlying problem of clearing the yeasts and healing the leaky gut and the liver to remove the general build-up of toxins in the whole body.

What happens if you get a leaky gut?

As mentioned above, the integrity of the lining of our gut wall is essential to our health. Effectively it is, along with our skin, a barrier between us and the outside world. When healthy, it does an amazing job of protecting us both from outside invaders (e.g. food poisoning bugs,) and from any internal saboteurs or toxins that they may produce. Our friendly gut flora is an integral part of a healthy gut lining and its immune capabilities and depleting it is the first step towards a leaky gut (or *increased gut permeability* as it is known in the trade).

Theoretically, it is possible to have a leaky gut without candidiasis as other parasites or food poisoning bugs such as Giardia can also damage the gut wall. However, since our modern lifestyle and overuse of antibiotics predispose us to both conditions and to gut dysbiosis generally, it is likely that if you have candida in its invasive stage, it is usually only a matter of time before you get a leaky gut, or vice versa. More specifically, if your diet has been mostly sugary food and drinks, refined foods, caffeine or alcohol for years, you are high on the risk list.

Dr Sherry Rogers from New York sums up seven results of a leaky gut or preliminary inflammation of the gut very clearly (Townsend Letter Feb/Mar '95):

1. The gut does not absorb nutrients properly, leading to fatigue and bloating.

2. Large food particles are absorbed into the bloodstream creating new food sensitivities and potential new targets for the storage of antigen and antibody complexes (allergies) such as in the lungs (asthma) and the joints (arthritis).

3. The proteins whose job it is to carry minerals across the gut wall are damaged, which makes multiple nutrient deficiencies possible.

4. The gut's ability to protect and detoxify is lowered or breached altogether, leading to new chemical sensitivities and possible overload of the liver.

5. The gut's protective coating of immunoglobulins is affected, meaning decreased defences against a host of invaders such as viruses, unfriendly bacteria and yeasts.

6. Since bacteria and yeasts can escape, infection can spread elsewhere in the body.

7. Auto-antibodies may form because of the leak of 'look-alike' antigens: these are implicated in rheumatoid arthritis, lupus, and MS.

Allergies, Food Intolerances and Food Sensitivities - is there a connection?

Though there is no hard data to support it, it is widely observed that people with food sensitivities often have candidiasis as well and vice versa. However in practice, their symptoms are so similar it is often not really possible to distinguish between the two. One of the most plausible connections, though again there is not enough supporting evidence to satisfy the scientists yet, is that while it is by no means the only cause, candida in its invasive form does the most damage to the gut lining. Once you have a leaky gut, more undigested food molecules pass through the gut wall, which the body reacts to as if they were foreign invaders, making food intolerance much more likely. But as Dr Brostoff points out, this doesn't explain the other common link with *chemical sensitivities*. He takes the broader view that we also find seems to fit with our experience with clients. He says "It is clear that candida interacts with the body in various ways, which are both complex and subtle - in particular, its relationship with the sex hormones and with the immune system. Perhaps the side effects unbalance the body's normal control mechanisms, and make food and chemical sensitivities more likely. Alternatively, there could be some underlying fault (in the control of the immune system, for example) that makes the body more vulnerable to candida invasion, on the one hand, and more apt to react inappropriately to foods and chemicals, on the other."

The point here is, as we will see in chapter 5, that to treat candidiasis effectively, one must remove all the strains on the body which includes looking at any sensitivities as well. Unless you identify these and stop eating the offending foods, they will inflame the gut lining even more, preventing its healing. If you continue to overload your system with these substances, the list of foods which cause a reaction in you will just grow and grow. (This is seen all too often in people who do not get proper treatment).

So what exactly are food sensitivities? I can do no better than give Dr Jonathan Brostoff and Linda Gamlin's definitions from their book *Food Allergy and Intolerance*. This is comprehensive, clear and practical and is essential reading for all candidiasis sufferers.

Classic allergy is defined as "any adverse reaction to food in which the immune system is demonstrably involved. A positive skin-prick test, is usually taken as adequate proof of immune system involvement." Classical reactions are immediate and violent and can be triggered by minute amounts of the allergen. They often get worse each time the sufferer comes into contact with them. They include the swelling of the lips, mouth and tongue (often meaning that the poor victim cannot breath within minutes), urticaria (nettle rash), vomiting and in severe cases, anaphylactic shock - which needs immediate hospital treatment. The most common foods are peanuts, shellfish and some berries. Other allergens (i.e. not food include bee and wasp stings and some chemicals whether inhaled or touched.)

Food intolerance is defined as "any adverse reaction to food, other than false food allergy, in which the involvement of the immune system is unproven because a skin-prick test and other tests for allergy are negative. This does not exclude the possibility of immune reaction being involved in some way, but they are unlikely to be the major factor producing the symptoms." Because food intolerance has long been thought of as an 'allergy', most research into its causes has centred on the immune system. It is only in the last [fifteen] years or so that other possible reasons for intolerance have been investigated."

12

There is no such thing as a 'typical' case of food intolerance. The symptoms are usually multiple (affecting any and every body system) and vague, and don't appear for several hours (or days in the case of bowel symptoms) after eating the food(s) and may need quite large quantities of to trigger any response at all. They also come and go and are not consistent, and often depend on the degree of underlying stress. This is the main reason why orthodox doctors doubt the whole phenomenon of food intolerance - as Dr Brostoff reminds us, "it is a fundamental part of the scientific approach to medicine that the same cause should always produce the same effect." However, he sees that "food intolerance is probably a result of many interacting factors" which explains why they can seem to be so fickle.

The symptoms include fatigue, digestive and bowel disturbances, bloating, wind, headaches or migraine, depression and anxiety, mouth ulcers, aching joints and muscles, water retention and in children, hyperactivity.   (Sound familiar don't they?) The offending foods are usually the very ones we eat most of and most frequently. Wheat and dairy (cow's products) are by far the most common in the UK (and corn in the USA, rice in Asia), but also oranges and tomatoes, coffee, eggs, other cereals. If you are intolerant to one type of food, say wheat, you are likely to react to other members of the same 'family', i.e. rye, barley and oats in this example. There are no foods that are completely 'safe' for everyone, though it is very unusual to see reactions to lamb, pears and brown rice (in the UK).

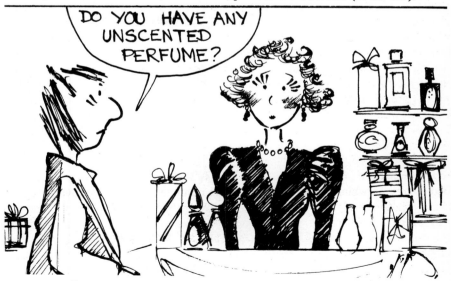

Sensitivities to chemicals and perfumes are also common

Because the offending foods are being eaten all the time, there is no obvious link between the food(s) and the symptoms, which is why intolerance is sometimes called *'masked food allergy'*.

Unlike allergies, food intolerances usually start to happen gradually, often building up in number and severity over years, usually accompanied by a general deterioration in health. However some people find they start more suddenly after a bout of 'flu or food poisoning, severe stress, or a course of antibiotics.

NB. Also unlike allergies which most people have for life, food intolerances may disappear if the food is not eaten for a few months and then only eaten in small quantities. So you are probably NOT stuck with them for ever!

Food sensitivity is the umbrella term used when there is both allergy and intolerance and any other adverse reactions to food, except where these are purely psychological.

Food aversion is simply a food that one doesn't like.

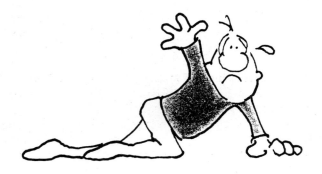

Food Addictions and Cravings

It is a quirk of food intolerance that about 50% of sufferers crave the very foods that are causing them the problems, some to the point of an 'addiction'. Some people are conscious of them, "Oh, I've just got this thing about Mars Bar Ice Creams" and others are not at all - though the look of horror or even panic on their faces when it dawns on them that avoiding bread and dairy products will mean their cheese croissants or whatever have to go, is a dead give-away. If not, a quick look at a 'diary' of the foods they eat over three days usually shows up the offending foods clearly. The explanation for this self-destructive behaviour is not fully understood, but seems to be that because eating the food makes you feel so 'good' initially, the connection is made between the food and the good feeling rather than the 'downer' you get a few hours or days later. Leon Chaitow mentions the research that Dr Orion Truss has done on Acetaldehyde. Candida can ferment or breakdown sugar into this form of alcohol in the body. It can be shown to react with a natural neurotransmitter in the brain, dopamine, to produce morphine-like substances which bind to special receptor sites in the brain, producing the many emotional and mental symptoms that are typical of candidiasis *including* addictions.

In the case of candidiasis, it is almost as if the yeast is demanding the sugar it wants. Sufferers often find it very helpful to know that their irrational and uncontrollable cravings are due not to their weak will but to the saboteurs in their guts, and that by starving them out, the cravings will disappear.

It is not just true of sugar that cravings do disappear surprisingly quickly once you eliminate the offending foods and those in the same 'family' completely. If you reintroduce them before your gut has healed and rebalanced, they will come back again all too quickly, but if you are patient, you'll find you can eat them again in reasonable quantities - but without the addicts' compulsion.

Be warned that 'food-junkies' often suffer withdrawal symptoms like any other junkie or alcoholic (though not as badly). Depending on your constitution, they can be pretty unpleasant but usually only last a few days, or be less severe but go on for several weeks.

There are several ways of diagnosing and treating food sensitivities which are outlined in chapters 5 and 12, and covered in Dr Brostoff's book in much more detail. One of the most widely used is the Elimination or Exclusion Diet. The suspected foods are cut out completely until the symptoms disappear . Once you have this "period of silence" you can start reintroducing the foods one by one, thereby identifying the ones to which you react and those that are OK.

Stress, Attitudes and the Immune System

Here are three facts:

- Stress suppresses IgA (immunoglobulin A) which forms a protective coating on the surface of our gut linings, allowing (bad) bacteria and fungi to grow and get through the gut wall
- Stress raises pH i.e. makes the gut and vagina more alkaline which favours yeasts

- Exercise reduces cortisol or stress hormone levels by a factor of 6 or 7

The role of dealing with stress in overcoming candidiasis cannot be overemphasised.

We all know that stress affects people's well-being. We also know that an identical work load can be an intolerable burden for one person and a stimulating challenge for another. In other words, it is our *attitudes* towards our various stresses, or how we handle them, that matter even more than the stresses themselves.

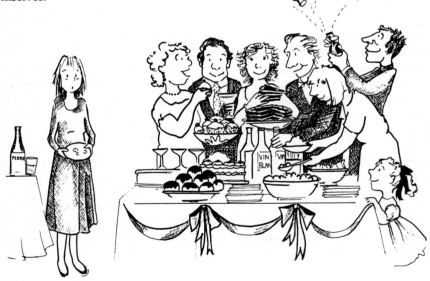

NOW I KNOW WHAT THEY MEAN
BY AN EXCLUSION DIET.

However, it is only relatively recently that science has come up with an "ology" to study stress and its effects on us. Psychoneuroimmunology (or PNI for short) was created when psychiatrists, neurologists and immunologists started talking to each other and each found missing pieces of their respective jigsaws. They discovered and have since shown repeatedly, that our mind/brain/nervous system, our immune system, our hormones, and every cell in our body, far from being separate, are actually all part of one intimately integrated whole. What this means in practice is that whether we think "I'm thirsty" or feel "I'm depressed", thoughts and emotions are instantaneously known or felt in every cell and vice versa. An "unhappy" immune system cannot function properly and will succumb to infections, whereas someone who is positive, in charge, and who loves life, will have very few things their correspondingly enthusiastic and vital immune system cannot cope with. As any naturopath or alternative practitioner will remind us, *happy cells do not malfunction*.

How does all this relate to the gut and candidiasis? In two major ways: One of the ways our immune system protects us is by providing a barrier (our mucous membranes) at which specific foreign invaders are trapped and flushed out by an antibody known as IgA (immunoglobulin A). Healthy individuals secrete between 3 and 7g (about a teaspoon) of IgA every day. This is spread thinly over our gut lining - 90% of it in the colon where there are most bacteria - and this acts as a powerful antihistamine which keeps any fungal overgrowth under control. Stress suppresses IgA, which explains the well known phenomenon of children getting tummy aches on Wednesdays if that is the day they do not like one of the teachers at school. Likewise, we might get the "runs" on a big interview day, or if we have a dental appointment. Similarly, people who suffer from allergies such as eczema know that these often flare up at or after a stressful time.

The change in levels of IgA was shown very clearly in an experiment with students at Tufts (one of the top medical schools in the United States). They took a series of samples from their guts 2 weeks before, during, and after, a week of exams. The IgA levels went from normal to low or *no* IgA during the exams and took 12 days to recover. So you can imagine what happens to the environment in our guts when we are under prolonged periods of stress, or if we have deeply ingrained negative feelings which, even if they are unconscious, are acting as stressors as far as our cells are concerned., around the clock, month in, month out.

A second important change that favours candidiasis when we are under stress is that acid production may be reduced in the stomach. The lactobacillus bacteria also makes lactic acid, so as your friendly bugs are likely to be depleted as well, the small intestine will become more alkaline which is the perfect environment in which the yeasts can thrive.

Tackling stress is easier said than done. If you are very ill, the illness itself will be a major stressor and you will have to start dealing with the physical symptoms first. Exercise, meditation or a combination of the two, such as yoga or Tai'chi, can reduce cortisol (stress hormone) levels dramatically, although overdoing the exercise can be just as bad for you while are ill. Visualisation and relaxation techniques are also very helpful. See chapter 5.

Standing Your Ground - tending your internal 'garden'

> *"Le terrain c'est tout,*
> *le germe n'est rien."*
>
> *Louis Pasteur 1885*

Louis Pasteur's germ theory, that specific germs cause specific diseases, enabled him to make discoveries that are vital to human health. However this got oversimplified into the implication that germs are the only factor in causing disease and this it has shaped much of Western medical thinking ever since. We have expressions like "my boss has given me his cold," in which there is a sense of the helpless victim. As we shall see however, naturopaths tend to look at things in a rather different way.

A contemporary of Pasteur's was Claude Bernard. He maintained that it is the state of *le terrain,* i.e. the ground or soil on which the germs fall, that determines whether or not the individual goes down with the bug or not. He said that if the immune system is strong and that you are in good health, germs simply "bounce off" and do not affect you because your immune system mounts an immediate and effective defence. This explains why, as everyone knows, thousands of doctors and nurses can work amongst people with contagious diseases without getting ill.

But as you can see the two approaches have very different implications. The germ theory implies that there is nothing you can do about it, apart from living in a bubble. If there is a germ about it will get you. But this does not add up when we consider there are germs everywhere - all around us and inside us - yet we are not constantly ill. Bernard's way of seeing it - and this is very much the view of naturopaths and alternative therapists - is that there is a great deal we can do about it. How strong and resilient your *terrain* is will depend on the quality of your diet, your environment, how fit and happy you are, and how fulfilling your job is. They all matter and make a difference. The quotation above translates "*it is not the germ (that matters), it is the ground on which it falls.*" It was said by Pasteur on his death bed, when he admitted that Bernard had been right all along.

All this is very relevant to candidiasis sufferers. T*he key to your getting better is to tend your internal garden or environment. Your internal ecosystem. Everyone has candida living in their guts. What makes the difference between it being harmless and it taking over and making you ill is the state of your internal environment.*

The human gut is one of the best illustrations of the metaphor of *terrain*, soil or territory. When friendly bugs are well established on the lining of the gut, the bad bugs and parasites do not stand a chance All the gardeners among you will appreciate that if you sow a patch of ground thickly with grass seed straight away and tend it until the lawn is mature, the weeds will not get a look in. However, if you do not sow it properly, the weeds will get a foothold and the lawn will never be healthy.

Similarly if you have a flower-bed infested with a weed such as ground elder, pulling the green tops off is a complete waste of time because within a few weeks the extensive root system lurking under the surface will have sprouted up many more weeds. Nor do weed killers work because they don't get to the roots. You have to sift through the flower-bed patiently and regularly, getting out every last little white root or it will simply grow back again. By the same token, antifungal drugs such as Nystatin kill any fungi they touch very effectively, but if the fungi has invaded your tissue it will not reach their "roots" at all. There is also evidence that the fungi develop a resistance to the drugs. Erica White, one of the leading candida practitioners in the UK, very appropriately calls the action of Nystatin and other anti-fungal drugs "the lawn mower effect".

Why antibiotics must be treated judiciously and with a new approach.

For most sufferers, antibiotics are the single factor most likely to perpetuate a candida problem. They have been treated as wonder drugs and 'magic bullets' since the fifties when they began to be widely used in family medicine. They have also made the fortunes of the drugs companies. It is true that they have saved many lives, but dishing them out indiscriminately, over several generations, is now causing its own problems. One only has to pick up Geoffrey Cannon's book, *Superbug* to see how drugs can compound the problem by making the 'badies' more resistant and the 'goodies' fewer and weaker, and setting up a dependency on the 'drug treadmill'.

However, these days whenever most people get an infection they nip down to the GP for some antibiotics and then they are fine, or so they think. What they do not ask, and are rarely told (and many patients won't be told), is that antibiotics, when taken orally, will also kill off drastic numbers of the friendly bugs in our guts indiscriminately, since these are often even more sensitive to them than the bad bugs themselves. This means that the territory on our gut lining is laid wide open to invasion by both undesirable bugs from outside and overgrowth by the opportunistic members of our normal gut flora such as our old friend, *Candida albicans* as well as *E. Coli, and Streptococci aureus* - one of the most antibiotic-resistant and tenacious organisms known to Man. All of these can cause serious secondary infections, particularly at a time when we are most vulnerable after an infection. This is why people should be warned to be particularly careful about food poisoning in the three weeks or so after taking antibiotics, or indeed whenever they know they are run down.

We have been brought up to believe that all bacteria and germs are 'bad' and that germ-free and sterile is 'best'. So we use an arsenal of chemical weapons, including antibiotics to control them, in the kitchen, the bathroom and in the food industry, and of course in hospitals - everywhere. Geoffrey Cannon calls this the "Domestos theory of human health". We think we need to kill *all* bacteria. Dead.

But eliminating bugs from our lives mean first, that we do not build up any immunity to them, so we are more vulnerable and second, that the bugs build up resistance to the drugs used to kill them, so that as fast a scientists develop new drugs, the 'superbugs' seem to be keeping a step ahead. This is particularly true in the livestock industry. Animals are fed low doses of antibiotics to make them grow faster and to make it possible to rear them in very cramped conditions without infecting each other. Most mass produced meat carries resistant strains of bacteria. (See *Superbug* again for more information.)

We need a radical change in attitudes and beliefs about how our defences and health work. The trouble is that patients have come to expect and demand antibiotics and there is no quicker way for the poor overloaded GP s to shorten the impossible queues in their waiting rooms than to write out a prescription for one. But in so many cases this is only a short term solution.

Professor Richard Lacey, one of the leading microbiologists and doctors in the UK says in the Afterword in Geoffrey Cannon's book, "In my judgement, evidence form modern medical and microbiological science indicates that in countries like the UK, antibiotics are grossly overused, and that they are appropriate in only in one in ten or less of the cases where they are now prescribed. Translated to individual patients, this implies on average a course of antibiotics not at the current rate of once or twice a year, mostly for trivial illness, but once or twice every ten years, or less for serious bacterial infections."

So it is up to you to take responsibility for your own gut flora and stay off or get off the drug treadmill! Provided the infection is not too serious, the way to strengthen your immune system so that it will simply shrug it off next time around is *not* to take any antibiotics. Instead, rest (an old remedy we seem to have forgotten about), and let the infection run its course. It should clear within a few days. More details are in chapter 4 under middle ear infections, cystitis etc. It is very important that you have your doctor in your side about this. If he or she is not sympathetic, see chapter 8.

Of course there are occasions when one would be very unwise not to take antibiotics, but if you *have* to take them, there are several things one can do to mitigate their negative effects and to restore your gut (and the rest of you) to its healthy balance as soon as possible. See under probiotics in chapter 11.

How long does it take to clear the candida and restore a healthy gut?

This is two separate questions. Clearing candida can be quite quick - 2-3 months, it is healing the gut that can take the time. Depending on how badly it is damaged and for how long, and the general state of your physical and emotional health and constitution, and assuming your treatment is appropriate and you stick to it, this may take anything from a further 3-10 months.

However, most people start to feel much better within 10-14 days of starting the programme, some even sooner. This is why people can stick to a programme for months on end - as long as you are feeling so much better and once you are in the swing of your new routine, it is no penance. However there will be a few downs as well as ups and you'll need some moral support to help you through those. It goes without saying that before stopping the treatment, you need to make sure that the balance in your gut is completely restored or the symptoms will simply return.

As you will find out, the secret of success is coming to understand and appreciate your unique needs for life - what suits you and what does not. So you could say that getting better will only take as long as it takes for you to find the foods and lifestyle that are right for you, and to settle into enjoying that new routine. Then it will simply be a matter of time and of enjoying the new adventure.

Will I ever be able to go back to my old habits?
This anti-candida programme is not about sticking to a "cure" for a few months. It is the first step to rediscovering how to listen to, learn about and respond to your unique needs for a healthy, happy life.

Clients never believe me (and you probably will not either) if I tell them that they will actually not want to go back to being a chocoholic, Big Mac junkie, or Pot Noodle freak, or that they will not miss their café au lait and croissant for breakfast. But then a few months later they tell me "I've noticed that now I can have one square of chocolate, and really enjoy it, and I don't have to eat the rest of the bar. Or, "I was offered a croissant and jam for breakfast, but I wanted to feel really good that day, so I enjoyed the smell while they ate theirs and I had my special muesli. I didn't miss the croissant one bit."

Of course you should be able to eat all the foods-to-avoid eventually, but you will not want them in the same frequency or quantities. This is because, by getting your gut back into balance, it will be able to tell you just what it does and does not want. And so long as you learn to give it 'silence', listen and respond to these messages, you will continue to feel better and have plenty of energy for the rest of your life. This book is designed to help you do this as effortlessly as possible.

CHAPTER 2

DIAGNOSING CANDIDIASIS

One of the problems with candida and the main reason why most GPs do not recognise it, is that it is present in everybody's gut, so there is no cut and dried method of testing for it in a laboratory. Secondly, since candida is an inextricably linked part of our astonishingly complex and finely balanced 'eco-systems' (our guts), candidiasis is both a cause and an effect of symptoms and it is very difficult to single it out as a strand that can be isolated in a lab. It is therefore woefully common for patients to be told by the orthodox profession "there is nothing wrong with you" or " it must be in you mind" just because their tests do not shown up positive. This is extremely distressing when you know there *is* something wrong but your friends and colleagues aren't so sure until a doctor has said so. If this happens to you, don't let it get you down - new tests are being developed all the time by the specialist nutritionally orientated labs.

There are two reasons for getting a clear diagnosis in syndromes like candidiasis. One is to get a piece of paper saying you have candidiasis, M.E., I.B.S. or whatever, so that you can get the medical certificate to get the rest and space, as well as the moral and financial support that may be crucial to your recovery. The second is to determine and fine tune your treatment. Of course the two overlap, but do be clear why you need whatever tests you are considering. If having a "proper" diagnosis matters to you, your boss or your insurance company, find a senior complementary practitioner who knows his or her stuff on the specialist lab tests that are available and is happy to feed back to your GP.

Gut fermentation, low stomach acid, blood sugar or thyroid levels, heavy metal toxicity, parasites, food intolerances and nutritional deficiencies can all be measured pretty accurately. However, many of these tests are difficult to organise through the NHS, so you need to be selective unless you are privately insured or are happy to pay what can otherwise turn into a large bill. However, there are several strong indicators which your practitioner can test for and some you can do yourself, which don't cost a penny extra and when taken together, can build up a pretty sure diagnosis. Many people only care about getting better and prefer to save the money and spend it on treatment. If it looks like straightforward candidiasis this is very sensible as long as the treatment is obviously working. It sounds very "unscientific", but to be honest, your gut and whole body-mind has miraculous powers of righting itself given half a chance. The seven point programme is designed to help them do so at every level, so you are likely to get better whatever was wrong in the first place. This has certainly been our empirical experience and once we have the funds for research we will be able to be specific. (In the meantime, keep trusting and listening.)

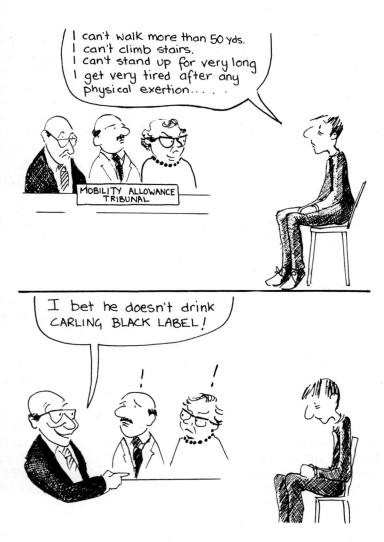

However if you are very ill, it will be some time before your body-mind is strong enough to pick itself up and tests are going to be necessary from the start to be sure that you get the most appropriate treatment. Since the various factors involved in your condition are likely to be much more complicated, you will save a lot of time and money by getting more specific diagnoses.

Having said that, the diagnostic capabilities of several of the alternative therapies can be quite amazing in experienced hands, particularly applied kinesiology, dowsing, iridology and the acupuncture pulses. In fact, when dealing with an entire syndrome such as gut dysbiosis that shows in such different ways between individuals, they usually get to the nub (or nubs) of a problem far more quickly and cheaply than lab tests. They can also show the extent of a problem, which can also be very helpful in monitoring your progress through recovery. In the end, a judicious combination of the two - "science based" and alternative, will probably be the ideal for you.

Primary indicators
Most of the authorities agree that if your symptoms include the following, it is highly likely that candidiasis is part of your problems. Particularly if you can date the onset to having taken antibiotics, the Pill or corticosteroidal medication or a very stressful time.
:
- unexplained fatigue
- abdominal bloating and/or flatulence
- food cravings, especially sugar and bread (sometimes causing binge eating)
- food and chemical sensitivities,

The other common symptoms are almost identical to those already listed for food intolerances given by Dr Brostoff , mentioned in chapter 1. Here they are again:

- headaches or migraine
- depression/anxiety
- recurrent mouth ulcers
- aching joints and muscles
- digestive and bowel disturbances
- rheumatoid arthritis
- water retention
- hyperactivity (in children)

In practice, in most cases it is not particularly helpful to try and distinguish between food intolerances and candidiasis since, as we have seen, they are intimately correlated and both need to be treated simultaneously. However if the following additional symptoms that specifically indicate fungal infection are either completely absent or very predominant, then you can gauge the relative importance of the two factors in your case:

- PMT and irregular periods
- recurrent thrush and/or cystitis
- itchy anus
- fungal skin or nail infections, athletes' foot, also psoriasis

If you are vomiting or have migraines as opposed to headaches this is usually an indication of food intolerance rather than candidiasis.

A more detailed analysis of your whole symptom picture coupled with pointers from your medical and life history has been used for 15 years by one of the pioneers in diagnosing and treating candidiasis, Dr William Crook. He has devised a questionnaire with a points system that is generally accepted as a pretty good indicator, and this is set out below. It will only take you 20 minutes or so to fill in, so do that now. I have added two more columns for you to score them again in six weeks and six months. Date each column as you will be glad to be able to look back at how much worse you used to be! It is amazing how quickly and completely we tend to forget.

Diagnosis by treatment
The next step, one of the best ways to confirm whether you have candidiasis for yourself, is 'diagnosis by treatment'. That is, to start the programme for 10-14 days (see chapter 5). If you feel better then you probably do have it, particularly if you get clear symptoms of die-off once you start taking anti-fungals. 'Reactions' to treatment when you might experience the symptoms getting worse for a few days, especially if you have lots of food intolerances, are explained in chapter 5.

If you reckon you haven't got candidiasis after all, there's nothing to lose because it is a very healthy diet anyway. In this case, some of the other checklists in this chapter might point you in the right direction. Fatigue, for instance, can be caused by several other imbalances from low thyroid function or diabetes to depression or nutritional deficiencies. I also have also included some brief indicators for some differential diagnoses.

Overlapping syndromes and masqueraders
I have already mentioned the similarity between candidiasis and food intolerances. It is also notorious for masquerading as other more serious conditions such as chronic fatigue syndrome (ME), fibromyalgia syndrome and multiple sclerosis *and vice versa*. Even experienced diagnosticians confuse these because they seem to be on the same spectrum, with many factors either in common or as precursors. So much so that boundaries between them get blurred (and can also change considerably with time) to the point of becoming almost meaningless. In these cases, the best policy is, as ever, to adopt a multi-disciplinary, integrated approach - to treat the candidiasis/gut dysbiosis *plus* whatever other specific problems you turn out to have.

DR CROOK'S CANDIDA QUESTIONNAIRE

William Crook is a paediatrician in the United States who first noticed a pattern in his young patients in the early eighties which matched that described as candidiasis by Dr Orian Truss. He devised the following questionnaire - which is in fact for adults not children.

Underline the questions below that are true for you and tot up the score at the end of section A. Make sure you have dated it as you will want to refer back in 6 weeks and 6 months time and re-score it to check on your progress. I have added a few symptoms in brackets.

Section A: History

Date...................

Point Score

1. Have you taken tetracylines or other antibiotics for acne for one
   month or longer?   35

2. Have you, at any time in your life, taken other broad-spectrum
   antibiotics for respiratory, urinary or other infections for two
   months or longer, or in shorter courses four or more times in a
   one-year period?   35

3. Have you taken a broad-spectrum antibiotic drugs - even a
   single course?   6

4. Have you, at any time in your life, been bothered by persistent prostatitis, vaginitis (thrush) or other problems affecting your reproductive organs?   **25**

5. Have you been pregnant:
    2 or more times?   **5**
    1 time?   **3**

6. Have you taken birth control pills:
    For more than 2 years?   **15**
    for 6 months to 2 years?   **8**
    (Have you been on an IVF programme? 25 points)

7. Have you taken prednisone or other cortisone-type drugs:
    For more than 2 weeks?   **15**
    For 2 weeks or less?   **6**

8. Does exposure to perfumes, insecticides,(dry cleaners or petrol stations) or other chemicals provoke:
    Moderate to severe symptoms?   **20**
    Mild symptoms?   **5**

9. Are your symptoms worse on damp, muggy days or in mouldy places?   **20**

10. Have you had athlete's foot, ringworm or other chronic fungus infections of the skin or nails? Have such infections been:
    Severe or persistent?   **20**
    Mild or sporadic?   **10**

11. Do you crave sugar?   **10**

12. Do you crave bread?   **10**

13. Do you crave alcoholic beverages?   **10**

14. Does tobacco smoke *really* bother you?   **10**

TOTAL SCORE, SECTION A

Section B: Major Symptoms

For each of your symptoms, enter the appropriate figure in the point score column:

If a symptom is occasional or mild:	3 points
If a symptom is frequent and/or moderately severe:	6 points
If a symptom is constant and/or disabling:	9 points

Add the total score and record it at the end of this section.

		Now	In 6 Weeks	In 6 Months
1.	Fatigue (unexplained) or lethargy			
2.	Feeling of being drained			
3.	Poor memory			
4.	Feeling spaced out or unreal			
5.	Inability to make decisions			
6.	Numbness, burning or tingling			
7.	Insomnia			
8.	Muscle aches (or tenderness)			
9.	Muscle weakness or paralysis (or cramps)			
10.	Pain and/or swelling in joints (Stiffness in the mornings)			
11.	Abdominal pain			
12.	Constipation			

No.	Symptom		
13.	Diarrhoea		
14.	Bloating, belching or intestinal gas (wind or farting)		
15.	Troublesome vaginal burning, itching or discharge (thrush)		
16.	Prostatitis		
17.	Impotence		
18.	Loss of sexual desire or feeling		
19.	Endometriosis or infertility		
20.	Cramps and/or other menstrual irregularities		
21.	Pre-menstrual tension		
22.	Attacks of anxiety (panic, depression) or crying		
23.	Cold hands or feet and/or chilliness		
24.	Shaking or irritable when hungry		
TOTAL SCORE, SECTION B			

Section C: *Other symptoms*

No.	Symptom	Now	In 6 Weeks	In 6 Months
1.	Drowsiness			
2.	Irritability or feeling jittery			
3.	Lack of co-ordination			
4.	Inability to concentrate			

		Now	In 6 Weeks	In 6 Months
5.	Frequent mood swings			
6.	Headaches			
7.	Dizziness/loss of balance			
8.	Pressure above ears, feeling of head swelling			
9.	Tendency to bruise easily (or heal slowly)			
10.	Chronic rashes or itching (or acne)			
11.	Numbness, tingling			
12.	Indigestion or heartburn			
13.	Food sensitivity or intolerance			
14.	Mucus in stools			
15.	Rectal itching			
16.	Dry mouth or throat			
17.	Rash or blisters in mouth			
18.	Bad breath (or foul taste)			
19.	Foot, hair or body odour not relieved by washing			
20.	Nasal congestion or nasal drip			
21.	Nasal itching			
22.	Sore throats			
23.	Laryngitis, loss of voice			

	Now	In 6 Weeks	In 6 Months
24. Cough or recurrent bronchitis			
25. Pain or tightness in chest			
26. Wheezing or shortness of breath			
27. Urinary urgency or frequency			
28. Burning feeling on urination (cystitis)			
29. Spots in front of eyes or erratic vision			
30. Burning in eyes, or tears			
31. Recurrent infections or fluid in ears			
32. Ear pain or deafness			
TOTAL SCORE, SECTION C			
TOTAL SCORE, SECTION A			
TOTAL SCORE, SECTION B			
GRAND TOTAL SCORE			

Scores will vary depending on whether you are a man or a woman:		
Women	Men	Yeast-connected problems are:
180	140	almost certain
120	90	probable
60	40	possible

Some other signs and symptoms we notice that are common are:
Score them out of ten for you

	Now	In 6 Weeks	In 6 Months
Can't lose/gain weight			
Dark rings under the eyes			
Dull, grey complexion			

How many hours sleep do you need / get?

If you are on medication or pain killers
make a note of the dose here

....

....

....

Make a note in your diary in 6 weeks and 6 months time to re-score this.

How much coffee / tea / fizzy drinks / alcohol / cigarettes / plain water do you have per day at the moment?
Next, make a list of the 6 symptoms (your own words) that bother you most with their level of frequency + severity out of 10.
For example.

      Can't get up in the mornings 9+8.
      Bloating after food   10+4

1. ....

2. ....

3. ....

4. ....

5. ....

6. ....

Differential and additional diagnoses

Candidiasis has many symptoms in common with the following conditions which is why it is often mistaken for them. One could write as much again on each of the following conditions, so I am just giving you the strongest *distinguishing* indicators and most common tests. You'll find more details in chapter 4 and some suggestions for further reading and useful addresses in the appendices.

BUT DO NOT ATTEMPT TO SELF DIAGNOSE OR SELF TREAT ANY OF THE FOLLOWING! ALWAYS START WITH YOUR GP.

I am giving you the following information because I believe that it may help you to find the right practitioner and to get better more quickly if you inform yourself well - not so that you can do a' DIY job' on what could be a very serious condition needing medical and naturopathic expertise!

That said, there is mounting evidence that gut dysbiosis (whether that involves severe candidiasis or not) is a precursor and perpetuating factor in a significant proportion of all the following conditions - which is why so many sufferers find that treating any candidiasis makes a dramatic improvement to their other symptom. So for treatment, keep thinking in terms of "both-and" rather that one single label.

NB: Because so many of these symptoms are so non-specific, you may well go down the lists, mentally ticking them all and ending up in a panic, convinced that you have ME, MS and schizophrenia all rolled into one! We all feel depressed, achy or can't sleep a wink from time to time - only 'tick' the following symptoms if they are severe and persistent.

Chronic Fatigue Syndrome (ME) Myalgic Encephalomyelitis
Also known as Post-viral Fatigue Syndrome, and " yuppie 'flu"

- Sleep disturbances, including sleep reversal i.e. being awake all night and sleeping during the day.
- Profound exhaustion for hours or days after quite slight physical exertion (e.g. climbing a flight of stairs) or mental exertion.
- Mental and cognitive disturbances - complete memory and concentration lapses, depression and anxiety.
- The unpredictability of symptoms from day to day.

The practitioners who are experienced in treating ME are marked in the directory.

NB The standard orthodox tests such as the Epstein Barr virus are not always conclusive.

Links with candidiasis/gut dysbiosis: Gill Jacobs, Leon Chaitow and Simon Martin all argue that viral infections are more likely to progress to M.E. when there is pre-existing candidiasis because the growth of viruses is enhanced by the presence of fungi and a damaged gut likely. Conversely, if ME is contracted the immune system will become depressed and unable to defend the body against any candida, so it is more likely to overgrow.

Bacterial Fermentation: Harald Gaier, who sees many people with severe CFS(ME) has observed high levels of various toxic alcohols in their blood plasma when they are tested for gut fermentation (see test below). These are not the more common ethanol or methanol produced by candidiasis. The propyl and butyl alcohols found are known to affect the nervous system and produce muscle tenderness, depressed respiration and reflexes with profound fatigue - all classic M.E. symptoms. Bacterial fermentation is usually associated with *"malabsorption syndrome"* caused by low or no stomach acid and/or the fact that the pancreas isn't producing enough or any pancreatin. Giving supplements to correct this can make a startling improvement that is maintained.
For more information and references, see What the Doctors Don't Tell You, vol 4. no 2.

Sick building syndrome and electromagnetic fields, and mercury toxicity have all been associated with CFS(ME). See chapter 9.

Dr Alan Stewart's book *Tired All the Time* covers all the other causes of fatigue and their diagnoses. See appendix 1.

Multiple Sclerosis (MS)
There are many cases of severe candidiasis being diagnosed as MS. This is a usually gradual but serious degeneration of the nervous system (the myelin sheaths in particular) with no cure really known, than can develop very quickly or over thirty years with long remissions in between. Dr Patrick Kingsley is one of the experts here. He finds that mercury toxicity is involved in most cases. (See chapter 9). The main symptoms initially, include persistent visual disturbances, sudden muscle weakness, numbness or tingling and loss of balance. In true MS, candidiasis is often present and clearing it may even put the MS into remission in

some cases. However, go *very* gently on the detoxification and anti-fungals or acute exacerbations are likely.

Hypothyroid
Low thyroid function causes fatigue and low body temperature, sometimes with a gain in weight (often around the chin and bust in women, "spare tyre" in men), and thinning of hair. The Broda Barnes test is something you can do for yourself. Simply take and record your temperature for 10 minutes before you get out of bed in the morning. If you are a women, ideally you should do this for a monthly cycle. If it is below 97.8-98.2F or 36.55-36.8C 9 (normal) then hypothyroidism is likely and you should get it properly checked by your GP.
The option for treatment is thyroxin (a drug) or supplements and kelp etc. from a complementary practitioner. The level and cycle of cortisol at the cell level controls thyroid production, so the Adrenal Stress Index test may well be worth doing as well. (See below).

Schizophrenia
Since observing that it was more common in people with coeliac disease (which involves a very leaky gut), this mental disorder has been strongly linked with food sensitivities, particularly gluten and dairy. Also nutritional deficiencies (see the ION's excellent little booklet *Mental Illness, not all in the mind*). Symptoms include paranoia, hallucinations (often with a sense of dual personality), acute depression and extreme mental confusion.

Laboratory tests to confirm candidiasis and associated problems

Diagnostech, a laboratory in the United States, run by Doctor Elias Ilyias, is making the three tests he has developed during his 14 years experience with candidiasis and gut dysbiosis available to us in the UK. They are non-invasive, relatively cheap and give a scale of severity, so they can be used to monitor your progress.

All three are available through qualified practitioners only, from Diagnostech Clinical and Research Services, Lakeside Centre, 180 Lifford Lane, Kings Norton, Birmingham, B30 3NT
(tests and prices will be available from September 1995)

Candiscan - Diagnostech
This promises to be a good test for the level of candida in your gut. More details from the address above.

Female Hormone Panel - Diagnostech

Severe menstrual and fertility problems are quite common in women with candidiasis. Dr Brostoff says that it is thought that this may be due to the fact that "the candida provokes antibodies which happen to cross react with some of the body's own proteins. Such antibodies have in fact been found, and they specifically attack the ovaries." The hormones are affected, hence the symptoms. In many cases, clearing the candidiasis clears the symptoms with it, but if they persist, a very specific new test from Diagnostech should identify which of the many possibilities is the culprit.

Unlike other tests for oestrogen and progesterone levels/imbalances which take a blood or urine sample on one day, the FHP uses saliva taken 11 times during a whole menstrual cycle. This means one can map the levels on a graph and see your total output and the complete pattern of ups and downs. The levels of hormones in your saliva match those in the tissues to 93% so it is very accurate. You simply take the samples on the specified days and post them to the lab. Your practitioner will be sent specific suggestions for your individual treatment with the results.

The test can also pick up any subtle effects that your lifestyle and the Pill may be having on your hormones levels, cycle and fertility.

The Adrenal Stress Index - Diagnostech

Stress and how our adrenals handle it is one of the key factors in so many health problems. (See also chapters 1 and 4). Our circadian (daily) rhythms are as important as the relative levels of adrenaline, cortisol and DHEA, but until this new test there has not been a convenient and relatively cheap way of monitoring them. Four saliva samples are taken in one 24 hour period which will give enough information to enable the lab to make many times as many options for treatment as the old blood and urine tests.

If you have any of the following symptoms, your practitioner will give you a stress questionnaire to fill in and discuss how this test may shed some light on things.

Lack of vitality and energy	Muscle and joint pain
Migraines	Stress maladaptation
Osteoporosis	Sleep disturbances
Poor memory	Alcohol intolerance
Low sex drive	Low body temperature.
Poor immune system	Poor thyroid function
Skin problems	

Individual suggestions for treatment will include one with DHEA (an adrenal drug supplement) and two nutritional protocols.

Gut fermentation test - Biolab £35 By post or in person.
This is one of the strongest indicators for candidiasis. After a 12 hour fast you are given 5g of a special glucose that is quickly absorbed into the duodenum. An hour later a blood sample is taken and analysed for the presence of a full range of alcohols. Ethanol and methanol (the type we drink socially) are produced by candida - but not enough to get you off a drink-driving offence ("but it's my candida offisher"). Dr John McLaren Howard from Biolab says the highest level he has ever seen due to genuine gut fermentation was 12 mg/dl compared to the breathalyser limit which is 80mg/dl. Other types of alcohol which also show up in this test can be produced by bacteria and can cause the tenderness and fatigue in muscles seen in ME and FMS.

Intestinal permeability (leaky gut) test - Biolab £35
A simple and reliable test developed by Biolab, which uses a special form of sugar that is not digested by mammals. Its chemical name is polyethylene glycol 400, so it is called the 'PEG test'. Having taken a small drink of the stuff, you collect all your urine for 6 hours. If any PEG shows up it means it has passed through your gut wall. Since PEG comes in 11 conveniently different sized molecules, the lab can measure exactly how leaky your gut actually is. NB This is not a test for candida as such as several other factors can cause a leaky gut. But is does show how well your gut is absorbing nutrients and how well its mucosal lining is working and will be independent of liver or kidney function or intestinal transit time. It is very important to note that this test can pick up problems in their early stages, and when caught earlier, they are must quicker to treat.

Low Blood Sugar (hypoglycaemia or glucose intolerance)
(See chapters 4 and 7)
30% of available glucose is used by the brain, so it is the brain that suffers when it drops. Symptoms include: fatigue, irritability and anxiety, depression, "foggy brain", weakness, faintness or dizziness, trembling, palpitations and blackouts. They often come over you quite suddenly (often before meals) and pass as soon as you have had something to eat - unless the glands are very weakened.
To correct it, it is crucial to clear any candidiasis and rest and support the glands which have resulted in the low blood sugar. These could be the pancreas, thyroid or the adrenals and you really must go to a qualified practitioner to find out which. A urine test will be suggested or a glucose challenge test at Biolab. The Adrenal Stress Index above, will show up any adrenal deficiency.

Nutritionists can give you specific supplements, enzymes, amino acids to help but all of them should recommend a refined carbohydrate-free diet. Food combining and stress management is particularly useful here.

Hair Mineral Analysis (includes mercury) - test by post.
York Nutritional Laboratories, see address below
Biolab £26
Ring for their kit and instructions.

Sweat Mineral Analysis, including Mercury - Biolab £37
Obviously sweat is a more recent measurement than using hair which will have taken several months to grow. However, you must be able to go to London for this one.

Food Intolerances and Candida - Nutron Laboratories £135
Tests 92 foods and candidal hypersensitivity.
Tel: 01483 203555 to book a test.
Food Sensitivity Testing - York Nutritional Laboratory
Cytotoxic test covering 74 foods, graded on a scale of 0-4.
Tudor House, Lysander Close, Clifton Moor, York YO3 4XB
Tel: 01904 690640

Biolab Medical Unit, The Stonehouse, 9 Weymouth Street, London W1N 3FF
Tel: 0171 636 5959 or 5905 Fax: 0171 580 3910
NB You must be referred by a doctor for tests at Biolab.

Alternative therapies which can contribute to your diagnosis

These medical traditions and therapies can be extraordinarily quick, detailed and cheap in giving you a diagnosis. See the second section in chapter 11 under each heading. AK and dowsing are both skills you can develop yourself.

Acupuncture pulses

Iridology

Applied Kinesiology

Vega test machine

Dowsing

CHAPTER 3

A DIFFERENT APPROACH AND PHILOSOPHY OF MEDICINE. WHAT TO EXPECT

If you have not been to a complementary practitioner before and are used to 10-15 minutes with your overstretched GP, you will find the whole process very different. While traditionally our family doctors knew most of us from when we were born, and took great pride in the social and personal role they played in our lives, now thanks to the speed with which we all move around the country and the inordinate pressure that the NHS system puts on GPs' time, they are usually unable to get to know most of us in any depth.

While there are definite signs that things are changing, most GPs' way of working is to diagnose the signs and symptoms and prescribe a drug, specifically designed to suppress those symptoms. This is a very time-efficient 'this pill for that ill' approach, and there is no quicker way to get on with the next patient than to write out a prescription. It is also a 'quick fix' for the patient as the drug usually means they can be 'back to normal' within a few days. This all works very well for most problems and of course the hospital system in the UK is still probably the best in the world for acute problems, life threatening illnesses and emergencies. However the conventional medical system rarely serves those of us with chronic, non-specific 'un-wellness'. In the case of candidiasis, because it seems to be caused by many factors including lifestyle,it seems that it can only be made better by a multi-level approach that includes looking at lifestyle. However, this needs far more time than the NHS system allows, which is why we see so many of you who have become absolutely exasperated with the whole medical system. Not because it *is* bad of course - far from it, just that it has totally failed you and your chronic problem. This is where the complementary or alternative approach can come into its own - and increasingly, this is being appreciated by doctors and public alike.

'Only Nature heals' (Hippocrates)
Whatever you call us - holistic, naturopathic, integrated, non-conventional, alternative or complementary, we all see your body-mind as the one that will be doing the healing, rather than the drug or the physician. Many of us include the 'spirit' as an essential part of your body-mind. We'll look at this in chapter 9.
Henry Lindlahr, writing in 1919 in true Edwardian style put it, 'the "great law of life" states that every living cell in an organised body is endowed with an instinct

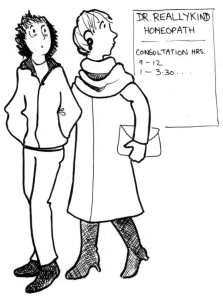

DR. REALLYKIND
HOMEOPATH

CONSULTATION HRS.
9 – 12
1 – 3.30 . . .

I THINK THEY CALL IT COMPLEMENTARY
MEDICINE BECAUSE THE OTHER TYPE IS OFTEN
SO INSULTING!

of self preservation which is sustained by an inherent force named *the vital force of life.'*. As practitioners, we see our job as simply to help your *life force* in its natural tendency to bring you back into inner balance, full health and *vitality* again. Ross Trattler expands on this very clearly in the introduction to his book. But the philosphy of naturopathic medicine is summed up by Lindlahr again:

'The natural therapeutic approach maintains that the constant effort of the body's life force is always in the direction of *self-cleansing, self-repairing and positive health*. The philosophy maintains that even acute disease is a manifestation of the body's efforts in the direction of self cure. Disease, or downgraded health, may be eliminated only be removing from the system the real cause and by raising the body's general vitality so that its natural and inherent ability to sustain health is allowed to dominate. Natural therapeutic philosophy also maintains that chronic diseases are frequently the result of mistaken efforts to cure, or attempted suppression of the physiological efforts of the body to cleanse itself.'

So we need to discover what the obstructions are and to help your body remove them in its own way. The rebalancing and fine tuning that can then take place and is *innate* in us all is really nothing short of miraculous. And this usually means that your body-mind will be the stronger and richer for the experience and better able to cope next time.

Obstructions or blocks can be anything from an accumulation of toxins, spinal misalignments or poor body mechanics (which also affect the nerves), imbalance in *chi* (the Chinese word for our vital energy), genetic traits or *miasms*, as the homoeopaths call them, imbalanced diets, nutritional deficiencies, disturbances in our electrical 'circuitry', negative emotional patterns, worries or attitudes, lifestyle factors such as stress and job satisfaction, your relationships, too much or too little physical activity - and those are just the main ones. The skill of the practitioner is to identify which are causing the problems in your *individual* case and how best to help you tackle them in a way that will fit in with your lifestyle and *unique* character.

Time and the healing process
The various therapeutic traditions each have their own methods of diagnosis and their models by which they determine the treatment. But they all involve understanding the whole picture and seeing you as a whole and unique individual. This takes *time,* which is why the vast majority of appointments with the practitioners listed in this directory are an hour or longer initially, and at least half an hour at subsequent sessions. Taking the time to really listen and observe is crucial - the practitioner should be skilled in picking up what is said as much as what is unsaid. And don't worry if we seem to be asking a lot of personal or irrelevant questions - they are all be necessary to build a complete picture of your unique blueprint. It also takes time to discuss and explain how to go about the changes you might need to make in your diet and everyday habits and to make sure you have understood fully. The language we use should not be mystifying or separate you from us in any way. Though a few new meanings might need some explaining such as 'energy, balance, and flow'.

Time is also crucial in the sense that we find that your body-mind needs to go at its own pace, with adequate rest and attention, and for deep seated blockages this can be months or even years. Healing is a life-long process and once set on the right track and supported in the right way, with the appropriate diet for instance, it will continue by itself, while always taking steps to maintain your health and prevent any future disease. We believe that this process and your body-mind's innate wisdom should be trusted and interfered with as little as possible. Drugs and surgery override your healing processes so thery should be judiciously avoided in favour of natural substances such as herbs and synergistic vitamins.

Reactions - learn to welcome them.
These days, we are used to sophisticated drugs and most people expect to be cured pretty quickly. However drugs don't actually cure anything. They suppress the symtpoms while the body sorts itself out. Drugs are not designed to get to the roots of the problem. In our view, suppressing symptoms is a bit like driving down the motorway with your oil light flashing and taking the bulb out instead of stopping to get more oil. But in the same way as we have been led to believe that absence of disease equals health, people still think that no symptoms equals a cure. But Nature doesn't work that way. Symptoms are actually signals that there is something wrong, and that the body is in the process of sorting it out. *Acute disease* is really the result of Nature's efforts to eliminate waste matter or poisons from the body and to repair injured tissues. Letting Nature take its course means encouraging these symptoms, some of which might be quite unpleasant, and rather inconvenient. They include inflammation, mucous, sweating, diarrhea, vomitting, pain, sneezing and coughing, local infections and even emotional outbursts. They may arise at any stage in the healing process in a way that is often described as 'peeling the layers off an onion'. It is well recognised that old problems or experiences reappear as they are being finally worked out of the system. However, continuing to suppress these attempts by your body-mind to re-establish equilibrium and positive health will eventually lead to chronic disease where 'vital organs are damaged and Nature's constructive and healing forces are no longer able to act.' So we always explain to new clients that they might feel worse before they feel better. In fact, generally speaking, the stronger and sharper your reaction, the more it is a sign that your vital force is in good shape. If your symptoms grumble on for days or more, it needs patient tender, loving care.

It's your health - it's your responsibility.
The other big difference between conventional medicine and 'us' is that in the former system you are not required to take any responsibility for your health other than to take the pills or whatever as directed. As you will have gathered by now, it is a different story in the alternative world where you will be asked to play a very active role and to make your own choices as soon as that is appropriate. Your well-being will become entirely your responsibility, whether directly or indirectly - though the practitioner is there as an equal partner in the process, to act as a guide as you learn (or re-learn) to listen to what your body-mind has to advise you. Nobody is pretending this is easy, particularly at the beginning. But hopefully with the right kind of support, you will treat these new things to learn as an exciting adventure.

Quality not quantity
These days things seem to be 'bigger and better' faster, more expensive or just more. But we believe we should try and hold on to qualities - and particularly our

quality of life because all the money or things in the world won't necessarily cure ill health, unhappiness, and loneliness. This should be reflected in the quality of your practitioner's attention and TLC (tender, loving care). We also believe that we should practise what we preach (well most of the time - and we try not to preach). If *our* vitality is low, our intuitive and communicative faculties will be impaired and we will not be able to help you so effectively. The other thing you will find is that unlike most doctors who become doctors out of a sense of vocation or because it is a good profession, and have often never had a health problem in their lives, alternative practitioners have very often 'been there'. Take me for instance. I used to sprint and ski competitively and thought I was indestructible until I put out my low back when I was 23. I literally couldn't move my head for three days. I know the sort of thing my clients with acute back pain are going through because I suffered it for nine months, with all the fear and wondering if I'd *ever* be free of it. I also know that for me, having tried several other complementary options, McTimoney chiropractic works brilliantly which is why I decided to do the four years training myself - and have never looked back! I also know what hell having food cravings and candidiasis is - and the experience of healing these also reinforced my belief in the quite amazing ability of our body-minds not only to rebalance itself, but to finish up the better for the experience.

The quality of intuition
Another thing you may notice about complementary practitioners is that we often act on intuition. I'm not saying that conventional doctors don't - far from it, but it is something that we actively develop and trust and we encourage you to do the same. You'll notice this particularly where hands-on work is involved. Many practitioners' hands just seem to 'know' where to go and what to do to relieve that tender spot or tension or blockage. In diagnosing too, whether dowsing, feeling your pulses or finding which bone is slightly out of place, or even just knowing that your father died when you were a baby, practitioners' sensitivity and acuracy is amazing and can't really be explained or measured by science as we know it today. It can be taught however, and it certainly develops with experience. So don't be put off if it all seems very low-tech and subjective, since intuitive powers are often in their own way as powerful as the latest piece of medical kit - and a great deal cheaper and non-invasive.

SO HOW DO I CHOOSE A PRACTITIONER?
Having mentioned a few of the qualities to look for, how about a balance of science and intuition? You can research the options with the help of the directory, and the introduction to it should answer most of the practical questions you may have. Trust what feels right.

The candida programme is quite a lot to cope with on your own, but once you have found a practitioner who is experienced and trained, it should all be pretty straightforward. What *does* matter is that you feel you have a good rapport with the person you choose, and can comunicate openly and build trust in each other. They also should enourage realistic but positive expectations. This is very important, so if you feel you are not quite on the same wavelength with the practitioner at your first attempt, do not feel embarrassed to say so. Be patient and persevere. A word of mouth recommendation from someone who knows you is usually the best route to finding a practitioner. However, if you are completely new to this field, I hope this directory will help you make your first contact happily. Practitioners should not mind at all if you ask to speak to them on the phone before committing yourself, or if you want to make your first appointment an exploratory one.

At All Hallows House where 16 practitioners work as a team, people often book a half-hour initial consultation to discuss which therapy would be most suitable for them. It is true that at first sight the bewildering array of therapies available in the alternative world can seem like a jungle. But remember that all of us, whether we are chiropractors, nutritionists or colonic irrigationists, will be looking at and treating you as a whole. Particularly where chronic or stress-related conditions such a candidiasis are concerned, your symptom patterns, while relevant indicators, are not nearly as important as your *unique* constitutional type, your past strengths and weaknesses, lifestyle factors and personality.

It honestly does not matter whether the *baseline* practitioner you choose is a nutritionist, herbalist, clinical ecologist or a naturopath. Their approaches will have different emphases, but all should have been thoroughly trained in an integrated, holistic understanding of candidiasis. Many of us are eclectic and have trained in several therapies over the years, or work at a multi-disciplinary clinic with a team of other practitioners, so we will have several disciplines to draw upon as appropriate.

Therapies for other related symptoms
You may well have other specific symptoms that have their roots in candidiasis, such as chronic neck pain or stiffness, irritable bowel syndrome, rhinitis or anxiety attacks. These are discussed in alphabetical order in Chapter 4. Sometimes they need more urgent attention than the candidiasis itself, and are best helped by other therapists who will not necessarily be trained in nutrition or the disciplines mentioned above. In fact, many people seek help for a related symptom long before they realise it may be candida-related (particularly if they

have never heard of it). Often the typical candidiasis symptoms are so mild in comparison that it is difficult to convince clients they even need treating at all.

If you decide to deal with a related symptom first, that is fine. The main thing is to start feeling better fast. But do realise that you should start dealing with the candidiasis directly as soon as you feel well enough, otherwise the problem will only recur, costing you more time and money. I frequently see this in chronic back pain sufferers for example. They are often reluctant to start making changes to their diets initially, but once they are better, they wish they had done so years ago.

Most therapies have their own systems of diagnosis and treatment, and many of them developed over thousands of years. But virtually all of them boil down to the principle of enabling your body-mind to release blocks, tensions, imbalances or toxins, and then to return to its natural state of homoeostasis and robust health. They all enhance each other and should prepare you for a speedier recovery when you do feel ready to start the anti-candida programme. However, a word of caution. In my experience, when I am treating people for back pain with McTimoney chiropractic, people with candidiasis are usually noticeably more sensitive to touch, and get stronger reactions to the treatment. So make sure your therapist is fully aware that you think you might have candidiasis before they start to treat you. (See reactions below).

Very broadly, therapies can be divided into four categories:

1.   *Physical body-work such as chiropractic/osteopathy or massage*
2.   *Bio-chemical, e.g. nutrition, homoeopathy, herbal medicine*
3.   *Listening/counselling and psychotherapy*
4.   *Self-help, e.g. yoga, relaxation techniques, and home remedies*

However, there are plenty of examples which straddle more than one. For instance, aromatherapy combines massage with essential oils which have very clear chemical properties, and biodynamic massage combines body-work with psychotherapy. Of course, listening and self-help advice with an element of emotional and spiritual care should be a key part of every complementary consultation.

What if I am already being treated by my GP with drugs?
Don't worry, it's not a problem. We do wish, though, that more people would realise that they can benefit from both approaches in parallel. So many people think they cannot do both - or are told so by their GP. Depending on the drug, the dosage, and the period over which you have been taking it, there is no doubt that

people usually respond better to naturopathic treatment if they are not already on drugs. However, you can work with natural remedies to build up your natural defences again *while you are continuing to take your drugs.* Eventually, you and your GP will agree that you can safely gradually cut them down to nothing. This usually works very well, and often surprisingly quickly.

When making your first enquiry with a complementary practitioner, do mention any drug treatment you are on, and bring any bottles of pills and creams with you to your first consultation. If appropriate, the practitioner will, with your permission, contact your GP either to clarify a few things, or simply out of courtesy to let him or her know that you are also consulting someone else. Many clients absolutely refuse to mention that they are seeing a complementary practitioner to their GP since they think he or she would be angry or ridicule them or whatever. Remember that GPs do pay a great deal of attention to what works for their patients, and until they start getting feed-back about the value of complementary medicine, they will be none the wiser. The 'us and them' situation we still have is not doing anyone any favours, so if you get help from a complementary therapist, do tell your GP.

What to expect
There is no typical course of treatment. As you can see from the directory, the length of sessions and charges vary considerably, and the length of treatment depends on how long you have been unwell, your system's abilities to adapt and bounce back, and how far you are willing or able to make necessary changes to your lifestyle. It also depends on the depth of your pocket and how regularly you feel you need the moral support from your practitioner. They should always be flexible and accommodating here, so discuss this openly at your first appointment.

Why trying to self-treat is a false economy (or worse!)
It is simply human nature that most of us do not learn from other peoples' mistakes. We have to experience them for ourselves, and even then it may take several attempts. So perhaps I am wasting my breath, but I'll say it anyway. PLEASE DON'T TRY TO SELF-TREAT. Candidiasis and gut dysbiosis is a complicated syndrome, full of red herrings, with no cut and dried rules. Like so many things in life, the more you find out about a subject, the more you realise how much you don't know about it. This one can be a minefield. Our record cards are full of tales of woe from people who thought they could read a book or two and do it themselves. However, there are also many who felt they were getting nowhere with orthodox medicine; they did not know where to look, failed to find a practitioner initially, and tried to treat themselves anyway. With this directory, this should no longer be a problem.

Common pitfalls in self-treating

The starting point for any treatment is to get the right diagnosis. If you have read chapter 2 you will appreciate that for candidiasis this is not unequivocal. Most people with candida have food intolerances, nutritional deficiencies or heavy metal build-up. It is much easier to start with a list of problems which have been identified by laboratory tests or a practitioner skilled in applied kinesiology, vega testing or dowsing, than to battle your way through an exclusion diet for weeks - or worse, not address these aspects at all.

Some people lose far too much weight because they are *too* rigorous and don't appreciate how many alternative foods there are, while others get understandably confused about which foods they can and can't eat or don't realise that many of the foods they think are fine contain lots of hidden substances such as citric acid, fermented foods and sugars - all going under other names.

Many spend months and not so small fortunes on supplements and remedies to treat a problem they never had, or miss those they do, such as parasites, or a faulty blood sugar metabolism. Another common one is to buy supplements piecemeal and end up taking 15-20 *different* pills a day. You would not believe the number of people I have spoken to who say 'I could open a shop with all the bottles I've got'. Not only is it much cheaper, but it is also much more effective to take them in the synergistic formulations or special combinations made up by the specialist manufacturers. We need to be sure that you have the co-factors or enzymes present that will enable you to absorb them and bear in mind that your absorption is likely to be impaired. Otherwise, you will simply be 'making very expensive urine'. Some doctors will take great delight in telling you this,

You need therapeutic doses which you will not find in the supermarket or over the counter in a chemist. The quality of supplements and remedies also varies enormously and has nothing to do with how attractive and expensive their advertising campaigns are - in fact the inverse is often the case. If you are not getting yours from a manufacturer recommended by an experienced practitioner, you might be getting poor to scandalous quality. This is particularly true of the probiotics. See chapter 7.

There is a strong move in the NHS to encourage patients to self-treat by making more drugs available over the counter (these are known as OTCs). But alternative remedies do not work in the same 'this pill for that ill' way as drugs. They are tailored to your unique self. In experienced hands, the whole of, say, a herbal mixture is a great deal more than the sum of its parts.

People have made great sacrifices to afford to have all their mercury fillings replaced, without knowing that one can go a long way towards the same result with chelation therapy and having the electromagnetic fields checked around their bed and work place first. This may cost £60-£100 instead of over a thousand pounds. See chapter 9 for more details.

After two generations of 'wonder drugs' and quick fixes, people no longer expect to get worse before they get better and would never dream that feeling grim for a couple of days is actually a very healthy sign - particularly when it happens out of the blue, just when they thought they'd really cracked it! But as I've explained above, all the natural therapies recognise that this is the way that Nature and the body works and a practitioner will prepare and advise you how to cope with 'reactions' and 'healing crises', so you can sail on through, rather than giving up in despair.

The most common mistake of all - and I am afraid to say that some inexperienced practitioners are guilty of this too - *to beat candidiasis, you need to focus on all fronts simultaneously and tenaciously.* It is not just a matter of wiping out a few pesky yeast cells. It is about rebuilding the environment in your gut and your immune system; spring cleaning your whole body, thereby creating the "silence" so you can hear its wisdom; and retraining your eating habits. The seven-point plan is outlined in detail in chapter 5. Go for it lock, stock and barrel and don't stop too soon. Getting it 70% right is often not enough, then you get disillusioned that all your effort come to nothing and the complementary approach gets a bad name. Too many doctors will be glad to tell you 'I told you not to meddle in alternative medicine'.

Beating candidiasis is often to plough a very lonely furrow especially if you have to sustain it for many months, so getting the right support from an experienced practitioner can make all the difference.

However.....
If your symptoms are very mild and you have had them for only a few months, you might well crack it by yourself, so by all means have a go, but only for three months. Hopefully this guide will help, but if it is not clear that your programme is working after that time, *seek help.* The vast majority of you should get better more quickly, more easily and more thoroughly - *and therefore more cheaply* - by seeing an experienced practitioner at the beginning. You might well not need to see them more than two or three times if you don't want to.

Do read as much as you can on the subject. Books and journals are listed at the back of the guide or under the sections to which they refer. And do join a self-help group and subscribe to our newsletter (see chapter 8.)

What if I am too ill or live too far away from a practitioner?
In either case, there are several nutritionists listed in the directory who do postal consultations. You can also get in touch with the Radionics Society for distant healing and diagnosis. However remote you may be, there are bound to be a few other sufferers nearby. Candida Support Groups will send you advice on how to contact them, or put you in touch with your nearest group if there is one. Details are in chapter 8.

If you are very ill, or if you have ME or MS, some practitioners will do home visits until you are well enough to travel, so ring them and ask, but do make sure you keep your GP in the picture.

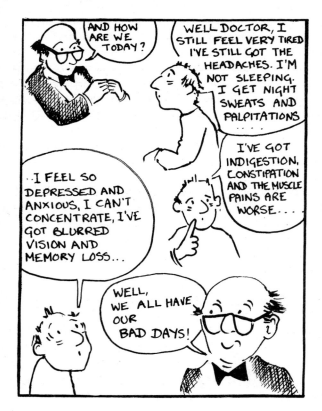

CHAPTER 4

TREATING OTHER SYMPTOMS OR CONDITIONS OFTEN ASSOCIATED WITH CANDIDIASIS

Suggestions for self-help using natural remedies, and useful therapies.

The aim of this chapter is to help you to improve the quality of your life as much as possible, and to give you plenty of suggestions for alleviating unpleasant symptoms *without resorting to drugs*. These will only add to your total toxic load, mask any healthy healing reactions or symptoms and may hinder your recovery. This is true for any problem, but it is particularly important in conditions such as candidiasis or gut dysbiosis and food intolerances because the liver is one of the main organs to need a rest and support. Drugs have to be processed by the liver and therefore simply put an unwanted burden on it.

Obviously it depends on how long you have had them but you'll find that most associated symptoms will melt away once you get the yeasts and toxins on the run and take the load off your system by eliminating the substances to which you are intolerant. This usually begins to happen within 5-40 days of starting the programme.
However, remember that you may get a 'healing reaction', i.e. an unexpected attack as your body is finally shaking off an old symptom.

NB the following notes assume you have candidiasis and gut dysbiosis, so they will not necessarily be complete for people who do not. All the suggestions below are in addition to the seven-point anti-candida programme outlined in Chapter 5.

Each symptom heading outlines:

• a brief explanation or description of the symptom or condition if not well known
• some self-help suggestions (only appropriate if symptoms are mild or very infrequent) or recommended books - but see general books below.
• some nutritional supplements or remedies that you should be able to buy for yourself (see chapter 7 for more details and where to find them, and chapter 2 for diagnostic tests).

- some suggestions as to which complementary therapies are most likely to help are in italics. But see the introduction to chapter 11 for why one cannot be dogmatic here - in practice most of the natural therapies will help most of the symptoms below.
- suggestions for a natural first aid kit, advice on natural remedies for travelling, pregnancy, children, giving up smoking, relaxation are also included at the end of this chapter.

PLEASE NOTE THAT IF YOUR SYMPTOM IS SEVERE OR PROLONGED YOU SHOULD SEE A PRACTITIONER FIRST.
DO NOT ATTEMPT TO SELF-TREAT ANY OF THE ASTERISKED CONDITIONS

GENERAL BOOKS ON TREATING SYMPTOMS HOLISTICALLY:

Overcoming Food Allergies, you don't have to 'live with it'. Gwynne Davies ND MTOS, Ashgrove 1993. Invaluable help for identifying food intolerances that might be the culprits for everyday symptoms.

You Don't Have to Feel Unwell, Nutrition, Lifestyle, Herbs and Homoeopathy, A Home Guide. Robin Needes ND SRN, Gateway Books 1994. An excellent and fascinating guide giving the full holistic picture.

Better Health through Natural Healing, Ross Trattler, Thorsons 1987. My old standby.

Food Allergy and Intolerance, Dr Jonathan Brostoff and Linda Gamlin, Bloomsbury 1989, will give you a detailed and clear understanding of this vast subject. It is well indexed.

Aromatherapy, A Guide for Home Use. Christine Westwood, Kerbina Ltd. 1991. A very clear and easy to use little guide.

Women's Bodies, Women's Wisdom, the complete guide to women's health and well-being. Dr Christiane Northrup, Piatkus 1995. A really remarkable book by a holistic physician trained in obstetrics and gynaecology. She gives sound advice at every level including how to heal yourself by listening to your body's wisdom and intuition.

The Complete Book of Water Therapy. Dian Dincin Buchman, Keats Publishing 1994. Hydrotherapy (using hot and cold water or ice, compresses, baths, enemas) is one of our the oldest therapies and one of the mainstays of naturopathic medicine. Since it is so cheap and easily available, and safe as long as you follow the advice here, I recommend you look at this book. Having explained all the principles, it lists symptoms alphabetically, giving recommendations for each.

Self help homoeopathy can be pretty hit and miss, but see the natural first aid kit at the end of this chapter. For minor complaints the *Family Guide to Homoeopathy* is a brilliant little booklet for £1.50 available from most health food shops.

Where *essential oils* are suggested, these can be applied either in the bath (6 drops), or diluted in a base oil (2-4 drops) and massaged either on to the painful area, or into the hands and feet, or on a compress (1-2 drops in water). They are also lovely as room fragrancers. See Christine Westwood's book above for more details.

Celloid Minerals are specially formulated minerals imported by Blackmores from Australia that we find particularly good, gentle and cost effective. (£3.99 for 84 tablets) The retail Compound range is given here, though you will find they are called something else if you get them from your practitioner.

ACHES (See under Muscles and Joints)

ACNE* & PIMPLES
The broad spectrum antibiotics prescribed for acne over long periods are a common cause of candidiasis. Then the extra load on the liver and interference with the hormonal system just make it worse. Make sure all your organs of detoxification are boosted (see chapter 5). Drink at least 2 pints of pure water a day. While the orthodox line is to deny it, we find that *nutrition* plays a key role in clearing all skin problems, as does *herbal medicine and homoeopathy*. Echinacea ACE. Chamomile oil for redness, Frankincense for scarring and Tea Tree for spots. Carrot, nettle, watercress and lettuce juices and kelp.
Celloids: Silica for blind pimples, Chloride for white heads, Sulphur for yellow heads, ZBM for scarring, Executive Formula B for nerve balancing. Vitamin C to bowel tolerance (see constipation).
Blackmores have an excellent Natural Skin Care and Skin Treatment Range for problem skin. See Katherine Marsden's book *Superskin*.

ALCOHOLISM*
It is a safe bet that most heavy drinkers will have a high level of gut dysbiosis. The tragedy is that candida can cause the craving for alcohol in the first place and a vicious circle is established. Once the individual has decided he or she wants to stop drinking, and not before, a combination of intensive vitamin and mineral supplementation to correct the deficiencies (particularly vitamins B and C, the anti-oxidants and Magnesium Compound

(Celloids), liver support and general detoxification will ease the process enormously. Specialist *psychotherapy* for the emotional and addictive aspects and/or someone to help restore your energetic body or 'electrical circuitry' is ideal. The Alcoholics Anonymous Twelve Step Programme has remarkable results. See under liver support in chapter 7.

If you cannot tolerate alcohol without a mother of a hangover, this is a sure sign that your liver needs extra support and you need a thorough detoxification. Rose, juniper and rosemary oils help if you have that hung over feeling, which you can often get without having drunk any alcohol.

ALLERGIES & FOOD INTOLERANCES
Allergy literally means 'altered reaction'. See chapter 1 for full definitions, chapter 2 for diagnostic tests and chapter 11 for therapists who can help you identify your culprit foods. Do read Dr Brostoff's book. So many people have been given strong anti-histamines or steroid drugs for years before realising that their sensitivities may be part of the bigger picture of gut dysbiosis. Treatment involves identification and complete elimination of the relevant foods with detoxification for several months. Rose and melissa oils help. Digestive enzymes can ease you through food intolerances (see chapter 11). If you suspect that air borne allergens are the problem (for hay fever or asthma), BioCare's Hystazyme can help, but you need to start taking it 2 months before the season starts. The house dustmite are a very common problem - suspect this if your nose is especially stuffed up in the mornings. Investing in a special vacuum cleaner (see appendix 2) can make a huge difference, although some people find that once the food allergens are eliminated, the dustmite is not longer a problem.

Homoeopathy, acupuncture and TCM often have good results for any allergy.

ANXIETY AND PANIC ATTACKS
These normally improve or disappear within about one month of starting the programme. In the meantime Celloids Magnesium Compound and Bach Flower Rescue Remedy are excellent. Natracalm is a herbal remedy that is easy to find. Blackmores Hypericum or Skullcap and Valerian. Bergamot oil is uplifting, and frankincense and lavender are good for panic attacks. If persistent, *autogenic training, meditation or psychotherapy plus herbal medicine.*

ARTHRITIS*
In many instances this may be related to a leaky gut and allergic or auto-immune reactions. Eliminate acid-forming foods. Ask to be checked for parasites. Blastocystis hominis is the most common implicated. Lavender oil and vitamin C reduce pain, and juniper oil any swelling. Rheumatoid arthritis responds to chamomile, juniper, ginger and lavender oils. We have found that *nutrition, acupuncture and gentle manipulation* is a winning combination. Take a look at any suppressed anger (Ylang ylang oil helps here).

ASTHMA* See also Allergies
This can also be related to a leaky gut and immune weakness. Antigen antibody complexes are stored in the lungs causing inflammation and smooth muscle spasm. Gwynne Davies' research finds asthma, sinus, catarrh and hay fever patients are intolerant to the following foods: cow's milk and white flour both in 90% of cases, cheese in 37%,

orange in 30%, and lemon in 28%. Maurice Hanssen lists 17 additives that are common triggers. Cedarwood, eucalyptus and cypress oils help when inhaled. *Homoeopathy or herbal medicine* both get good results. Try BioCare's Candicidin first. Mycolyte and garlic supplements can be effective if catarrh is bad. Many people using steroid inhalers find they get thrush in their mouths and throats. Swilling some warm water around after using them can help. The liquid anti-fungals used as a gargle or nasal spray can keep it clear (see chapter 7)

ATHLETES' FOOT

A fungal infection, usually between the little toes causing scaling, itching and cracking - which can then also get bacterial infections. Keep clean and dry always. Fresh air and sunlight help. Wash with vinegar or Tea Tree oil (the Blackmores Anti-bacterial Face Wash is great). Boric acid soak. BioCare Dermasorb, Vitamin E or calendula creams or aloe vera will improve and soothe. Celloids Sulphur, garlic supplements, Vitamin A and Zinc. Like fungal nail infections, this can last for months and is unlikely to go until you have cleared the candidiasis in the gut. BioCare's Candicidin has been shown to clear problems that months of drug therapy have not shifted

BACK & NECK PAIN (see Joint aches and Pains and Posture)

BLOATING (see Gas/wind and Fluid Retention)

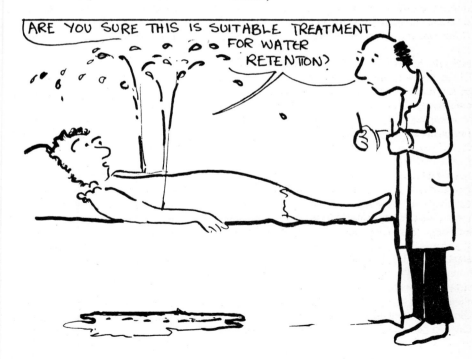

BODY ODOUR AND BAD BREATH

Any nasty smells mean either there is something wrong internally - though if you are seeing a practitioner and following the programme this should be being addressed (don't be embarrassed to raise it if you don't think it is, as this mustn't just be covered up and ignored). Or it can mean that your body is ridding itself of accumulated wastes - which is obviously an encouraging sign, though unpleasant. Either way, here are some practical tips to help until things rebalance again. apart from soap and water deficiency, BO can be due to a poor diet, zinc deficiency, eating too many saturated fats, or a liver or kidney disorder. If you are sweating a lot as well, don't suppress it with powerful chemicals. Several natural antiperspirants are available from health food shops. Washing with natural anti-fungals or with Blackmore's anti-bacterial face wash (all over) twice a day if necessary. Epsom salts baths are great - see hydrotherapy. For bad breath, have your dental hygiene and gums checked and gargle with one of the liquid anti-fungals listed in chapter 7. Constipation, digestive deficiencies, liver overload, respiratory problems and stress (which interferes with your digestion) can all cause the problem. Don't resort to mints as they'll be full of sugar. Chew on some fennel, anise or cardamom seeds, parsley, or cloves. Peppermint tea and Echinacea will also help.

CATARRH

An intolerance to dairy products is often behind any build-up of mucous. Eucalyptus and pine will ease any congestion and sandalwood is good inhaled. Blackmores Super Horseradish & Garlic, Celloids Chloride, BioCare's Mycolyte. *Acupuncture, herbal medicine and homoeopathy.*

CELLULITE

Many clients are amazed and delighted to find that their cellulite disappears without having to diet.. This is because cellulite is not ordinary fat but the body's way of disposing of waste and toxins that it otherwise cannot deal with. Dry skin brushing, rebounding, detoxifying generally (drink lots of water and no coffee) and regular *massage or aromatherapy* with cypress, fennel and lemon oils will speed it on its way. *Manual Lymphatic Drainage* see under massage in chapter 11.

COELIAC DISEASE *

Severe intolerance to gluten causing pale foul smelling stools, mal-absorbtion and stunted growth. Obviously this needs specialist treatment, but there is no reason why you cannot diagnose and treat the food intolerances gut dysbiosis that underlies it while receiving orthodox treatment if your GP is open to this. See Brostoff and Gamlin's book. Celloids: Sodiphos, Magnesium and Calcium. *Herbal medicine.*

COLD HANDS AND FEET

Found in 98% of CFS(ME) sufferers. A combination of dry skin brushing, regular stretching/exercise including breathing, several small meals per day, and hydrotherapy should help, as will massage with rosemary, ginger and frankincense oils. Blackmore's Ginko Forte is great for improving circulation, Magnesium and Vitamin E. Check thyroid function (see chapter 2) *Naturopathy, reflexology or acupuncture.*

CONSTIPATION

This is very common with candidiasis, and getting bunged up is the last thing you want as you will absorb more toxins, so I'll go into some detail. Ideally we should go at least once a day (preferably twice) and our stools should float (to show they are not too compacted), and they should not be too dark (vegetarians' will tend to be lighter). Many people say when first starting the diet, they cannot give up their prunes or figs or their strong coffee fix for breakfast without getting constipated. The following tips to follow daily should prevent this, although bowels often take a week or so to settle down when you change habits.

All the general advice in chapter 5 on detoxifying and diet will help.

The most common food intolerances are wheat, dairy and tea/coffee. Avoid laxatives and all refined foods. Increase your dose of acidophilus or take Replete for a week. A herbal colon cleanse done for at least 4-8 weeks (e.g. Higher Nature's Coloclear, BioCare's Colon Care) and/or a course of *colonic irrigation* will get your candida programme off to a flying start as well as helping your constipation. Or see a *medical herbalist.*

Sip a mug of hot water with a slice of lemon first thing (and later on too). Drink *plenty* of water - at least 2 pints a day. Raw juices are also excellent.

Seeds, especially linseeds (flaxseeds). Start with 1 teaspoon per day and build up to 2 tablespoons - preferably freshly ground and soaked overnight in a little water or apple juice, and served on muesli or yoghurt.

At least 2 tablespoons of virgin olive oil, and flaxseed oil is also good (available from Higher Nature - but it must be kept in the fridge.) Use in salad dressings or in cooking.

Pre soaked oat bran (e.g. Mornflake) NOT wheat bran (in most 'high fibre' cereals e.g. All Bran) - the latter is equivalent to using a brillo pad on your insides and causes food intolerance in many people. Many sufferers improve on making this change alone.

Olive oil cream rubbed slowly but firmly in big circles into the stomach (down on the left, up on the right). Try adding rosemary and black pepper oils. Dry skin brushing twice a day. Regular exercise. Most women I ask confess that they don't allow themselves any time to just sit on the loo and would never disappear with the newspapers for half an hour every morning like their menfolk. Make a regular time that is yours and not to be disturbed!

Vitamin C powder *to bowel tolerance* - Everyone needs different amounts, and this will vary according to how much stress you are under, exercise and how well you have been eating. To find the right amount for you, start with 1 level teaspoonful twice a day with a large glass of water, ideally first thing in the morning and last thing at night, and increase by 1/4 teaspoonful each time until you get a runny tummy, then cut back by 1 teaspoon and maintain the dose. Biocare's Magnesium Ascorbate (vitamin C) is excellent.

Check thyroid and take kelp if low. Tone the liver with Blackmore's Dandelion, their Cape Aloes and Cascara is a gentle laxative. Celloids: Magnesium Compound to help nerve depletion, Calcium Compound if you have elastic tissue problems.

Shiatsu Point: Lay your thumb straight alongside your fingers and a little mound of flesh will appear at the base of it. Take your other thumb and gently press across this mound (with the first thumb relaxed) use firm, deep but gentle pressure as you breathe out. Repeat on the other hand. Do not use this point if you are pregnant.

Look at whether you are "holding on to things" emotionally.

CRAMPS

These should also go quite quickly, but are very unpleasant at the time. Shorten the muscle immediately and rub it hard. Do not take salt - a multi-mineral or Celloids: Magnesium and Calcium Complexes should do the trick and make sure you are getting at least two pints of water a day. A massage with juniper oil will help, or rosemary, marjoram and lemon grass if it is following too much exercise. Dry skin brushing will help any after-effects.

CROHNS DISEASE* / ULCERATIVE COLITIS*/ SPASTIC COLON*

We find that emotional factors, which may be profound, are often the key to recovery in these conditions. *See autogenic training, meditation, psychotherapy.*

When the mucosal lining of the colon has ulcers, it has been shown that this linked with low production and absorption of butyric acid. (See BioMed, Feb. 1990: Dr Torben Neesby). Vitamin U (cabbagin), slippery elm and raw juices before meals help. Grated apple that has been allowed to brown is good. Millet porridge is very soothing, since it is alkaline. Eliminate wheat, dairy, and acid-forming foods (including coffee) and sometimes all gluten. Gwynne Davies frequently finds eliminating the 4 C's (chocolate, citrus, cheese and coffee) plus wheat and milk is the solution, in which case he suspects "gut migraine". Celloids: Magnesium and Chloride Compounds. Anti-oxidants plus zinc. Vitamin C must be buffered *Herbal Medicine, Western or Chinese* has a great deal to offer here.

CYSTITIS

This is a burning feeling when you pee that can be agonising. It is caused by infection and inflammation of the urethra (the tube from the kidneys). Get this checked by a GP to make sure other infections such as chlamydia are not around, but if it is straight forward cystitis DO NOT TAKE ANTIBIOTICS! (see alternatives to antibiotics below) It may be the last thing you want to do at the time, but it is important to drink plenty of filtered/mineral water or fluids (but nothing containing any sugar) and to empty your bladder completely to flush out the infection.

Unsweetened cranberry juice neutralises the pH (acid) very effectively. Or try homemade barley water: Boil 1/3 bag pearl barley for 20 minutes and drink the barley water (you can use the barley for supper). Repeat 2-3 times per day for 2-3 days. Fresh homemade vegetable juices are also excellent. Try one pint daily of: 10oz Carrot juice, 3 oz Beetroot juice, 3 oz Cucumber juice, or 10oz Carrot juice and 6oz Spinach juice, or 9oz Carrot juice, 5oz Celery juice and 2oz Parsley juice. Keep to a low acid diet.

BioCare's cranberry Extract followed by UR 228 is very good, also Magnesium Ascorbate (Vitamin C is an alkaline form). Celloids: Sodiphos and Silica Compounds, Blackmores herbals: Bilberry 2000 or Cornsilk (to line the urethra), Juniper and sandalwood oils help. Use lavender oil for the pain and eucalyptus if you have a temperature.

Angela Kilmartin's book on Cystitis is the classic (though resist the temptation to resort to antibiotics).

DEPRESSION

Far from being the cause, you may well feel that depression is the result of candidiasis and the emotional and social isolation that too often goes with it. The chemicals made by the yeast such as acetaldehyde can certainly be a cause. Either way, the negative feelings will

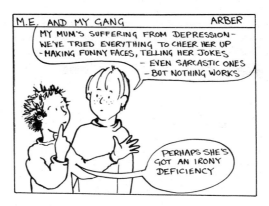

not be helping your immune system recover, so it is vital that you do whatever you can to alleviate or counter it.

True depression tends to be worse in the mornings, whereas the ghastly low feeling one gets with candidiasis may come and go and is worse after eating certain foods, when you are tired or if your blood sugar is low (see low blood sugar). Gwynne Davies finds that coffee, milk cheese, colourings, and sugar are the most common culprits. Eliminating them should make you feel better within days, and it means that the pancreas will start to produce the amino acids again which are essential for balanced mental function. See chapter 9 on negative feelings, electromagnetic fields and mercury toxicity. Any daily exercise you enjoy is essential. Even if you do not feel like doing much, spend 10 minutes stretching and breathing every morning (see chapter 5). Clary sage and bergamot oils are very uplifting (try them on a room fragrancer as well) Vitamin B complex, Celloids: Magnesium Compound. Blackmores Hypericum. *Bach Flower Remedies.* Depression can often be stress related or suppressed anger or fear, in which case if persistent, *psychotherapy or autogenic training* will help you deal with both. Check hormone imbalance (FHP Panel) and Adrenal Stress Index, both from Diagnostech.

DIARRHOEA
If accompanied by blood, mucous or pain, note the times of day and the foods it follows. Diarrhoea for a few days is fairly common during the first few days of the programme and is a good sign. If emotional factors are involved *Bach Flower Remedies* can be marvellous. Start with a high dose of probiotics or Replete.
Raw juices: equal parts of apple, carrot, beetroot and celery, twice a day on an empty stomach, but build up slowly from 1/2 a cup diluted, to 2 cups. Fresh papaya and pineapple is good for poor assimilation and pancreatic weakness if you can take it. Grated apple is also good (allow it to brown a little so the pectin develops) especially with live yoghurt, or Blackmores Apple Fibre Complex and Slippery Elm Tablets. Celloids: Sodiphos and Calcium. See a *nutritionist, herbalist or naturopath* if persistent, and check with your GP as it could be parasites or several other factors. (See also under IBS and travelling.)

DIABETES*

This can be related in some cases to the sugar cravings and damage to the endocrine system associated with candidiasis, poor diet and stress. But it needs very careful professional/medical handling until you can get the system back into balance. Avoiding all refined foods is essential, while exercise improves insulin take-up by 30%. See supplements for blood sugar levels in chapter 7. Multivitamins and minerals especially B and C. Blackmores Ginko Forte. Celloids: Magnesuim Compound. *Nutrition and stress management/relaxation techniques.* Diagnostech's ASI index may be worth checking out..

DIVERTICULITIS*

This can be caused by food and debris getting caught in little pockets in the intestine which then inflame. It may take several months to heal, and it may make the candida programme more difficult as your gut will be extra sensitive and you will have to make changes to your diet more slowly than others, so be patient - it will be worth it. Start by identifying your food intolerances and getting your diet and *nutrition* right. Juices are great, particularly in the early stages.

Probiotics and digestive enzymes will be very helpful. Celloids: Silica, Calcium and Magnesium Compounds. Blackmore's Slippery Elm Tablets. General digestive enzymes and remedies.*herbal medicine.*

EATING DISORDERS (Anorexia*, bulimia and binge eating)

Candidiasis and gut dysbiosis are virtually inevitable with any eating disorder and will in turn make any food cravings even worse (see chapter 1). Whether your eating disorder was originally the cause or an effect (the latter is more likely) does not really matter as, either way, you will probably be feeling trapped on a very lonely roller coaster. Knowing that it is very common and that the cravings have a physical/chemical cause makes a huge difference, so get your trigger foods identified and start on the programme as soon as possible. You may well need some professional support to unravel the emotional knots that you may have been tying yourself into, if this has been going on for some time. Overeaters Anonymous ia a good place to start especially if there is a support group near you. (see appendix 2) It is highly likely that there will be some fellow sufferers at a Candida Support Group, so try them too (chapter 8) as the moral support will help you enormously. Read the sections here on negative feelings and low self esteem in chapter 9 and see under and overweight below. Mention the problem before booking with your baseline practitioner as most of us have had quite a bit of experience with eating disorders or are ex-sufferers. *Bach Flower Remedies, nutritional supplementation* (especially B complex) will all help. Celloids: Sodiphos and Magnesium Compounds. Digestive enzymes. If feeling distant and detached, try jasmine and ylang ylang oils. *Aromatherapy/ massage* will help you to get to like your body again.

Anorexia is more complicated and professional help is essential. In our experience the holistic approach is usually more sympathetic and better at getting to the true underlying emotional causes - and they work well alongside any orthododox treatment. *Reflexology, shiatsu, herbal medicine, nutrition and psychotherapy* will all help enormously

60

ECZEMA (Atopic)* See also Allergies

Gwynne Davies' research reveals intolerances in the following percentages of clients with eczema and psoriasis: cow's milk 74%, white flour 70%, orange, cheese and lemon all 37%, and egg white 27%. NB if you are breast feeding and your baby has eczema, you will have to be tested and eliminate anything that will reach the baby in your milk. Lavender oil is marvellous, chamomile for itching or burning, frankincense if the skin is weeping. Most people find the non-biological or eco-friendly washing powders much better. Resist the temptation to use cortisone creams from your GP. Miasmic and constitutional prescribing from a *homoeopath* can work 'miraculously', especially if the problem is caught early on. *Herbal Medicine* to cleanse the lymph and tone the liver, Blackmores Dandelion and Sasparilla. *TCM* gets particularly good results - a cream by Phytopharm is available through your GP. Vitamins A, C, E, BioCare's Mega GLA. Celloids: Chloride and Silica Compounds.

FATIGUE (see also CFS (ME))

Fatigue is almost universal for candidiasis sufferers particularly where food intolerances are involved as well. It will usually start to lift in less than 2 weeks, but may come straight back as soon as you lapse or overdo things. It will be the benchmark for how much stronger you are getting. Blackmores Ginko Forte is good and Magnesium Compound and the anti-oxidants and B vitamins will pick you up. Try clary sage and lavender oils with orange. Rosemary, juniper and jasmine for lethargy. Rosemary and bergamot is a good combination for that Monday morning feeling. Dry skin brushing and a warm-cold-warm shower never fails! CoQ10 is a special enzyme that is plays in integral role in our ability to 'recharge our batteries' (ATP production), BioCare's Lipoplex is a good synergistic source. See chapter 9 for mercury toxicity and electromagnetic fields. See Dr Alan Stewart's book Tired all the Time for other possible factors. Leon Chaitow's beat Fatigue Workbook is very practical. Kathryn Marsden's All Day Energy, and any of Leslie Kenton's books will pick you straight up!

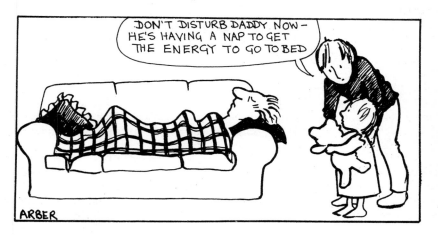

61

FIBROMYALGIA SYNDROME (FMS) or 'fibrocytis'*

More research is needed, but we suspect that, like ME(CFS) and IBS, severe candidiasis is behind much of the intense suffering and muscle pain that can go on for years. The pain is described as diffuse aching or burning. Positive diagnosis is 'official' when 11 out of 18 specific sites on the body are very tender to the touch and when the widespread pain has been present for more than 3 months. Leon Chaitow wrote in the Journal of Alternative and Complementary Medicine in June 1995 that "FMS and CFS (ME) have a wide range of identical symptoms ranging from fatigue through impaired cognitive and memory functions, to muscular pain, digestive disturbances, headaches and sleep disturbance." In children, it often starts with flu-like symptoms, and later involves Attention Deficit Disorder (ADD) and allergies. They may also have over-flexible joints. American statistics show that it occurs mainly between 26 and 35 years old and that 86% of sufferers are women. It is as common as rheumatoid arthritis, in that there are up to 1.5 million sufferers in the UK, 25% of whom are too disabled to work.

The most commonly prescribed drugs for FMS are tricyclic drugs. While these may be useful in extremis in the short term, they may lead to dependency.

I shall not mention any self-help remedies here as it is best to see a *nutritionist, naturopath, gentle manipulator or acupuncturist* first.

The Fibromyalgia Association UK, 8 Rochester Grove, Hazel Grove, Stockport, Cheshire SK7 4JD, have a newsletter, video and books. They will put you in touch with support groups and helplines throughout the UK. Fibromyalgia Network 5700 Stockdale Highway, Suite 100, Bakersfield CA 93309-2553 USA.

FLUID RETENTION

This is another unpleasant and common symptom that should go within a month or two. BioCare's Celery seed and Potassium Ascorbate (vitamin C) or Blackmores Herbal Fluid Balance works well with Celloids Sodiphos. Rebounding and dry skin brushing followed by a massage with juniper and fennel oils is great. *Manual lymphatic drainage* is particularly helpful. If monthly, check hormone imbalance with Diagnostech's FHP test (see chapter 2).

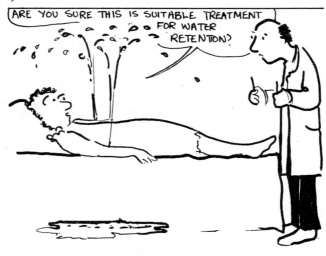

FOOD INTOLERANCE (see Allergies and chapter 1)

"FOGGY BRAIN" (see hyperventilation)
This is quite the most infuriating and embarrassing side effect of candidiasis. It may get even worse during die-off as it seems that the acetaldehyde produced by the yeast is the main cause of it, but it will clear after that - permanently once the gut is healed. When it strikes, basil and grapefruit oils will clear the fog, while rosemary will help blurred memory. If accompanied by a dread of effort, try sandalwood. All these work well in a room fragrancer and by massaging your temples and scalp. Blackmores Ginko Forte is excellent, as is their Executive B Formula (vitamins) and Celloids Potassium.. BioCare Candicidin has been shown to get good results with mental symptoms like this. Read the section about mercury toxicity and electromagnetic fields in chapter 9 if it persists.

GAS / WIND (see also Irritable Bowel)
This can be painful and embarrassing, but while there will be some ups and downs as your gut rebalances, this is usually one of the first symptoms to abate once you stop eating any sugar, alcohol or yeasty foods. Fennel oil is great, whether in the bath or rubbed gently into your tummy (up on the right and down on the left - the direction of the gut). Probiotics, BioCare's Tanicidin, digestive enzymes and Blackmores Ginger tablets will all help, as will Dr Stewart's Peppermint tea made very strong.

HEADACHE and MIGRAINE
Please try to resist the temptation to reach for the Paracetamol or whatever until you have tried Celloids Magnesium Compond taken with hot water every 15 minutes and rubbing your temples, forehead and jaw with lavender oil (this oil can be used neat on the skin), and under the base of your skull, neck and shoulders with one drop of peppermint oil. (This must be diluted in a carrier oil). Basil oil helps sinus headaches and rose and juniper if it is an allergy. Rosemary helps with pressure and migraines, but do not try to massage during an attack. Food intolerances are often behind headaches, so identify and eliminate them and drink plenty of water. Many clients have found that sticking to a more even routine, i.e. eating and sleeping and waking at the same times every day, makes a significant difference. Remember that headaches are a common aspect of 'die-off'. See also posture below and check mercury toxicity and electromagnetic fields in chapter 10. In the case of migraine, if you are on the Pill, this has a direct action on the blood vessels and is a well known cause of migraine. See alternatives to the Pill at the end of this chapter. *Acupuncture, reflexology, colonic irrigation, herbs and homoeopathy* will all help. One of the most common causes if frequent, is poor alignment in the neck and spine, so see *gentle manipulation and cranial osteopathy.*

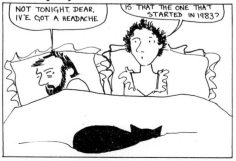

HEARTBURN (dyspepsia)

Another common one to go within a few weeks as it usually caused by poor diet and lifestyle, though it can be due to other factors, so seek professional help if it persists. Celloids: Sodiphos every 15 minutes. Digestive enzymes and *Herbal Medicine.*

HYPERACTIVITY (see also under Children)

This is a stage which commonly precedes the crash into chronic fatigue. If you recognise that anything is 'wrong' at all, it is very difficult to resist the temptation to carry on rushing around getting lots of things done. Drinking lots of coffee and caffeinated drinks and frantic work-outs in the gym every day will only precipitate the crash. Book up some *autogenic training or relaxation techniques* now. Invest in some regular *aromatherapy.* Clary sage, lavender and marjoram oils are wonderful to help you wind down and rebalance. Celloids: Magnesium and Calcium Compounds. If you are on tranquillizers, see Jill Tricklet's book (Thorsons).

HYPERVENTILATION

People who are anxious or under stress may get into the habit of breathing too fast all the time, which means the carbondioxide levels in their blood will fall, altering the pH and producing a wide range of mental and physical symptoms. Many of these are very similar to those seen with candidiasis and food intolerances - but the most characteristic are felling 'spaced-out', numbness and tingling. The trouble is that most people don't realise they are doing it. To test yourself, next time your symptoms are bad, hold a large, clean paper bag over your mouth and nose and breathe normally for a few minutes. By rebreathing your waste CO_2, you'll raise its level in the blood again. If you start to feel better, you've found the problem. It may clear up on its own within a few weeks of starting the programme, but it could be a contributory factor in itself. A *physiotherapist or stress management counsellor* should be able help you to retrain your breathing.

HYPOGLYCAEMIA (low blood sugar) and SUGAR CRAVINGS

The *last* thing you need is any sugar - or any refined carbohydrates for that matter as this will just put more of a strain on your system. See also "Losing your sugar cravings" in chapter 5 and supplements in chapter 7.
Celloids Magnesuim Compound. BioCare's Chromium Polynicotinate, Zinc and a *low* dose of B vitamin complex (or it will overstimulate your appetite). Digestive enzymes.

IMMUNE DEFICIENCIES (AIDS, HIV+ , Rheumatoid Arthritis, Lupus)

This is where complementary medicine can come into its own. You will need close orthodox supervision, and you will need to do everything possible to lighten the load on your immune system, by detoxifying, supporting the liver, eliminating allergens and optimising nutrition. Drugs such as AZT (for AIDS) have been brought into question. Many people are finding that an HIV+ state can be maintained for a normal life span with complementary therapies, without the need for drugs. *Herbal medicine or TCM, naturopathy, acupuncture and nutrition* are all very powerful. *Relaxation techniques and group therapy* are also vital.

INFECTIONS (see alternatives to antibiotics)

INFERTILITY /RECURRENT MISCARRIAGE (see pelvic inflammatory disease)

Please try natural therapies for one year before resorting to IVF (in vitro fertilisation) as we find candidiasis is frequently present in infertile couples, and IVF involves huge doses of hormones that will make any candidiasis present far worse. Clients of ours have become pregnant even after mechanical damage. See a *nutritionist plus a herbalist (Chinese or Western), reflexologist or psychotherapist* (all for both partners if appropriate). Learning aromatherapy and massage for couples can also work wonders. A low acid-forming diet (if the vagina is too acid it will kill sperm). Vitamin E and zinc.

INSOMNIA

Most candidiasis sufferers sleep like logs, but insomnia and sleep reversal can affect some people, particualarly if you have CFS(ME) or suffer from anxiety depression or pain. It is really important to try and sort this out as you need your REM sleep for your healing process (and sanity). *Herbalists, autogenic training, psychotherapy and relaxation techniques* can be very helpful. If mild or infrequent, try Celloids: Magnesuim and Calcium Compounds, B complex, Blackmores Valarian. Natrasleep is available in chemists. Relaxation tapes are well worth a try (see appendix 2).

IRRITABLE BOWEL SYNDROME

IBS shares almost identical symptoms with CFS and FMS (*ibid*) and is another label or general dumping ground for when a diagnosis cannot be pinpointed. It is usually caused in part by a leaky gut leading to local inflammation and smooth muscle spasm. Check food intolerances. Parasites are often implicated, such as *blastocystis hominis*. It usually involves very tender spots on the abdomen, is worse for stress and changes in the weather. High dose probiotics, slippery elm and Magnesium Compund will all help. if you suffer with low back ache, get some *gentle manipulation. Homooepathy, herbal medicine, reflexology, stress management, autogenic training, yoga* are all effective. See also Constipation, Diarrhoea, Gas/wind.

JOINT ACHES AND PAINS (see also Arthritis, posture)

I have lost count of the number of people I have seen who think their chronic pains must be structural, only improve partially or temporarily with manipulation and get completely better once on the candida programme as well. Detoxification, food combining and a low acid-forming diet are all essential. Celloids: Magnesium (for spasm), Silica and Sodium Compounds. See stretching and breathing in chapter 5. For pain, Vitamin C, Blackmores Salgesic, Lavender oil. *Gentle manipulation, reflexology, acupuncture/shiatsu yoga and homoeopathy* are all likely to be helpful. Get a member of your family to massage you with an oil (Weleda Massage Balm is the one I use) with some extra Lavender, Marjoram and Juniper Berry in it. They want to aim to both ease out any tense or tender spots and to stimulate the circulation around the joints. Dry skin brushing is also excellent (see chapter

5). If there is swelling, see the *Water Therapy Book* and use some Chamomile oil. NB People with candidiasis generally are much more sensitive and have stonger reactions to the treatments above than other people.

LOW SEX DRIVE and IMPOTENCE

This is hardly surprising when you are feeling so lousy, but will usually improve once the candidiasis is on the wain, as it seems that acetaldehyde directly affects the hormones. You may feel more like it in the mornings. The general lifestyle guidelines in chapter 5 are important for you. See 'thrush' and 'prostatitis' if appropriate. If persistant, some *psychological* help may be needed. See notes on self-esteem in chapter 10. Celloids: Magnesuim Compound. B complex, zinc Blackmores Ginseng. Bach Flower Remedies: Larch, Mimulus (for fear). *Aromatherapy (for both of you), reflexology, counselling.*

MENOPAUSE & HRT

We have observed that women whose body-minds are strong and well balanced prior to reaching their change usually sail through with only minor or no symptoms, or do very well on HRT (hormone replacement therapy), while those whose systems are out of balance, find that HRT makes them even worse. Gut dysbiosis and exhausted adrenal glands are common in the latter. Osteoporosis (calcium deficiency in the bones) is also due to hormonal and mineral imbalance and absorption problems that can be treated nutritionally. Exercise is essential here. Celloids: Silica for bone density and Chloride Compound for the ovaries. BioCare Femforte is a special multimineral-vitamin for women. Mega GLA, Dong Quai for hot flushes. Royal Jelly for exhaustion. See anxiety or tranquilizers. Natural progesterone can be a lifesaver for some women, but should be used in conjunction with all the nutritional changes recommended here so you shouldn't need to take it for long. Contact the Higher Nature Nutriline in the directory. Geranium and lavender oils help to rebalance things. Chamomile and Geranium are good for hot flushes.

The menopause can come at a cross-roads in your life when you need to reassess your relationships and roles in your family and/or career, and particularly to ensure you have an outlet for your creative and individual expression. (See Dr Northrup's advice)
Reflexology, acupuncture, homoeopathy, herbs (Western or Chinese), naturopathy and nutrition.

ME (Myalgic encephalomyelitis) or CHRONIC FATIGUE SYNDROME (CFS)*

Formerly known as 'chronic Epstein-Barr syndrome' or 'chronic mononeucleosis' or 'neurasthenia'. Sometimes called by doctors 'masked depression'. For some people the fatigue is worse and for others it is the muscular pain and weakness. Approximately 90% of all ME sufferers probably have or subsequently develop candidiasis. See Chapter 2 for diagnostic factors. *Nutrition, herbal medicine, psychotherapy, stress coping skills and graded exercise* are all likely to be needed. See the whole of Chapters 8 and 9 and the entry under 'healing' in chapter 11. See also FMS. Contact Action for ME who support the need to tackle candida as a priority - not all doctors do.

MUSCULAR ACHES AND PAINS (including fatigue) (see also Fibromyalgia)

These often have no apparent physical cause and can move around - baffling your GP. Again acetaldehyde may be the culprit, and if so, things will improve within a few weeks of starting the programme. A low acid diet is important. Magnesium Compound and vitamin C for the pain. Blackmores Ginger tablets. Too much exercise is as bad as too little. See also posture.

Stiffness in the mornings will improve after detoxifying. Marjoram and Juniper Berry oils and Rhus Tox. (Nelson's is stocked by Boots), skin brushing, breathing and stretching (see chapter 5) will all help. See also electromagnetic stress in chapter 9. *Gentle manipulation, shiatsu, massage, yoga.*

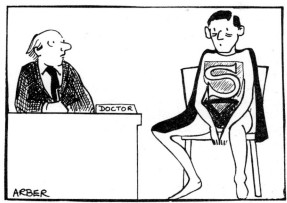

OVER THE LAST FEW WEEKS I'VE ONLY BEEN ABLE TO LEAP OVER SMALL BUILDINGS AND TRAVEL AT THE SPEED OF A SLOW BULLET.

NAUSEA

This can be a good sign of yeast 'die-off,' but it can also indicate a sluggish liver, pancreatitis and pregnancy. Celloids: Sodiphos and Magnesium Compounds, Blackmore's Dandelion Complex will help the liver and Ginger tablets. Peppermint oil or tea (Dr Stuart's, made strong). Bach Flower Rescue Remedy and Hornbeam.

NUMBNESS (see hyperventilation)

This is another of those symptoms that may well just disappear once you start the programme. Nerve interference can be involved, and if you have had any back or neck problems, injury (e.g. whiplash) or repetitive strain in the past, *gentle manipulation* might help. *Nutritional supplements or herbals* to support the nervous system.

OVERWEIGHT (See also cellulite, eating disorders, low blood sugar and anxiety)

Calorie counting and scales are *banned* at All Hallows House! The diet food industry and most GPs tell us that 'calories in minus energy out = weight', but in our experience it is almost always simply the gut (and therefore usually the hormones) that are out of balance - and *not* because you have been raiding the fridge at 1 a.m. The diet food industry feeds off this misconception. Masked food intolerances, and poor liver and pancreatic function are usually to blame for the build-up of toxins in the body. If you have subjected yourself to years of low calorie diets, you will probably need some hefty *nutritional supplementation.*. See the section on low self-esteem in chapter 8. Take heart, many of our clients find that as soon as they stop worrying about being fat and start eating for their health, their whole metabolism changes and weight ceases to be an issue. A good mulit-mineral vitamin plus Mega GLA and Chloride Compound. *Nutrition and herbal medicine. Ayurvedic medicine* has a very interesting approach (see Depak Chopra's Perfect Weight)

PARASITES

If you understand that our gut is like a mini ecosystem, you will not be surprised to hear that when a gut is out of balance, it provides a friendly home to a wide range of gut parasites should you come into contact with them. Symptoms vary according to the parasites, but the following should make you suspicious and suggest the need to get properly tested straightaway: Watery diarrhoea (usually 5-10 days after contacting Cryptosporidium), weight-loss, signs of unexplained malnutrition and malabsorption, dehydration, loss of appetite, blood in the stools, hypersensitivities, tenderness over the liver are all signs. Other symptoms such as fatigue, nausea and abdominal pain and flatulence are similar to candidiasis, so do not get alarmed unless you have some of the above, or you know you may have come into contact with the faeces of a child, animal or your partner who has had parasites diagnosed, or that the water supply is infected. However, if your candidiasis or leaky gut is severe or long term, or if it does not appear to be improving, parasites are a real possibility and should be checked anyway. Most of the drugs used to treat parasites are toxic in varying degrees, so the treatment of choice for a candidiasis sufferer is herbs, which marry very well with the candida regime you will already be on. BioCare's Eradicidin or Candicidin are highly effective or *see a herbalist.*
Tannic Acid binds (i.e. takes out of commission) the iron which the parasites need (unlike the friendly bugs). It can also precipitate proteins, thus rendering many parasites, such as the house-dust mite, non-allergic.
Beware of die-off effects, as for candidiasis, see chapter 5..
Dr Alan Hibberd has written a very good leaflet all about gut parasitic infection available from BioMed Publications .

PELVIC INFLAMMATORY DISEASE*

This is a most insidious condition since it can leave you infertile, often without your knowing there is anything wrong. Infection can spread from the vagina into the uterus and fallopian tubes. Parasites, fungal infections, poor diet, and sexually transmitted diseases are all causes. See 'Thrush', 'Endometriosis', 'PMS' and 'Infertility'. Surgery is usually the only option offered, but remember what amazing powers of healing you have given a chance. You will need a multi-leveled approach: *Herbs, nutrition, reflexology, healing, relaxation techniques, and often help exploring your feminine and spiritual side will all contribute.*

PRE-MENSTRUAL SYNDROME & PAINFUL PERIODS

Symptoms include depression, tearfulness, irritability, anxiety, fatigue, bloating and severe tummy cramps, back pain, headaches, fluid retention, swollen and tender breasts, and spots. PMS often occurs in women who are quite reasonable and charming people for the rest of the month.

NB: do not go on the pill for this condition until you have tried the following plus the anti candida programme first. Just as thrush usually flares up during the 1-4 days before a period, PMS does too. If candidiasis is present this will be for the same reason. That is the rise in progesterone raises our pH which favours the yeasts. Gwynne Davies shows that the '4 C's' (coffee, chocolate, citrus and cheese) plus white flour are the most common allergens. (These have to be avoided all the time rather than just when symptoms are worst.) General nutrition and how you deal with stress are key factors, see Chapter 5.

Vitamin B6 to rebalance the progesterone/oestrogen levels and pituitary gland and for the metabolism of essential fatty acids (all good for the sex hormones.) Evening Primrose is known to be effective, but needs to be taken in large quantities. *BioCare's* Mega GLA provides the full spectrum in a much more cost effective form.

See a *herbalist* for *Agnus castus* plus a host of help for all forms of menstrual problems. Blackmore's Viburnum Complex and Dong Quai. Echinacea complex for lymph congestion. The *Bowen Technique and reflexology* are recommended. Celloids: Manesium and Iron Compounds.

Go back to your GP if these do not help within 3-6 months.

PROSTATITIS & ENLARGED PROSTATE*

Candidiasis is usually present. Zinc deficiency is also directly related. A low acid diet and lymphatic cleansing is essential.

Celloids: Iron and Chloride Compounds

Any of the 'baseline' therapies, acupuncture, reflexology, stress management skills or counselling will help.

SKIN RASHES, ITCHING, URTICARIA

These are usually a sign that the body is trying to detoxify itself through the skin, so they should not be suppressed with steroidal medication. Depending on the severity and type, it can take several months to clear the toxins and get the liver and lymph systems going again. But *herbal and homoeopathic* ointments can soothe the skin in the meantime. Exercise, drinking plenty of water, giving up smoking, and *breathing techniques* are all essential.

Dermasorb, a cream containing tea tree oil by BioCare is good.

SEASONAL AFFECTIVE DISORDER (SAD)

If your symptoms are worse during the winter or if you work night shifts, this may be worth looking into. See under *light therapy* in Chapter 11.

Melatonin is worth a try - it is very effective for jet lag, a similar problem.

THRUSH   Vaginal Candidiasis (candidosis) or Monilia*

Itching and soreness to burning in the vagina or vulva, and/or discharge. This may be thick and white, "like cottage cheese" or thin and prurulent and can drive you mad. Thrush has been on the increase since the end of the sixties and is now one of the most common infections seen by GPs. It is also one of the surest signs that you have candidiasis in the gut. However, you can have candidiasis without ever getting thrush. In studies, between 80% and 95% of women with recurrent vaginal infections have *candida albicans* isolated in their swabs. Thrush is much more common in pregnant women, women on the pill and in diabetics. It is well known that it tends to begin during the week before one's period (when there is a more alkaline environment in which the yeasts thrive) and that broad spectrum antibiotics predispose us to it. However, as yet, British GP s are not in the habit of prescribing probiotics after antibiotics, as they do in France.

A recent article in the British Medical Journal does note however that patients with recurrent thrush often suffer from depression and may already have or will develop psychosexual problems. Therefore recurrent thrush is a "difficult problem to manage". Sadly most GPs still do not recognise a significant connection between candidiasis in the vagina and the gut. Treatment is as for candidiasis in the gut, but the following douches and creams will make life bearable until you are better.
Use Biocare Cervagyn twice a day (contains friendly bacteria) or insert a Bioacidophilus capsule into the vagina night and morning or French ovules (contains hydrastis and calendula - very soothing.)
Douche 2-3 times daily with: 600ml distilled water (or equivalent), 3 dsrtsps Cider Vinegar, 3 drops Tea Tree Oil, 3 drops Lavender Oil, 3 drops Rosemary Oil, (Ask a pharmacist for a plastic syringe or use a meat baster!) Douching with live yoghurt is often recommended, but not only is this incredibly messy, it is not nearly as effective as the suggestions above as the strain of bacteria cannot get established on human mucosa. It is better to eat it, if you are not dairy intolerant. Freezing yoghurt in small ice cube boxes and inserting them can be very soothing - as can plain ice cubes for the pain.
Celloids: Sodiphos and Chloride Compounds
Relief should be fairly rapid if certain other guidelines are followed: avoid nylon underwear and tight, warm clothes and wear stockings rather than tights. To prevent infecting your partner, or him reinfecting you, use a condom. Avoid bubble baths, soaps, hot baths - use unscented soaps and warm baths or shower.

UNDERWEIGHT (see anxiety, parasites)
Again your weight should improve as your absorbtion recovers. See your GP about the possibility of worms (garlic is very good if so) Digestive Bitters and Celloids Calcium Compound will help. *Any of the baseline therapies* will help. Obviously you must make extra sure that you eat enough while on the programme, particularly if you can't take too many carbohydrates. Take several small meals a day. Food combining will help enormously.

URTICARIA (see Skin rashes)

VAGINITIS and URETHRITIS*
While these are not nearly as common as thrush, and if you have thrush, you are less likely to have any of these as well, they can potentially lead to pelvic inflammatory disease or scarring in the fallopian tubes or infertility. SO IF IN ANY DOUBT, SEE YOUR GP!
CHLAMYDIA: a sexually transmitted parasitic bacterium that often has no symptoms, which is why regular checks are a good idea if you know your immune system is low and you want a family. Any discharge is a thick mucous and there may be some burning when spending a penny (like cystitis). If antibiotics are needed, take a strong probiotic such as BioCare's Replete as you finish the course, and see a *herbaist, homoeopath or nutritionist*

to prevent recurrence. TRICHOMONAS: A sexually transmitted protozoa, which also causes itching and burning, but with a frothy yellow/green discharge that sometimes has a fishy smell.

OTHER TIMES TO USE NATURAL REMEDIES

ALTERNATIVES TO ANTI-BIOTICS (see also Cystitis)

As explained in chapter 1, far from being the benign panaceas generaly believed, antibiotics are to a certain extent immunosuppressants and probably one of the main reasons you have candidiasis in the first place. If you have or are planning children, for goodness sake try and start their developing immune systems on the right foot and use natural alternatives wherever possible. Find and develop a relationship with a good local *homoeopath or herbalist.* If you are on or have been on the recurrent infection treadmill, it is vital you break the cycle - and ironically the best way of doing this is to help and rest your way through your next infection, using the suggestions here. This process will give your immune system the opportunity to build up its natural defences again. You'll need a sympathetic GP already in place (see chapter 8). Unless you have one of the life threatening conditions listed, you should stick to good old fashioned rest, loving care, plenty of fluids (hot filtered water is best) and little, if any food (NOT glucose!) The plant world have plenty of natural antibiotics to offer us, that are suprisingly powerful. Echinacea, Eucalyptus, Garlic, Goldenseal and Propolis (from beeswax) are the best known. Blackmores Echinacea Complex includes the anti-oxidant vitamins as well. Take extra vitamin C (eg BioCare Magnesium Ascorbate) to bowel tolerance (see constipation). Lavender and Tea tree oils are useful.

It is fine to take a few pain killers if necessary (avoid any with caffeine in them), or use Blackmores Salgesic (natural 'aspirin') and Lavender or Chamomile oils. Hops Valarian, Skull cap, Dong quai are all analgesics. Vitamin C is also a strong pain killer. It is best to see a *homoeopath, herbalist or acupuncturist.*

BABIES AND CHILDREN

Breast feeding The best possible start you can give your baby's health. Aim to breast feed for at least 6 months and use goats' milk formula ('Nanny') if you have to. However it is crucial to clear any candida and food intolerances you have. For sore, or cracked nipples don't use any antibiotic sprays. Fennel and Geranium oils or calendula cream massaged into the nipples will be enough. Royal Jelly and Evening Primrose both help.

Children Roman Chomomile for colic,. Blackmores Ordourless Garlic and Parsley for any infections. For ear infections *don't* accept antibiotics - Hopi candles (from Health food shops) and a decongestant, herbal nasal spray will ease it. Note that most of the supplement supliers have special formulations for children. (See chapter 7) *Homoeopathy* really comes into its own with children - many of the miasms (inherited tendencies) can be corrected at this early stage. Read Susan Curtis' *Handbook of Homoeopathic Alternatives to Immunisation* (Winter Press1994).

GIVING UP SMOKING

Don't necessarily try to do everything at once, but if you have candidiasis there are two very good reasons to give up smoking as well as the ones we all know about. First, nicotine is a stimulant, so your blood sugar will be raised every time you have a cigarette, feeding the yeasts. Second, you are just adding to the load of poisons that need to be cleared as part of treatment. Everyone knows that giving up nicotine is difficult because it is so addictive, but it is also because withdrawal enables the body to detoxify which can cause as many of the unpleasant side effects. If however, you only cut down on your cigarettes while you give your body a thorough spring clean for 4-8 weeks and *then* give up (while continuing to encourage detoxification) you will probably find it is relatively easy - and you'll feel great afterwards! Extra anti-oxidants and B vitamins will be needed plus magnesium to help the cravings, so Blackmores Executive B Stress Formula and Bio ACE will be ideal. Their Liquorice Complex will help you through any lung infections.

Gillian Riley's excellent little book *How to Give Up Smoking and Stay Stopped for Good.* is very clear and includes a good section on, the emotional side of giving up which I recommend you read even if you don't think you are emotionally hooked!

Acupuncture before and during withdrawal makes all the difference for most people. *Hypnosis* is also successful as long as it is part of an integrated programme. One offs rarely work long term. Alan Carr's programme in London is a good one.

NATURAL FIRST AID KIT

Since many of the following are not as easily available as things you get in a pharmacy (particularly the good quality versions) it would be wise to buy them for your medicine cabinet now rather than waiting until you need them.

Homoeopathic creams:	Calandula to soothe sore skin
(Nelsons or Weleda)	Hypercal for cuts
	Arnica for bruises
	Rhus Tox for stiffness
Drops	Apis for bee stings
Rescue Remedy	cream and drops for any of those panicky moments
Supplements	Vitamin C for the adrenals (ie exhaustion), pain and infections
	Vitamins B and C for hangovers
	Bioacidophilus (keep in the fridge) for tummy upsets
Herbals	Echinacea for bacterial infections or immune weakness
Essential oils	Lavender for most things (see under symptoms)
(Neals Yard	Tea tree for infections
or Tisserand etc)	Peppermint for headaches, tummy upsets, travel sickness
	Geranium - balancing
	Marjoram for stiffness and aches
	Rosemary to pick you up
Massage Balm	*Weleda*'s is a lovely all rounder.
Celloids (Blackmores)	Sodium Complex for tummy upsets
	Chloride Complex for inflammations
	Magnesium Complex for nervous balancing

POSTURE (see breathing and stretching in chapter 5)

Good posture is crucial for the proper functioning of all your organs. Bad posture will exacerbate any muscle and joint pains and stiffness. McTimoney does a very good, simple leaflet on correct sitting and lifting. See chapter 11 for address Please send an s.a.e. and an extra first class stamp. If you are sitting for long periods, your chair seat must tip forward so your spine can support you with no strain. See appendix 2 for good back shops. *Manipulation, Alexander Technique, Yoga and connective tissue work (massage)* are all very effective.

TRAVELLING

Travelling even relatively short distances can be exhausting for some people and make others sick, so it pays to plan ahead so you can enjoy whatever you are travelling to!

Sickness: Peppermint and ginger help. Try Blackmores Ginger tablets and their Digestive Aid.

Going abroad: especially if your immune system is below par, you may be susceptible to the unfamiliar bugs abroad. Acidophilus, garlic and echinacea tablets are essentials. See alternatives to immunisation book mentioned under children.

Long haul flights: the much greater radiation levels at high altitude cause free readical activity which can cause more jet lag than the time change. BioCare's Jetzyme and homoeopathic anti-radiation drops from Ainsworths help. Lavender and geranium oils are great, with Rosemary for when you need perking up at the other end. Bring a big bottle of mineral water and drink at least half a pint per hour (*not* the orange juice they hand round continually.) Rescue Remedy, Bergamot or Chamomile oils are all good for anxiety.

Back and neck pain: It is essential that your back is supported comfortably when you are travelling any distance - and of course seats in trains and planes, even cars never seem to fit. Blow up lumbar supports and neck pillows (so you can go to sleep without waking up with a stiff neck) are available from Boots and the Back Shop. Rolled up jumpers and little pillows are good, but bulky to carry. Make sure you wear loose, comfortable clothing and shoes made of natural fibres. Get up and stretch and walk around every hour.

See Ainsworths under Homoeopathy, who sell travel kits including anti-radiation drops for long haul flights.

See Biocare (supplements suppliers) for Jetzyme enzymes to mitigate the free radical activity during long haul flights.
Melatonin

CHAPTER 5

TACKLING YOUR CANDIDA ON ALL FRONTS,
treating change as adventure and discovering your habits for life

Most people find the treatment programme outlined in this chapter very clear and logical. It makes sense - in theory at least. However, whether you actually find it easy to do, to make the changes necessary and to stick to them, varies enormously. It always depends ultimately on your attitude, and just how fed up you are with feeling so lousy and that life is passing you by, weighed against the considerable effort and determination it can take for some of you to stick to the programme. Experienced practitioners can almost always spot the ones who will really go for it and will be bouncing back to the clinic in a few months or less, full of their old energy and feeling wonderful about life again!

Before getting into to the practicalities, here are four key points to remember:

1. *Put yourself first for a change. You must take charge and ask for help (see chapter 8 if you find that difficult)*
2. *Remember that you are unique biologically and emotionally, so only your rules apply. The general guidelines that follow will help, but you will have to discover what these are for yourself.*
3. *Treat your body-mind with the respect it deserves. Nurture it as well as you would a child and appreciate and support its amazing powers of healing.*
4. *Understand that life gets its "fizz", not from outside stimulants, but from your inner balance, love and truth. (Sounds 'heavy' but see for yourself...)*

As you read through the programme below, if you feel negative voices and excuses nagging away at your resolve, stop and read the section on negative feelings in chapter 9. Then try again, keeping a note of your feelings, "can'ts" or "buts" in the margin or at the back of the book.

Enough talk. Let's get down to business!

THE SEVEN POINT ANTI-CANDIDIASIS PROGRAMME

Dr Jeffrey Bland, one of the foremost nutritionists in the world has, in typical American fashion, a 4-step programme for treating gut dysbiosis. Each step starts with R, to make a good mnemonic or memory jogger. I have added the last three to make it up to a "heavenly seven".

---

1.   *Remove* - *the toxins*
                    - *the yeasts' food source (sugars)*
                    - *your individual food intolerances (yeasts plus...)*
                    - *and kill the yeasts*

2.   *Replace* - *the nutrients with fresh, whole foods and supplements*

3.   *Re-infest* - *the gut with friendly bacteria*

4.   *Repair*   - *the damage to the gut lining (this may be stage 2)*
                    - *and to your liver (if applicable)*

5.   *Release* - *your stresses*

6.   *Restore* - *your belief in yourself*

7.   *Rest*   - *to allow your body-mind to get on with healing itself*

THE "BASELINE" TREATMENT SCHEDULE

I am giving this to you now as a simple framework, so that as you read the rest of this chapter you will be able to prioritise things and slot them into place in a way that will work for your schedule, commitments and lifestyle, your finances and your resolve and energy levels.

Please note that this is for the hypothetical middle-of-the-road candida suffer (who of course does not exist) and that you must modify it according to how ill you are. It does not include any of the other associated problems individuals have, nor the many "optional extras" that will speed your recovery. See chapter 7 for the appropriate supplements - or use herbs.

THE "BASELINE" TREATMENT SCHEDULE

- *Diagnosis (see chapter 2), including your food intolerances*
- *Detoxification either with a fast from over a long weekend to 10 days, or an elimination diet (under professional supervision only).*
- *Keep to the sugar and yeast free diet plus exclusion of your personal intolerances rigorously and completely for 3-8 weeks. Reintroduce foods one by one after that.*
- *Start taking the probiotics (see chapter 7) - Replete (20 billion microbes per day) for 1-2 weeks for major imbalance, followed by 4 billion microbes per day. Plus Fructooligosaccharides (FOS) Start with 4 billion for a minor imbalance.*
- *Don't add the anti-fungals until you have been on the programme and detoxified for 1-3 weeks Build up dose gradually and see "reactions" below.*
- *Support the liver and heal the gut lining. Preferably, start early on or wait until yeasts are clearer (after 4-8 weeks) if funds are limited. Use herbs and Mega GLA.*
- *Stick at it! The yeasts/fungi should be back where they belong within 2-3 months, but healing the gut and liver takes longer (2-9 further months plus). It is fine to relax your regime occasionally if you feel okay but you are aiming for a complete rebalance, not having to "control" yeast overgrowth indefinitely.*
- *Maintenance for life! Take 1 billion microbes of probiotics every morning if ever you are under pressure (see chapter 7). The habits that suit you should be well established by now, so have fun with your new energy, but keep clear and listening to maintain your health and balance.*

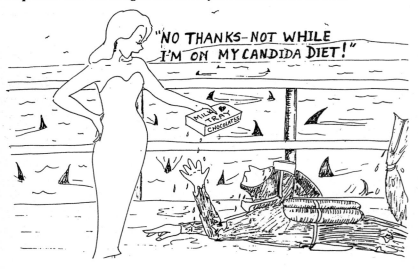

An asterisk by a symptom indicates that you should refer to it in the alphabetical listing in chapter 4; by an item means it will listed under 'useful addresses' in appendix 2. An asterisk by a therapy means see the notes in chapter 11. (These are also listed alphabetically.)

LIGHTENING THE LOAD
The importance of getting rid of your body toxins (pollutants) and irritants (food intolerances)

Anyone who has had candidiasis in their system for a while is best advised to give their system a good spring clean before they do anything else. Otherwise when the candida starts dying off as you withdraw its food and start the treatment with the anti-fungals over the following few weeks, the extra toxins produced *in addition to* those already being carried in your system will probably produce some nasty side effects. If this still happens, see 'reactions and die-off' below.

The more you can lighten the load of both general pollutants and your personal irritants and allergens, the more spare energy your digestive, endocrine and immune systems will have to focus on healing and rebalancing things again.

Above all you will feel less exhausted and have the energy and the will to go for this programme.

As long as your system is full of toxins, your vital communication lines (life lines) that tell you which substances suit you and which do not, will be 'fuzzed', like interference on a radio. As Dr Brostoff emphasises, you need a 'period of silence' so your body can 'speak' to you clearly.

HOWEVER SPRING CLEANING AND CHANGES MUST BE DONE GRADUALLY, particularly if you are very ill or have had a lousy diet. So the sooner you start the better.

Environmental toxins are unlikely to decrease in the foreseeable future, so getting into good habits now will stand you and your family in very good stead for the rest of your lives.

Naturopaths believe that the most important underlying factor in all degenerative disease is the fact that everyday waste products and toxins build up in an individual's system faster than it can clear them out. Cancers, heart disease, arthritis, MS, ME, Alzheimer's, can all be attributed to years of toxic build up and high free radical activity, causing tissue degeneration. Equally attributable are the more mundane problems such as headaches, putting on weight and not being able to lose it (especially cellulite), spots and skin rashes, general aches and stiffness, bad breath and the ageing process. Since a toxic load puts such a strain on the immune system and the liver, the auto-immune diseases and allergic conditions such as asthma, eczema, arthritis, urticaria and so on are also understood to be products of this same fundamental problem.

Candidiasis can be one of the biggest single contributors to your toxic load because the toxins are being made inside you, like internal saboteurs. It also involves a leaky gut, low digestive acids and liver overload that makes everything so much worse. But do not despair. It is reversible. Even the ageing process can be slowed significantly. By following these guidelines and making most of them habits for life, you will 'live long and die young'.

Further Reading:
Leslie Kenton's book the "Ten Day Clean up Plan" is an excellent little book which covers this subject in detail. See also "All Day Energy" by Katherine Marsden," You Don't Have to Feel Unwell!" by Robin Needs and "Natural Healing" by Ross Trattler.

MINIMISING THE RUBBISH YOU TAKE ON BOARD
Water: filter all the water you use whether it is for drinking, tea, cooking or steaming vegetables. (Filters* only cost about £13-£16) Even better but not essential, buy bottled water for drinking as it should be purer, and mineral water (as opposed to "spring" water) will have beneficial minerals present as well. If you can afford it, consider plumbing in a water filter under the sink, or buying a reverse osmosis machine. If your company does not do so already, get them to supply spring water. People tend not to drink tap water as it tastes so nasty these days, but drinking enough water (2 pints a day) will much improve everyone's concentration spans and mental acuity.

As for the following advice, you obviously cannot cut everything out comprehensively, but having the information will mean you can do as much as is reasonably possible. Take it step by step.

Chemicals in and on our food: these days very little reaches our plates having escaped the agrochemical industry. The average apple or lettuce for instance will have been "enhanced" at least 16 times with different chemical sprays and processes to make them pest free, look uniform and perfect. Many foods are also irradiated to prolong their shelf life. (If you have ever returned from holiday having left something like a punnet of strawberries in the fridge for 10 days, to find them beaming at you "as good as new", you will have wondered what has been done to them). Livestock, including farmed fish, are fed sub-clinical doses of antibiotics and hormones to make them put on weight faster and given vaccinations to delay any diseases. These also get into milk. Even though they are supposed to be withdrawn from the antibiotics so there will be no residues before they are slaughtered, some of these will be stored in their tissues especially in their fat, so we end up getting some too. Admittedly these are (or should be) minute amounts but the effect is cumulative, year in year out.

Wash your fruit and vegetables. Many of the toxins stay just under the skin so peeling helps, but most of the goodness is there too. Grow your own, or buy organic when you can.

When choosing food, bear in mind that the more "mass produced" it is and the further it has travelled, the more likely it is to contain unwelcome "enhancers". So patronise your local growers and organic farmers, and pester your supermarkets to stock more organic food.

Airborne pollutants: you obviously have less control over what you breathe, but it is very important. Whatever goes up our noses directly affects our brains and most of the things that get into our lungs will filter into our bloodstream. Choose the household chemicals and cleaning fluids at home with care. Are they necessary at all? Avoid dry cleaners, petrol stations, traffic jams, wear a mask if you cycle. (In fact, in cities it is the pedestrians and drivers who need masks far more than cyclists, who are emptying their lungs again by breathing properly after 20 minutes exertion.)

Heavy metals: it is not just the lead in exhaust fumes you need to watch. The *aluminium and Teflon* in aluminium and non-stick cooking pots leach into the food, especially if lemon juice, vinegar or salt is present. Most restaurants use aluminium pots and pans, and of course take-away food and ready-made meals are usually packed in foil. Invest in one or two stainless steel or enamel (e.g. Le Creuset) saucepans and they will serve the entire family well. Aluminium is also in most anti-perspirants and toothpastes. There are several delicious natural ones available at health food shops, e.g. Blackmores and Weleda.

Any *mercury fillings* in your mouth are obviously not as easy to get rid of as your old tin pots. Mercury apparently 'affects' only 1-2% of the population, but if you are one of those, you will almost certainly have candidiasis as it loves the environment methyl mercury creates in the gut. Having mercury fillings replaced by a dentist who is experienced in this kind of work can literally transform people's lives. But before you rush off to the dentist, read the section in Chapter 9. However, and this goes for everyone, if you need fillings in future, insist on the mercury-free, white ones.

Drugs: if you are on any prescribed medication, then whatever you do, do not stop taking it without discussing it with your GP. See "What if I am already on drugs?" in chapter 3. Before you reach for any over the counter drugs for a headache or indigestion or whatever, read about the relevant symptoms in chapter 4, and try the natural alternatives first. Otherwise, not only will you be adding to the toxic load for your poor old liver to deal with, but you will be suppressing the natural 'progress reports' or warning signs from your body.

Electromagnetic fields and radiation: this is obviously a little more tricky since most people cannot tell when they are being affected, but it is known that more free-radicals are produced in 'hot spots' or areas of high electromagnetic fields and radiation, which explains why there are clusters of deaths from leukaemia, brain tumours, and cancer in certain areas. Power lines, sub-stations, radio transmitters, faulty domestic electrical appliances, microwave ovens, VDUs (particularly if the back of somebody else's is pointing at you in an office) fluorescent lighting, electric blankets, all of these are potential culprits. Clearly you cannot easily move house or job, but see chapter 9 and the entries on dowsing* and long-haul flights (chapter 4)*, for what you can do quite cheaply to mitigate their effects. As your system becomes clearer, you may well become more sensitive to these harmful fields and you will 'just know' when to avoid particular places.

Holidays and long weekends: Remember that giving your system a rest from any toxin or stress will mean it will enable it to recharge its batteries and have more strength to cope with these when it has to. Choosing remote spots in the country, by the sea or up in the mountains for your holidays, and taking long weekend breaks when you can, will do wonders. People in full time jobs find that taking a Monday and Friday off, giving them two four day weeks in a row gives them a rest that is out of all proportion to the two days holiday allowance they have taken. Commuting is, we observe, a far greater drain than people recognise. Nowadays with communications technology, it is perfectly possible to work from home - and during the train strikes for example, all my clients who had to work from home said that they got three or four times as much done as usual! Put your needs first and discuss the possibilities with your colleagues of working from home one day a week.

MAXIMISE THE EFFICIENCY OF ALL YOUR EXCRETORY SYSTEMS

Our bodies get rid of their rubbish via five excretory systems: bowels, liver and kidneys, the lymph system, skin, and lungs. Here is how to ensure they are all working our best for you. But first let us look at the three essentials that will help all five systems at once.

1. Drink at least 2 pints of plain, filtered or bottled pure water a day, but not with meals as this will dilute your digestive juices. You will need more if you work in an air-conditioned environment or if it is hot and you have been sweating. If I were asked what single thing would contribute most to the health of everyone in the UK this would be it. We are - or should be - about 70% water. Virtually every bodily process, particularly our detoxifying processes, depends on having plenty available. As Kathryn Marsden reminds us in *"All Day Energy"*, we are 90% water when we are born, but most people are down to around 60% in "wrinkly" old age. It makes you think, doesn't it? I am convinced that loss of concentration at work or in the car for instance is often caused simply by dehydration. Any professional model will tell you that drinking plenty of water is the secret to keeping your skin supple, line-free, and young looking.

Keep a bottle of mineral water on your desk and in your car and take a swig whenever you remember. Little and often is ideal, still water is preferable, but ring the changes. It is better to drink it at room temperature than straight from the fridge. A mug of hot water with a slice of lemon in it is a very good way to start the day and I find plain hot water very refreshing, particularly if there is only canteen tea or coffee around. Most ancient healing traditions recommend sipping very hot water (plain) at half to one hourly intervals over several days either when you need to detoxify or if you are ill. Do this particularly during candida 'die-off' and after any treatment session. It really works, and gently too.

2. Exercise

Take some regular exercise, whatever you enjoy and feels good. Stretching and breathing first thing in the morning, and aerobic exercises at the end of the day. If aerobic exercise tires you at the moment, DON'T do it! Skin brushing, hydrotherapy* and breathing will have the same effect for you until your systems get stronger, or try Yoga*. See the section on exercise below.

3. Rest

Make sure you get enough sleep and rest particularly in the first 3-6 weeks of your programme. After that, if you think you do not have enough time, practising "active relaxation", i.e. meditation*, or autogenic training*, can act as turbocharged rest.

THE SIX EXCRETORY ORGANS

1. Bowels
Particularly if you have candidiasis and general digestive imbalances, your bowels are likely to be coated in old debris and mucous, such that they are unable to do their job properly. Changing your diet and food combining will help significantly here, but it may take as many years to clear as it did to build up, so a course of cleansing herbs* and/or some colonic irrigation* will go much deeper more quickly. If constipation* or irritable bowel syndrome* has been a problem for you in the past, read these sections in chapter 4 and make them a priority to deal with.

2. Liver and kidneys
The liver is responsible for processing any metabolic toxins (i.e. our body's waste products), chemicals or drugs in our system. It also rebalances hormone surges. Avoiding alcohol and coffee will make a huge difference, as will drinking plenty of pure water.
Some books or natural therapists recommend a liver flush, using olive oil and lemon juice. We think this is rather too drastic for most people with candidiasis, but by all means use it occasionally when you are better. See Ross Trattler and Robin Needes.

3. The Lymph System
Our lymph is the dear friend which collects most of the waste from our cells (mainly lactic and uric acid) and transports it to the liver for processing. It also carries some essential nutrients. Unlike the cardio-vascular system, it does not have a pump, but relies instead on the movement of our large muscles and our breathing to a lesser extent, to move lymph around the body. This is why you will really feel the difference, particularly if you have a sedentary job or spend a lot of time resting, if you give the lymph system a bit of extra help. It also stops you from getting stiff after exercise.

The best way to do this is by *dry skin brushing*, before your bath or shower for 2-4 minutes a day (first thing in the morning is ideal). Buy quite a strong, natural bristle brush from a health food shop. (The Nutricentre will send you a good one with a long detachable handle for about £7.) If your skin is very sensitive use a raw silk glove. Start gently for the first few days, and your skin will begin to look forward to it. Both you and your brush need to be dry. Tone up the lymph node in the right groin with a gentle circular action, then with long firm strokes, always towards the heart, cover the whole of your right leg, front and back, starting with the thigh. Include the top and sole of your foot as this stimulates the reflex points and nerve endings. Repeat this for the left groin and leg, then do the same for the arms and hands. The lymph nodes for your arms are just under the breast muscles. Do as much of your shoulders, buttocks and back as you can reach (not your face). Finally do your tummy with gentle downward strokes on your lower left abdomen, then make circular movements coming up on the right and down on the left. This is the direction of the bowel and will help with elimination there too. You will find that there is no better general pick-me-up than a brisk skin brush followed by a shower. Make it warm, then cool-to-cold for just 30 seconds which will stimulate your circulation, then warm again. I use this trick at the end of a hard day when I know I am expected to be scintillating that evening! You will find that the quality of your skin improves, and any cellulite is reduced.

4. Skin

People tend to forget that our skin is an important organ of excretion. The Chinese call it the second lung, although in the UK we get very few opportunities to use it in this capacity. Interestingly, iridologists* will tell you that British people tend to have stronger 'skin signs', i.e. toxins accumulated under the skin, than our antipodean counterparts.

To keep our pores open and breathing well, we must keep them clear of dead skin (skin brushing is very effective for this). Have a regular sweat, either by exercising or with an Epsom salts bath, or hydrotherapy*. Be careful not to smother your skin with body lotions. Saunas are great for some people but others find them enervating, so don't be pushed into taking them by some zealot if they don't suit you. If your skin tends to be dry, you may need to eat more oil, or your hormones may be out of kilter. (Stress can affect your skin, consider the Adrenal Stress Index test in chapter 2.) See "Superskin" by Kathryn Marsden. Antiperspirants are best avoided too, partly because most contain aluminium and partly because they are designed to suppress a necessary function. In a month or so, when you have detoxified, any BO should be less of a problem too. You may find that your skin breaks out as you start to detoxify. If so, don't panic, it is a good sign! See under acne and pimples*.

5. Lungs

You have probably taken air for granted like everyone else, but just consider that virtually every cell in our body needs a good supply of oxygen to be healthy, and our brains use six times as much as any other part. Candida albicans, free radicals, and unfriendly bugs, including malignant ones, thrive in oxygen-less (anaerobic) conditions. So how much oxygen we get through the system, as well as its quality, is crucially important. If our muscles are all stiff and short and we sit in slumped positions, our ribs and lungs are unable to move and function properly. With 2 minutes simple stretching and deep breathing exercises first thing in the morning you can increase the movement in your ribs and chest significantly (see exercise below). By learning to relax your tummy properly when you breathe (see Yoga*) and by making sure your chair or car seat is properly designed to support you (see posture* at the end of chapter 4), you will find that you will be using your lungs effectively all day without even thinking about it. You may need to rethink your wardrobe a bit if you tend to wear tight fitting clothes.

COPING WITH DIE-OFF

All the advice on detoxifying will stand you in good stead if you get any symptoms as the yeasts start dying off in large numbers. The significance of healing reactions and why you should welcome them as a good sign was explained in chapter 3. Even so, die-off can be pretty unpleasant in some cases, so you need to soften the effects if you can.

First cut back on your anti-fungal supplements for the next few days and don't start building up the dose again until all the symptoms have abated. Drink plenty of water, get some rest and follow all the other advice in this chapter to speed the toxins through and out of your body. Refer to chapter 4 for advice on any specific symptoms.

Die-off usually happens as you start the anti-fungals, but it may reoccur at times that you increase the dose or if you get a surge of progress in your healing at a later stage. If you feel it is appropriate you can fast or do a vegetable juice fast for a day, sipping hot water every hour or so.

FOODS TO EAT IN PLENTY

Fresh, vitality-packed fruit and vegetables

These contain the enzymes, vitamins and minerals essential for our repair work and for cleansing our system. They are rich in anti-oxidants which scavenge the damaging free radicals.. These days, most people judge the quality of fresh food more by how it looks than how it smells and tastes - with the inevitable result that most 'fresh' supermarket fruit and vegetables look perfect but taste of nothing, and we can never be sure how much nutritional value it has. I am writing this bit in France, where every town has a market where one can still get ecstatic about plump, sappy vegetables with real mud on them that snap when you break them. This poor, deprived little Brit had to bury her face in the piles of fruit so she could smell the sunshine! ('Elles sont foues, les Anglaises'.)

We Brits seem to have forgotten that food is a living substance (or should be) and that we need its vital energy to live - and even more of it if we are to heal. So sniff out suppliers of local and or organic foods and squeeze and smell everything before you buy it.

Cooking your vegetables for optimum vitality:
The less you do to your food the better in terms of maintaining its nutrients. This may mean you need to completely revise your cooking habits, but it will be great fun discovering new recipes - see chapter 6. This way also saves an awful lot of time and is very satisfying. However, this is not to say that raw food all the time is necessarily best for you and your fellow candida sufferers. Leslie Kenton wrote several really marvellous books in the eighties such as *"Raw Energy"* and *"The Bioenergetic Diet",* expounding the virtues of raw everything. Do get hold of copies as they are packed with information that will help you here, but remember that eating 80% raw as she recommends is not for everyone, all the time. Candidiasis, being fungal, is a 'damp' condition (as acupuncturists and ayurvedic practitioners would say), so it often needs warming and drying food to balance it. Again this depends on you and your body type, so stop and listen and experiment with soups, luscious vegetable and bean stews, and stir frys with ginger and gentle spices, particularly in the colder weather.

Fruit
Many candida books and practitioners ban fruit altogether because of the high fruit-sugar (fructose) content. While we agree that this is essential in the first three or four weeks for everyone, it is quite difficult to sustain and not always necessary. You would also be missing out on certain important nutrients and cleansing properties. So find out what your safe level is. It is probably not more than two pieces of the less sweet fruits (apples, pears, and bananas) per day. Always eat fruit separately, i.e. not at meals with other foods. This will mean you will digest and absorb it well instead of it fermenting inside you.

Get hooked on juicing!
The time you definitely do want raw fruit and vegetables is for juicing. Fresh, home made juices are packed with vitamins and enzymes in an easily absorbable form and you can have a great time inventing new combinations - and glasses of jewel-like colours. Do not underestimate its healing properties. The Gerson Therapy, which is based mainly on juices, has had consistent success in reversing cancer in patients who had been given only a few of months to live.

A good juicer* costs £38-45 but it is well worth it as bottled juices are very expensive and never as good for you as the absolutely freshly made, organic, homemade stuff. If you have apple trees or vegetables from the garden, a juicer is a must as you can enjoy even the biggest glut. Wash and cut your ingredients into pieces then push them all through in one go, cores, skin and all. I find putting an ice cube and a drop of fresh lemon juice in the glass stops the juice oxidising so quickly. Drink, or rather sip your juice immediately - you can feel the vitality running right down your throat. Yum! Always rinse out the machine straight away, or it will be a real fiddle to do later. For convenience and packed lunches, V8 (8 vegetable juices) comes in cans and bottles and carrot juice is easy to find in packets in supermarkets.

Nature's candida-killers:
Garlic, onions, leeks and chives, particularly garlic, are all powerful fungicides and will kill off fungi, moulds and viruses but not bacteria. So our friendly bugs are safe. If you are worried about your breath smelling, nobody will notice once your system is used to it, and you are eating it daily and the rest of the family is getting their fix too. Fresh parsley eaten with it means you can even get away with raw garlic. However, if you really cannot stand it, we do recommend that you take one garlic supplement a day (see chapter 7). If you take it at the beginning of your main meal it will not repeat on you or smell.

Sprout Your Own Nutrients
Sprouted seeds, beans and grains produce more nutrients ounce for ounce than any other natural food known. You can grow them yourself in a jam jar in the airing cupboard and they will be ready to eat in 1-6 days and cost next to nothing. Leslie Kenton gives a very clear step by step guide to DIY sprouting in *Raw Energy*. Her sprouting chart gives the soaking and growing times and tips and notes on each of 16 different types. She gives examples of the phenomenal increases in the vitamin content of seeds when they germinate: the vitamin B2 content of oats, for example, rises by 1300% when they germinate and by 2000% by the time little leaves form. Biotin (needed to prevent yeasts damaging the gut lining) increases by 50%, and the vitamin C in soya beans multiplies 5 times within three days of germination. In fact, two tablespoons of soya beans contains the entire recommended daily adult requirement of vitamin C. They contain a synergistic balance of amino acids, fatty acids, natural sugars and vitamins and minerals, so that they are actually capable of sustaining life on their own. They also don't seem to produce any gas unlike some ordinary beans and pulses. And by the way, they are absolutely delicious - in salads, in stir-fries, in nut cutlets and even in bread. So give them a try. If you have children, they will love growing them for you.

Whole grains
Generally, our bodies do best on whole foods because:
a) our systems can digest, absorb and excrete them far better in their whole form;

b) their energy is released in a steady, sustaining stream, in contrast to any refined carbohydrate or sugar which bursts upon the system, causing it to have to release a chain of hormones to rebalance the blood sugar levels;

c) the goodness has not been stripped out of them by processing and refining and they even contain natural antibiotics. Whenever you can, *buy organic*.

However, candida sufferers need to be careful because:
i) yeasts feed on carbohydrates so you need to go easy on quantities. Some sufferers can barely tolerate any at first

ii) *gluten*, found in wheat and to a lesser extent, in rye, barley and oats, is a sticky, mucous-forming protein that can cause havoc with many people with candidiasis and a leaky gut. Even if it does not cause allergic reactions in you, it will slow down or even prevent your detoxification process. Many practitioners recommend eliminating gluten altogether for the first 3-4 weeks. Do this if you can, and then one by one, try reintroducing oats and rice first, then rye and barley, and wheat very cautiously, if at all.

iii) the major mass-produced grains (i.e. mainly wheat and corn) have been genetically engineered to increase the gluten content, but it has also made their husks more permeable to fungal toxins *(mycotoxins)* and the agrochemicals used. Fungal toxins usually grow while the grain is being stored, especially if it has not been dried thoroughly. They are heat stable, i.e. once they are there, no amount of grinding or baking will get them out again, so they become part of the food chain. The answer is to stick to *oats, millet and rice* for the most part since they are the least susceptible to mycotoxins and chemicals, and contain relatively little gluten. *Oat bran and oat germ* contain no gluten at all as it is found only in the middle of the grain. *Oatcakes, porridge and homemade muesli, rice cakes, Ryvita with sesame seeds* are all delicious, although, since we are such a wheat-orientated culture, you will need to plan ahead a bit when you are eating out (see below). See also 'alternatives to sandwiches' in chapter 6.

Pasta is one of many candidiasis sufferers' passions, and is a common example of an 'allergy addiction' or food craving. Those people who cannot tolerate wheat are sometimes OK with a little pasta because it is made from durum wheat which is a much harder variety from further south which harbours fewer mycotoxins. However for most people, it is better to stick to the huge range of buckwheat, vegetable and rice pastas that you can find in the health food shops. *Kemut and Spelt* is pasta made from special un-tampered-with wheat which is fine for most people. You can get Spelt flour as well.

Get your Fats and Oils Right!

One of the areas of greatest controversy and double-talk in the food and food-advertising industries must be around fats and oils. So let's get it straight as it is important. Fats have generally been labelled 'bad', but we need fats and oils to be healthy, and this includes cholesterol. Our brain and nervous system and all our hormones are made of the stuff. We need plenty of omega-3 and -6 essential fatty acids (deep sea fish, salmon, mackerel, herring, linseeds, and flax seed). So very low fat diets are dangerous. Mega GLA from Biocare is a good source of the full spectrum of EFAs, (see chapter 7). As for the calories, bodies in good balance will take care of them (see over/underweight*). And don't forget that anything labelled 'low fat' or 'lite' is likely to have more fats that have been damaged by processing and more artificial ingredients - so will do us more harm than good. Very low fat diets are dangerous!

Trans and cis-fatty acids: there has been a big fuss about saturated and polyunsaturated fats when what really matters is whether the fat molecules are intact, as in their natural form *(cis fats),* or whether they have been changed during processing and heat into damaged molecules *(trans fats).* Our bodies cannot recognise the latter and therefore cannot deal with them, so they cause great free radical activity and harm. Trans and cis-fats are only just beginning to be marked on food labels, but the rule of thumb is that highly processed foods, including foods labelled "low fat" or "light" and hydrogenated margarines will probably contain a high proportion of trans fats. As far as I know Flora margarine is the only commercially available spread to date to have quietly changed its formula to one free of trans fats. Vitaseig and Vitaquell from health food shops are good.

The *cis fats* are those in virgin, cold pressed, unheated oils and you need to keep them all in a cool dark place (in the fridge if you have room).

Mono unsaturated fats - olive oil and butter are not harmed by heat, so these are the ones to cook with. Olive oil (which contains *oleic* acid) actively helps to restore the balance in your gut, so spend the money you are saving on all those processed foods, to get the best quality virgin oil (yum) and have lots!
Butter is very low in milk sugar (lactose), so even people with an intolerance to dairy products (meaning cows' in this case) can usually eat butter with no problems. Nor are there any trans-fats in butter.

Other sources of essential fats and oils:

Seeds: sunflower, pumpkin, sesame and linseed together make a whole protein. They are delicious on porridge or muesli, in yoghurt, on fruit salad, and in stir-fry vegetables. Mix up your own and keep them in an airtight, light-proof jar. Grinding them fresh every other day makes them more absorbable, but keep any left over in the fridge or they'll go rancid.

Avocado pears are a wonderfully nutritious food, convenient and *not* fattening once your diet is right.

Nuts: do make sure they are very fresh as old nuts can go rancid (free-radicals again) and harbour moulds. Peanuts (which are not actually nuts) and, I'm sorry to say, pistachios are the worst culprits. Almonds are best. Again, ideally keep nuts in the fridge.

Fat in meat and fish: many chemical toxins and heavy metals are fat-soluble, so anything which we humans cannot excrete immediately will get stored in our fat. High concentrations can build up which may explain why people often get signs of detoxification when they lose weight. It is just the same for livestock (particularly pigs and beef) and fish. In other words, whenever livestock or fish has been intensively farmed agrochemically or has been living in polluted waters in the case of sea fish, it's fat will probably be full of unwanted toxins. Cut off as much fat as you can before you cook it, then use olive oil for cooking. Game and organic meat and poultry will obviously be much better for you.

What if you cannot digest fats?

Some people find that fatty foods give them indigestion. Depleted levels of friendly bugs directly interfere with our ability to break down and absorb fats. Bile is produced in the gall bladder and is crucial for our ability to absorb fats. Our friendly bugs are able to recycle bile acids and therefore conserve them. A bonus is that the recycled bile acids also favour the friendly bugs by improving the environment for them. Do not take indigestion tablets - instead, see a nutritionist or herbalist, who will be able to help you get your gall bladder back into shape. In the short term, digestive enzymes and/or Replete will help (see chapter 7)

Find the right protein levels for you.

Many candidiasis sufferers find they cannot tolerate many carbohydrates, especially in the early stages, so they have to eat more protein. This is fine as long as you are getting plenty of vegetables too. It is important to explore new vegetable sources of protein (pulses, beans, nuts) as well as to know the pros and cons of meat, dairy and eggs, so you get plenty of variety. The average westerner eats far more protein than he or she needs. 4oz per day maximum is a rough average for what most people need. However the amount of protein that you feel right with will be quite different from the next person. It depends on your metabolism.

Meat or vegetarian?

Strict vegetarian diets can be disastrous for some people, though most find they feel much livelier on less or no meat. Even organic meat puts more of a strain on the digestive system, particularly if it is eaten with carbohydrates (see food combining below). Non-organic meat contains higher levels of toxins than most other foods. White meat is generally thought to be 'better' for us. Perhaps this is true if we are talking about organic meat, but remember chickens are probably the most intensively farmed of all livestock. Sadly, the same now goes for salmon and trout. The 'Real Meat Company' supplies organic meat reared under approved conditions, mainly through independent butchers. See Appendix 2.

BEWARE OF IMPORTED POULTRY The laws restricting the use of the most powerful antibiotics are much more lax on the continent than in the UK. So imported poultry is likely to contain *resistant* strains of bacteria. When your colonies of friendly bugs are depleted, (so this goes for anyone just after they have taken antibiotics as well), you are more susceptible to food poisoning because they normally kill off any potentially harmful bacteria as soon as they reach the gut. If you get food poisoning from one of these birds with resistant strains, it could be that only the most powerful antibiotics will help you.

Protein from vegetables - peas, beans, lentils, chick peas:

I am one of those lucky people who thrive on a vegetarian diet and I just love experimenting with the fantastic variety of pulses and beans that one can get. When combined with rice or other grains, they provide a complete protein and, mixed with vegetables, they make a satisfying, sustaining meal that still leaves you feeling light afterwards - and is very light on your pocket too! Combining them with aubergines and nuts (and mushrooms later) can make them taste surprisingly 'meaty' (see recipes). We have no hesitation in serving them up to our 'committed carnivore' friends, who then confess that they will now consider lentils with a new respect and ring up for the recipe. Admittedly, nut roasts do still have rather a reputation to live down - of sitting like a brick in the pit of your stomach, but far from being only for funny people in macramé sandals, these days, lentils and pulses are very 'foodie', so you'll have no problem finding great recipes.

The pros Quite apart from their image and how delicious they are, they are very cheap, store well, come in infinite varieties, and organic ones are easy to find. They are much more eco-friendly than animal sources of protein and as yet, have not been taken over by the agrochemical industry. They *don't* cause wind as most people think, as long as you chuck the soak water away and cook them in fresh water. Adding a strip of seaweed seems to make them cook faster and are more digestible.

The cons Their only disadvantage is that they need some forethought as most need soaking overnight or they will take ages to cook. I have to confess that I resort to tins and bottles when I've not planned ahead. Not ideal, but life is too short. A pressure cooker can help you out in emergencies, but do not buy one specially, because they are not too good nutritionally. If you are food combining, pulses do need careful treatment as they contain both carbohydrate and protein.

Dairy - go for goat and sheep
The milk sugar (lactose) in cow's milk is the most difficult for humans to digest,. particularly after it has been pasteurised (UHT is even worse). Mass produced milk also contains some drug residues. This is why cow's milk is, with wheat, by far the most common food to which people are intolerant. The constitution and size of the molecules in goats' and sheep's' milk is much more akin to those in human milk, and they have probably not been as intensively farmed as cows. Sheep's milk freezes very well, so you can buy it in bulk, and it has a delicious creamy taste. However, more significant for you is the fact that candida thrives on undigested milk sugar, and dairy products, like gluten, are mucous-forming, so they slow down or prevent detoxification.

While some people do very well on *soya milk*, others cannot stand it, so try it and see. Make sure it is unprocessed so the isoflavo molecules are intact, since these regulate your hormone levels. (However, while some women whose hormone levels are low thrive on soya, other people can get too much, so beware.) Even if you do not like soya milk, try other products such as soya ice cream, tofu in blocks to go into stir-fries, and silken tofu for sauces and dips

Yoghurt: the lactobacillus and bulgaricus strains are the friendly bugs we need to keep our gut 'ecosystems' healthy. Live yoghurt is full of them. It is no coincidence that Bulgarians are known both for their longevity and their yoghurt eating. It is also an excellent source of protein for you as the milk is 'pre-digested', but to do you any good, those strains must still be alive when you eat them - so forget most of the supermarket brands, unless they are plain, natural, the label says 'live', and they taste tangy. The best yoghurts are those sold in good health-food shops - or home made. If you have any problem with cow's milk, even though most of the lactose will have been pre-digested, it is wise to stick to goat and sheep's yoghurt most of the time. If you want thick Greek style yoghurt that you can use like cream cheese, just put it through a sieve with a square of kitchen paper. The whey is very refreshing to drink and good for you too. You can also make lassi, a delicious and refreshing drink from India which is simply yoghurt, whey, water and a pinch of salt, mixed to a smooth liquid consistancy.

Kefir

If you can get a starter culture, this is a delicious and very nutritious way of making your own fermented milk - particularly good if you have a dairy intolerance. You simply keep feeding the culture with fresh milk every night, keep it in a warm place and lo and behold, it's ready to drink next day. The culture grows and grows (it looks a bit like cauliflower) so there'll be plenty to give away to friends. The only snag might be for some people is that it is like having a pet. (Dr Anthony Fox's family calls theirs Phyllis). You can't just abandon her for a few days, though if you are going away, you can either give her to friends or put her in the freezer, like sending her to kefir kennels!

The Case for Organic Food

As well as all the advantages mentioned above of avoiding the chemicals and hormones used in producing non-organic foods, there are many other points in its favour. Crops are grown in healthy soils that are built up and balanced by natural composts and manure and by rotating the crops. Livestock are raised in plenty of space, meaning they will be much happier, and they are less likely to fall prey to the diseases that are rife among their unfortunate, intensively-farmed cousins - so they are less likely to need drugs. They will also carry less fat. But above all, organic food tastes so much better!

Waitrose, Sainsburys, Tesco and Safeway all carry organic foods, though sometimes their ranges are limited. Do keep pestering the managers to stock more, otherwise they will not appreciate how great the demand is. If anyone complains that organic food is more expensive, I remind them what they are saving by not drinking coffee and alcohol, and not eating ludicrously overpriced processed, convenience foods, with their seductive packaging. Contact the Soil Association* for your nearest growers or suppliers as they will be far cheaper - and it is good to support the locals and small businesses. See also *"How to be Green"*, page 73, for a list of organic outlets.

I will not go into all the ecological, wildlife and ethical reasons for buying organic food. You can read about these for yourself in Nigel Dudley's *"This Poisoned Earth"* (Piatkus 1987)

Enhancing the value of your food even more

Have you ever wondered why monks and yogis say grace and eat in silence? Of course I am not suggesting you should do the same, but there is no doubt that you benefit more from your food, and your digestion will be much smoother and more effective if you pause before you start a meal and do not rush through it, and resist eating standing in front of the fridge or in the car, as we are all prone to do occasionally!

From a purely mechanical point of view, chewing your food thoroughly will enhance your digestion significantly (remember the digestion of starches actually starts with the saliva in your mouth), and sitting quietly during and after your meals will free your blood to go to the stomach where it is needed at that time. Eating while stressed however means that your sympathetic nervous system will actually be diverting your energy away from the task of digestion in hand. On an esoteric level, there is plenty of anecdotal evidence that making a point of pausing to appreciate or bless your food and thanking everyone involved in bringing it to your plate actually has an effect on the vital quality of the food, enhancing its benefit to you. If you think this sounds crazy, see Dr. Leonard Laskow's book *Healing with Love*. He gives several experiments you can do yourself, cutting an (organic) orange in two or splitting a bottle of wine into two jugs, and focusing love and appreciation on one half and not on the other. You simply will not believe the difference in taste and smell - and it gets stronger if you leave them for another half hour. Everyone can tell the difference blindfold. It is not the sort of thing one can do a controlled scientific experiment on, but Larry Dossey the best-selling author of *Healing Words,* which is full of evidence that prayer can help people heal to an amazing extent, is convinced that people who say grace before their meals (i.e. pause and appreciate their food) benefit significantly by doing so. My favourite grace is from the Bulgarian master, Beinsa Douno (1864-1944)

The Love of God brings Abundance of Life. (Said three times).

TREATS

Most people were rewarded with food, especially sweets, when they were children, and when we grow up many of us perpetuate the pattern on behalf of the little child still inside us. So we buy ourselves chocolate or a pastry, whether it is because we have done something well, or because we have not done something well enough and so need cheering up - or anything in between! But once you start appreciating real goodness in food again, you will find yourself treating yourself instead to a particularly luscious smelling punnet of raspberries or a wonderfully fresh bunch of organic asparagus.

In the middle stages of combating candida (i.e. after the first 3-6 strict weeks) it is fine to treat yourself to some of your 'foods to avoid' occasionally. We are all human for goodness sake, and how else can we check our progress if we do not challenge our systems with some of the old culprits occasionally? The important thing is that having 'lapsed' at one meal, you get straight back on the straight and narrow at the next meal. Otherwise the yeasts will start to get the better of your system again. Some of the most difficult times for anyone trying to stick to a programme is at parties, when eating out or when staying with friends, but even these situations can be smooth if you plan ahead a little and have a positive attitude. (See chapter 9.)

FOODS TO AVOID AND WHY

Many people coming across an anti-candida diet for the first time immediately latch on to all the foods they can't eat and have got to give up - and start making excuses. But with all the delicious foods above (and you haven't even got to the ideas and recipes in chapter 6 yet), who needs sugar and junk? This is why I always look at what people CAN eat first.

No, it is NOT a life sentence to self deprivation and weird behaviour in restaurants!

People also assume they have to give up bread, chocolate and wine for ever! Many of us do find we feel better if we avoid one or two foods for several years afterwards, but by that time it is a choice rather than a chore and it is a tiny price to pay for feeling so well. If you do have rather a list of foods to which you are intolerant, it can seem very hard at first, but sticking at it for a month or two is not much to ask for the years of health and energy you will enjoy afterwards. Within a few months you will find that most of the intolerances will be okay again. The point is that by giving your system a complete holiday from all the substances that have been putting it into turmoil, it is able to heal and strengthen itself - hopefully for life. The only other option, if you can call it an option at all, is to take anti-histamine drugs indefinitely to suppress your body's allergic reaction to those substances. (For special occasions or Christmas, you could take some digestive enzymes, see chapter 7.)

But, most precious of all, having been through that 'period of silence' when you eliminated those foods, you will have learned to stop and listen, and found out exactly what are the right foods for you, and just how much you can eat of the not so good ones and how often, without upsetting things. These foods and levels will probably change subtly over the years, and there may be times when you feel set right back, but you will always have that gift of 'just knowing' if you choose to use it.

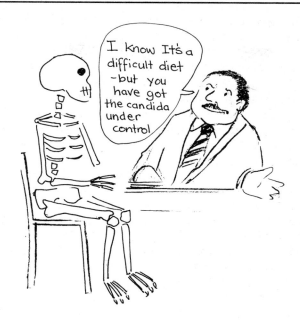

OTHER THERAPEUTIC DIETS

Food Combining speeds recovery significantly. See page 128.

Low acid-forming diet
This is the simplest principle and should be put into practice by everyone with candidiasis. It is that certain foods form acid 'ash' in the body and others alkaline, and we need a balance - particularly when we are trying to heal. Stress, toxins and free radical activity all produce acid. As do sugar, meat, stimulants (coffee and tea), alcohol, condiments, drugs, eggs, flavourings, tobacco. Honey and kelp are alkaline.
The dairy alkaline foods include: yoghurt, *raw* milk and whey - all other dairy foods produce acid.
Almonds, fresh coconuts and roasted chestnuts are alkaline, the rest are acid.
All cereals are acid -forming apart from millet
All flesh, fish, fowl and gelatine are acid.

Fasting
Complete fasting (i.e. taking water only) has gone out of fashion, but it is still one of the most powerful ways we have to allow the body to redirect its energy towards eliminating toxic wastes and other obstructions to its life force and vitality. Animals and babies have not lost their instinct to refuse food when they are ill.

However, practitioners have noticed that over the past twenty years or so, adults seem to respond differently to fasts. Three day fasts are fine for short, sharp fevers that put you in bed, but anything longer needs careful supervision. The reactions or healing crises that accompany fasting include headaches, a coated tongue, flu-like symptoms, diarrhoea and fatigue as the toxins are eliminated. While in generally healthy people these are then followed by tremendous mental clarity and abundant energy, if you have been sapped by years of illness, you will have a much higher level of toxins to offload and less vital force with which to do it. The major metabolic changes that occur both during the fast and when you reintroduce foods afterwards can themselves produce symptoms. You must be particularly careful if you are underweight, very toxic or have blood sugar problems.

For candidiasis sufferers it is therefore wiser to use more gentle, gradual methods. Eating just one type of food (e.g. apples) can be an effective compromise. A three day water and fruit or vegetable fast, *under supervision* can get your anti-candida programme off to a flying start. Short 'mono' diets (e.g. raw carrots and carrot juice rather than fruit) can also be very helpful at certain points later on in your programme, particularly it times that you feel 'stuck'.

One of the big problems these days is that rest as a therapeutic tool has gone out of fashion along with fasting. It might not feel as if anything much is happening, but your body will be spring cleaning furiously in there and we all know how exhausting that is. So you need plenty of rest! Always choose your time to fast with this in mind.

Fasting therapeutically is a real science and an art and, as I have said, tremendously powerful in skilled hands. Ross Trattler's book is excellent here, but do seek proper supervision from a naturopath for your individual needs.

Elimination diet
An elimination diet is not a treatment, rather a means of identifying any food intolerances, which as I explained in chapter 1, are likely to be a significant factor in candidiasis and gut dysbiosis. And one must be aware that it can sometimes be difficult to disentangle whether a symptom is due to the yeast, die-off or a food intolerance. As Dr Brostoff puts it so clearly, 'the purpose of the elimination diet is to ask your body questions about the foods it has to cope with, and give it a chance to tell you which ones make it ill. In order to hear the answers, you need a period of "silence" - that is, a period with no symptoms at all. This is why you must exclude all foods that are likely to be causing problems at the outset.' This he calls the *exclusion phase*. Once the symptoms have cleared, then you are ready

to move on to the *reintroduction phase,* in which foods are eaten again one by one, with about two days in between and in the reverse order of likelihood of their causing a reaction. Unlike other diets, you cannot take a day, or even a meal 'off', or you will not get a clear result.

Most patients will be sensitive to 2-5 foods. For them, a rigorous exclusion phase is not necessary - they simply need to avoid the most frequent offenders, such as wheat, milk, eggs, citrus fruits, yeast, chocolate and additives.' This very much concurs with our experience, and to add some detail: we find oranges the most frequent culprit of the citrus, with lemon rarely being a problem, eggs less commonly mean trouble. The stimulants, it goes without saying need to be included in this list, i.e. coffee and tea, caffeinated drinks and cigarettes.

Rotation diets

There are two understandings of the term rotation diet, which have arisen from the observation that people are often able to get away with eating foods to which they are sensitive, as long as they are not in too great quantities, not too often and not at the same time as several other sensitive foods.

The first is a way that people can eat foods that are'borderline' for them, and is a means of checking that they don't eat them too often. The second is for people who find they get new sensitivities easily, and involves putting all the foods they can eat into four columns, separating those in the same 'family', and only eating foods from each list once every four days. This is even more restrictive than a straight elimination diet and many social events become impossible. As Dr Brostoff quite rightly says, 'the costs have to be weighed against the benefits. Loneliness and isolation can be as damaging to the health as eating the wrong sort of food.'

TO EXERCISE OR NOT TO EXERCISE?

Just walking for 20 minutes a day reduces stress cortisol levels by 6-7 fold. The breathing and raised circulation helps all the systems in your body-mind to function well and to clear any debris. Equally important is that it gives you a break mentally. Particularly if you have a demanding job, or are rather a worrier, making time for physical re-creation (in the true sense of the word) will bring your body-mind back into balance again, and you will find you will sleep and be able to relax much better. It is also an opportunity to be with friends, learn new skills and have fun - or if you get plenty of these anyway, to have time and space entirely for yourself, preferably in beautiful surroundings

It might take some time, effort and self-discipline to organise - particularly initially - but it will be worth every ounce of that effort, and be an essential part of your getting better.

Exercising regularly should keep you feeling light, energetic and full of life. However, if it leaves you feeling exhausted, and only fit for sitting in front of the TV with a pint of chocolate ice cream, then DON'T EXERCISE until you are getting better again - by which time your body will be telling you it wants to anyway.

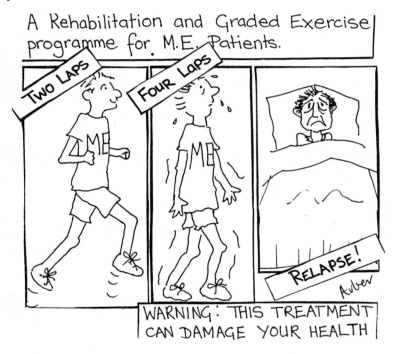

A Rehabilitation and Graded Exercise programme for M.E. Patients.

WARNING: THIS TREATMENT CAN DAMAGE YOUR HEALTH

This will be the case for many candidiasis sufferers. Unfortunately, a common pattern among many sufferers, who always used to rely on a good work-out to pep themselves up whenever they were feeling sluggish, pent up, or out of condition, is to carry on driving themselves to take more exercise long after their bodies are past coping with it. They think: 'It never failed me before. It must be because I am not taking *enough* exercise that I'm feeling so lousy.' Many candida sufferers go through a hyperactive stage for several months or even years before their systems 'crash' and they get so dreadfully tired. They often get hooked on a daily adrenalin fix from very strenuous aerobic exercise during this time, and it takes a while to realise that it is no longer doing them any good.

Exercise is another example of having to overcome the crazy ideals and idols foisted upon us by modern culture and the media. 'No pain, no gain' is one of the most harmful ideas going. Exercise should be fun and relaxing. It should be something you look forward to, and it must fit comfortably into your daily routine. It honestly does not matter whether you walk, swim, cycle, or go belly dancing, as long as it is fun and it makes you feel you good.

But don't skimp on breathing and stretching
However much you don't want to take any exercise (i.e. aerobic exercise) and however ill you are, gentle breathing and stretching for 5-10 minutes once or twice a day will make a huge difference to how you feel and how quickly you get better. If you ever feel depressed, anxious or can't sleep, exercise is one of the best rebalancers. Incidentally, even if you are taking regular aerobic exercise, you need to breathe and stretch *as well*.

You will not believe how powerful Yoga or T'ai Chi are until you try them - nor how wonderful you feel afterwards. This goes for professional athletes right through to near invalids. (See chapter 11.)

TRY THIS EXERCISE
In the meantime, here is a very simple, but powerful breathing exercise that everyone can do in two minutes. It is best first thing in the morning, but of course you can do it at any time, and as many times a day as you like. It is fine to do it sitting on a straight chair if standing tires you.

Start by giving yourself a gentle wake-up stretch or shake like a dog or cat does when they first get up. Have a good yawn, opening your jaw as wide and pulling as funny a face as you can.

Stand square, with just your big toe joints touching. Pull your knees back, then tighten your buttocks as if you are holding a tennis ball between them. Settle your low back, shoulders and head so that it feels as if your head is right over your centre of gravity (i.e. between those big toe joints) but is being supported by a thread coming straight up out of the top of your crown. (This feeling will come with a few day's practice.) Release your neck and shoulders so your fingers can fall low down your sides.

1. Now close your eyes and take a full breath in, through your nose, as you lift both arms above your head, palms inwards, stretching up as far as you can through your little fingers. Aim to get your arms back over your ears. Feel the breath filling every corner of your lungs, back and under your side ribs. As you go up, think *'LIFE'*

2. Hold your breath and your stretch and think *'STRENGTH.* Feel the space growing between each rib.

3. Then gently lower your sides as you let your breath out, through your mouth, imagining all your tensions and worries flooding out with it, and think *'HEALTH'*.

Do this ten times. Each sequence should take between 8 and 15 seconds according to how much puff you have. You will find that the space in your ribs becomes bigger and more flexible each day. If you feel at all dizzy, go more gently and don't hold your breath for so long. If you find breathing so slowly difficult, see hyperventilation in chapter 4.

General suggestions for stretching.
As with breathing, stretching is best done every morning, before you get dressed - but this depends on your routine. Just after the breathing exercises above is ideal. Many people only stretch after exercise, finding they can do it 'better' when they are warm - but the whole point of stretching is to prepare you to move more freely and gracefully, whether on a squash court or just going about your daily life. Therefore the time to do it is first thing in the morning, before taking exercise (this should also prevent any injuries) and after exercise for just two minutes to 'warm down' rather than slumping straight on to a bar stool!

Aim to develop a routine that suits you, so that once established, you can switch off and relax your mind.
Take the phone off the hook or put the answering machine on and put on some relaxing or classical music - rather than the news.
Go systematically through your body starting at the top, stretching one group of muscles at a time. The whole thing should take between 5-10 minutes. If you are very busy and spend more time than this, you will end up not doing it at all, so keep to 5 minutes plus the 2 for breathing at the very most.

Take each muscle group to its comfortable limit, take a breath and stretch a little further as you breath out. It is more effective and safer to do only two or three stretches per muscle and hold them for longer (10-15 seconds) rather than lots of repetitions. Never 'bounce', just hold and grow longer. I find it helps to picture your muscle fibres all separating and becoming smooth and lined up like an embroiderer's new skein of silk.

Don't forget to breathe! This is the most common problem we all have, particularly when learning new exercises.

This should be no effort - tight muscles cannot stretch. Think of letting each muscle feel 'soft' as you work on it.

When you are standing on one leg, make sure you always have something to hang on to like a chair-back or a wall. And above all when you are stretching your hamstrings for instance, don't have your whole body weight pulling on the muscles (i.e. don't just touch your toes from standing). Sit on the edge of a firm bed with one leg along the edge of it and stretch one leg at a time. Make your low back hollow by tilting your pelvis forwards and then lead with your chin - or you'll do your low back in.

Anyone with a sedentary lifestyle needs to spend extra time on stretching the whole length of their abdomen and their quadriceps (the muscles on the front of our thighs.) Lie on your tummy with your hands under your shoulders as if you are about to do a press-up. Keeping your hip bones in contact with the floor, push up gently with your arms. Think of elongating your front rather than trying to arch your back. For your quads, stand on one leg and aim to pull the heel of your other one to your buttock with your hand, so that your knee goes vertically down. If you can't reach at first, hook a small towel around your foot and pull up on that.

The Squat

This is a superb exercise for anyone with a low back problem, stiffness in the mornings, constipation, problems in the reproductive area and candidiasis. As well as freeing up the muscles in your low back and sacral area, it gets all the energy flowing down there. If I have time to only do one stretch, this is the one. NB. If you have dicky knees, this may well not be suitable for you. You can get a similar effect by lying on your back and hugging your knees.

Stand with your feet shoulder/hip width apart at arms' length from something solid such as the edge of the bath. Feet pointing straight ahead (don't let them splay out). *Keeping your weight going down through your heels*, drop down into a squat, aiming to get your bottom as close to your heels as you can. You should feel a stretch and a broadening across your lower back and sacrum. You will probably feel you will fall over backwards and need to hang on to the bath at first, but will find you get more supple surprisingly quickly. Once you can do this comfortably without hanging on, gently drop your head and clasp your hands behind your neck. You should feel a stretch going right down the length of your spine. Breathe out and go a little deeper.

I couldn't do this to save my life at first, but got there within a week or so. Now it feels great! If you find it very difficult at first, keep your shoes on or put your heels on 1"-2" of books.

Rebounding
Perhaps the best way to get your lymph system and breathing going in a small space is by getting a rebounder. This is like a mini trampoline (under three feet across) that you can walk, hop, skip or jump on. 2-5 minutes a day will really get you going. Available from The Wholistic Research Co, see Appendix 2.

Integrated exercises for the Body, Mind and Spirit
There is a set of six very beautiful and powerful, but simple exercises from the Bulgarian mystic, Beinsa Douno, whose grace I mentioned earlier. They connect you to the powers of Nature and align you with Love, Truth and Wisdom - while stretching and breathing. They are best done outside, first thing in the morning and take about 10 minutes. *If you would like a sheet explaining how to do them, please send an s.a.e. and extra first class stamp to: Beinsa Douno Exercises, Lesser Halings, Tilehouse Lane, Denham, Bucks UB9 5DG.*

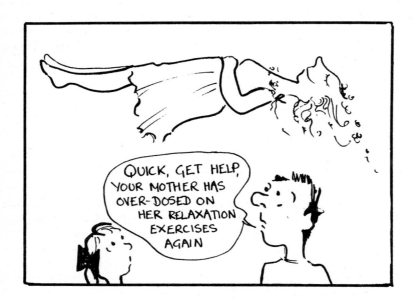

CHECKLIST OF FOODS TO AVOID AND THEIR ALTERNATIVES.

All these alternatives are easily available from good health food shops and increasingly from supermarkets. See notes on where to find them opposite. Foods in brackets mean you may have them later on in the programme (ie after 3-6 weeks) in small quantities, if you have no reactions.

AVOID	*ALTERNATIVES*
1) All foods containing **yeast** or derived from yeast: **Bread**, pitta bread, pizza, **marmite** Yeast free stock, spices, monosodium glutamate (MSG) Soya sauce, **citric acid** (citrus drinks), (Care on foods containing breadcrumbs e.g. sausages, burgers).	Yeast-free breads, Ryvita **Rice cakes, Oat cakes, rye pumpernickel.** **Use garlic, onions & ginger to flavour.** matzos, soda bread, chapattis
2) All fermented foods/drinks: Alcohol, wine, beer, ginger ale, all vinegars (olives, pickles, mayonnaise, dressings)	Herbal teas, Yogi Tea, Dandelion coffee, Water - 2 pints plus daily.
3) All foods rich in **sugar** or containing any sugar: Sweets, cakes, biscuits, pastries, canned foods. Look out for fructose, sucrose, glucose, syrup, dextrose, lactose and molasses - all sugar. Artificial sweeteners	(Use apple juice to sweeten.) Sugar free spreads and jams. Hazelnut & cashewnut butters, (honey)

NOTES ON YOUR NEW ALTERNATIVES & WHERE TO FIND THEM

Many of the alternatives mentioned are now being stocked by supermarkets..
However DO CHECK ALL LABELS as sugars, yeasts, vinegar, citric acid and
wheat turn up in all sorts of foods.
Further details of anything mentioned below are in chapter 6.

1. Bread contains both yeast and wheat, so it is best to start enjoying other staple foods. Good healthfood shops stock an increasing number of special breads and a delicious Russian yeast-free rye bread is now available in Waitrose - by lots and put in the freezer. Pumpernickel keeps well and is great toasted. Paterson's oatcakes or Waitrose own brand are OK unless you cannot take *any* malt. (Sainsbury's own brand, Nairn's or Walker's contain sugar and wheat). Sesame Ryvita is delicious; avoid the malted variety. Supermarkets even have rice cakes these days.

2. Cold drinks: fizzy water with a squeeze of fresh lime or lemon is much nicer than G&T! There is nothing to beat freshly juiced, organic vegetables, but V8 and packet carrot juice (from supermarkets) are good standbys. 'Diet' drinks contain artificial sweeteners and citric acid, so avoid them.
Hot drinks: try hot filtered water with a slice of lemon and/or fresh ginger. Tea made with a sprig of fresh thyme, rosemary or mint from the garden is delectable. and will pick you up. Parsley is very cleansing, Yogi Tea is very warming, and Barley cup or Rooibsch tea are good.
2a. Relishes and sauces: most contain vinegar, yeasts and sugars. Either find the special ones in health food shops (e.g. Good Earth) and/or make your own .

3. Breakfast cereals. This can stump people initially, particularly as milk is discouraged as well, but soya milk, or water with a dash of apple juice is delicious in muesli or on rice bubbles. Rice Dream (like milk) is great, though rather expensive and some people find it too sweet. Avoid wheatbran (which may be added to oats) - Mornflake oat bran is good. Most supermarket brands of muesli have sugar and wheat in them, so make your own. Wild Oats make a fantastic muesli mixture for candida sufferers.
3. Sugars. Are *everywhere*, so read the labels! Health food shops stock *masses* of sugar-free foods, but they often contain concentrated fruit sugar (fructose).

4) All **refined carbohydrates** (which are essentially sugar): All types of white flour, white pasta & white rice. Anything with 'startch' or 'filler' on the label	**Brown rice, whole grains** Vegetable, barley, corn & rice pastas & flours **Baked Potatoes**
5) **Cows' milk** (contains lactose) and milk products e.g. cheese/yoghurts. You may be OK on butter (see your practitioner). Watch for casein, lactalbumin, or whey on labels.	**Sheeps & goats milk & yoghurts, Soya milk**
6) All **fungi and moulds** **mushrooms,** truffles, blue cheeses, buttermilk, soured cream, dried herbs Make sure nuts are very fresh. Peanuts and pistachios usually contain mould.	**Eat plenty of fresh salads & vegetables** Fresh nuts, **& seeds, eg sesame, linseeds sunflower, pumpkin,**
7) **Smoked foods** (fermented or dyed), **Salt.** **Snacks** avoid very spicy foods (they inflame the gut)	Naturally smoked foods Kettle chips, blue corn and corn chips, roasted chickpeas
8) Meat or fish containing **antibiotics/hormones** (Most poultry, pork, red meat and farmed salmon).	**Free range eggs, chicken, Game, fresh, tinned tuna organic meats, beans & pulses**
9) **All stimulants**	Avoid 'natural' substitutes eg Guranna-

10) **Avoid fruit for the first 3-4 weeks** and then add back one at a time, taking care to note any adverse reactions. Tomatoes and oranges should always be avoided (too acidic) and dried fruits and grapes (too sweet and yeasty/mouldy). Start with apples and pears and bananas (lower fructose). Wash or peel all fruit unless it is organic and never eat it if is over ripe as it will be mouldy.

4.   Refined carbohydrates and starches. Also used all over the place as thickeners and fillers, so check labels. Stock up on Kemut and Spelt flour and pastas from healthfood shops. See recipes and health food shops.

5.   Dairy products. Sheep and goats' yoghurts and cheeses are now widely available. Fewer people are sensitive to sheep's milk and it freezes well and has a softer taste than goats', but soya milk keeps better. Butter is fine for most people but if you want a margarine get Vitaseig or Vitaquel, not the hydrogenated spreads. Waitrose does a good goat cheddar that is also good for cooking, but you may find that cooking makes all cheeses less digestible.

6. Flavoursome foods: people often complain about not being able to cook with mushrooms. Brown your vegetables a bit more and include lightly toasted nuts and seeds. Aubergines also have a "meaty" taste. Eden shake (sesame seeds and a seaweed) from healthfood shops livens up salads, stirfries and pasta.

7. Nuts and seeds: The quality of seeds is far better in healthfood shops. Buy organic if you can. Check the sell-by date if you are buying shelled nuts.
Salt:. Do not add to anything, use sea salt if you must as at least this has a full complement of minerals. Celtic salt is best if you can get it.

8. Organic/free range meat, fish and poultry: you are more likely to find good meat in the small independent butchers. People think white meat is "good", but poultry is most affected by antibiotics in their feed - lamb, least and of course game is good. Bear in mind that some tuna fish has traces of mercury in it and the brands that are 'dolphin friendly', are marked

9. Stimulants.
Avoid caffeine alternatives containing gurrana as this is a stimulant too.

10. Fruit and vegetables: buy as fresh and organic as possible - though of course organic foods do not have as long a shelf-life as pesticided and irradiated foods. Organic carrots, potatoes and onions do keep well and are now often sold in supermakets. So are bean sprouts. Frozen foods are very high in nutrients and good standbys, especially peas (but check for added sugar), spinach and sweetcorn. The texture is impaired in many of the other vegetables.

Chapter 6.

THE CANDIDA FREE COOK
Recipes, menus and ideas for making good food.

While the variety and availability of convenience foods that you can fit into your new diet is increasing each year, there are no two ways about it. *You are probably going to have to change quite a few of your ideas about food and cooking.* This chapter is designed to make this as smooth, easy and enjoyable as possible.

There are a few very good recipe books, specifically for Candida sufferers, which are listed at the end of this chapter, so the following recipes are just a small selection of our favourites to get you started. I have also listed some ordinary recipe books that have some particularly good ideas that you can use or adapt for your new diet. However, try not to be hide-bound by recipe books. Use them for ideas by all means, but as soon as you are confident enough, it is much quicker and more creative just to do it your way.

You don't have time to cook?
Neither do I, which is why none of these recipes will take more than 2-20 minutes to prepare (plus cooking time). The general rule is to *start with good, fresh ingredients and cook them as little as possible.*

You may need to get to know some new shops, and try some new cooking equipment, so the sooner you start exploring the better. And the better organised and uncluttered your kitchen is, the less time you will need to spend in it.

You 'can't cook'?
That's great - you won't have any bad habits to unlearn and you'll have much more fun discovering a fascinating and creative new art and science rolled into one. Over the years, and particularly in our Candida Support Groups, I have taught many people to cook who had been convinced that they couldn't cook to save their lives. With a bit of encouragement and confidence, every one of them has discovered how easy and creative cooking can be. In the Groups, I'd show everyone a few quick recipes, which we'd eat together. Everyone said 'I had no idea cooking for candida can be so quick and easy and *so delicious.*' For the moment, I am assuming that every one reading this chapter is clueless in the kitchen and starting from scratch.

Getting started

Start with a visit to a good health food shop and look at the 'kit list' at the end of this chapter. Next, ask a practical friend who loves cooking or a fellow sufferer from your candida support group for help. Ask them round for the evening and get him or her to go through this chapter and the checklist of foods at the end of chapter 5 with you. (It is a good idea to photocopy the checklist and notes and keep it in your shopping basket.) If they will come shopping with you for the first time, even better. If they are a vegetarian or grow their own vegetables, that's ideal - not because there is anything wrong with being a carnivore, but rather because vegetarians and gardeners tend to have a much better appreciation and understanding of the importance of good, fresh, organic ingredients and how to cook them.

Good, fresh, simple ingredients - and perfect timing

If you start thinking of food as medicine and as the vital constituent for rebuilding your health, you will soon get the hang of this way of cooking and eating. The best chefs in the world cannot do much with tired old ingredients or even fresh but agrochemically produced ones. They know that what makes their clients ecstatic about their food is the flavour, crisp texture and *vitality* of their ingredients before they have even touched them. Their skill is how they bring out and marry those flavours in their cooking, keeping the combinations subtle and simple. Another critical skill is *timing*. Most would-be cooks get hung up on the timing, so they prepare and cook everything in advance which means their food loses its edge - or loses its flavour and texture altogether if it is left standing around for too long, like one of those ghastly catering buffets where everything is kept under lights for hours. Virtually all the following recipes except the breads and pastries should be done at the last minute and eaten immediately. But they are so quick and simple that once you have made them a few times for yourself, you'll feel quite relaxed about making them for friends and the family. If you are entertaining, remember that friends would far rather wait ten minutes for something fresh and delicious with mouth-watering smells wafting out of the kitchen, than have something on time, but tired and overheated, from the hostess trolley.

So to recap:

To maximise the goodness and flavour and minimise candida-feeding foods
- store as much fresh food in the fridge as you have room for. Remember that organic food will go off more quickly than its treated counterparts.
- wash and scrub fruit and vegetables thoroughly, rather than peeling them. Doing this leaves more essential fibre and goodness and is much quicker. However, any chemicals are most likely to be under the skin, so it is best to peel them in this case. If in any doubt, or if you are very sensitive to moulds,

all fruit and vegetables can be washed in a couple of drops of antifungals e.g. Citricidal or Paracidin.

- whenever possible, prepare and cook everything immediately before you eat it. All you need is a good sharp knife and a large chopping board. If you are cooking for more than two, do experiment with a food processor for grating things or making pates and a liquidiser for homemade soups.
- steam briefly rather than boil. Things are improving, but many British housewives boil their vegetables to death and then tip the goodness down the sink! Try drinking any vegetable water - it's delicious, or you can keep it in the fridge and use it for making soups later.
- discover stir-frying. It is quick, fun, delicious and nutritious.
- use olive oil or butter (or some nut or seed oils for a change) rather than sunflower or corn oils for cooking.
- if you use good oils, fresh herbs and lots of garlic, ginger and gentle spices, (all of which are good for your gut in their own right) you will not need the time-consuming and cloying sauces which candida is so fond of.
- *learn to chop vegetables fast and efficiently.* It really is worth mastering the art of chopping as it saves so much time - with a bit of practice you will soon be like a pro! You need a big board and a large *sharp* knife. You'll have to learn to sharpen this properly with a stone or steel, like the chefs do. Serrated knives are also good, but they won't work for the tricks below as you have to pull them across the fibres. For onions, cut in half through the root, peel the two halves, *leaving the roots on* as this will hold it all together while you chop. Make slices 1/4-1/2in apart with the tip of the knife towards the root, but just missing it, then slice at right angles to your last cuts. For garlic, the cloves are much easier to peel if you squash them with the flat of a large knife and your fist first. For carrot-shaped vegetables, guide the blade with the finger tips of your other hand tucked under, so you can get even, thin slices. For chopping/dicing anything finely (e.g. herbs), hold the point of the knife with your other hand, chopping and moving the broad part of the blade over the pile of herbs or vegetables. Of course if you are food processing things, rough chunks will be fine as long as they are vaguely the same size so they cook evenly - top and tail and wash the vegetables, line them all up on your board and chop right across in one go.
- last but not least, if you enjoy cooking it, the food will taste even better.

The figures on the right of the recipes give the preparation and cooking or standing time, e.g. 4+20 means this will take 4 minutes to prepare and 20 to cook/stand.

BREAKFAST

Biercher-Muesli.   *2-4 mins + overnight.*

Dr Biercher-Benner was a famous Swiss doctor who invented this much loved start to the day. Have plenty, and it will see you through the morning and keep your blood sugar levels nice and stable. It can either be made just before you eat it or soaked overnight, in which case it will have a lovely soft, sticky texture that is actually a lot easier for you to digest.

In a bowl, mix a handful of organic oats (with some oat bran and oat germ, e.g. Mornflake) with any other grains that are OK for you such as rice flakes, millet, barley or rye flakes, with 2-3 tablespoons of the mixed seeds and nuts below, preferably ground, some filtered water and a dash of apple juice or soya milk. This is delicious as it is, but once you are eating a little fruit again then you can add whatever you like, such as some mashed banana or some fresh strawberries (citrus fruits do not mix well with muesli). Grated apple is particularly good for sensitive tummies, if you are soaking it overnight, put the grated apple in then so the pectin develops. Flaked coconut is another popular addition.

Nuts and Seeds Mixture

Take equal quantities of sunflower, pumpkin, sesame and linseeds and either almonds or walnuts and keep this mixture in an airtight jar in the fridge. Daily or at the most every other day, grind some of this mixture in a clean coffee grinder or mini-food processor. Keep any left over in the fridge or it will go rancid very quickly. This combination provides a full protein and a balanced source of essential fatty acids. By grinding them up you will absorb the goodness from them even better. Mixed with yoghurt it makes a delicious meal in itself.

N.B. This mixture can also be used in savoury dishes such as stir-frys or stews and on salads (unground looks better). You can also sprinkle the ground seeds on buttered oat cakes or rice cakes for tea. By grinding them for longer, you can make a rough seed "butter". Try roasting the nuts or seeds lightly first. The bought nut and seed butters are smoother, but more expensive.

Porridge.   *1+12 mins + overnight to soak.*

Many English folk think that porridge has to be made with milk and sugar but of course proper Scottish porridge is made with water and a tiny pinch of salt. Use organic rolled oats or even better pinhead, though this needs soaking overnight before you cook it. Experiment with different grains to make some delicious porridges which will warm you up and see you through the whole morning in winter. Try millet, (the only alkaline forming grain), quinoa, rice flakes or buckwheat (try roasted and unroasted).

Try different flavourings such as cinnamon or nutmeg and ring the changes between a dollop of sheep yoghurt or unsweetened soya milk or brown Rice Dream (though some people find this too sweet). Oatbran can be added to any of the above if you tend to get constipated.

Before anyone starts whinging about the pan being too difficult to clean, don't even attempt it! Leave it to soak and it will all come clean in one satisfying skin later.

Crunchy muesli.   *1+20 mins*

Make up a mixture of oats and other grains with unground nuts and seeds. Melt some butter (and a little honey later in the programme) with some nut oil (hazel nut, walnut, sesame, almond oils). Mix it into the dry ingredients and spread on a large roasting tin in the oven. Roast at a medium heat turning once or twice until it is just brown and crispy. Store in an airtight container.

Eggs

Any way you like. .

If you are frying them use butter or olive oil. Scrambled eggs work very well with butter and a dash of water in the place of milk.

Oeufs en Coquettes   *1+10 minutes*

Break one or two eggs into a ramekin or a little oven proof-dish. Put a dash of sheep or soya milk and a generous knob of butter on the top with a sprinkling of pepper (and nutmeg if you like) and bake in the oven on a medium heat until just set round the edges. Some people put these in a *bain Marie* or dish of boiling water (in the oven). If you like a softer texture, fine, but it is not worth the hassle otherwise.

For bread recipes see the end of this chapter

LUNCH/SUPPER

SOUPS: QUICK, SIMPLE, NOURISHING AND DIFFERENT

You can make wonderful soups out of virtually anything, so here is an opportunity to be really inventive with your combinations. If you don't already have one, invest in a food processor or liquidiser and you'll never want to buy another packet or tin of soup again. See the kit list for recommended brands and prices.

Start with the base and add whatever you like - or whatever was looking good in the market. If you want a creamy soup, use extra butter and sheep or soya milk -

111

or add sheep's yoghurt at the last minute (don't boil it or it will curdle) - this looks great if you only mix it half in to the bowls.

If you want a rich, brown soup, brown the onions and root vegetables for longer, stirring all the time, before adding any liquid. And if you want a pale and interesting one, or one that keeps its fresh green colour for instance, use a lower heat and cover it so nothing browns.

Stocks

A good stock gives soup body and a velvety finish. They freeze very well - but make sure you freeze them in manageable batches and label them clearly. However when you are pressed for time the Swiss Marigold yeast-free stock powder is excellent.

Whether you are using the bones of meat, chicken or fish, the principle is the same: cover with cold water with an onion, carrot and bunch of herbs (including their stalks). Cover and simmer for 1-2 hours (less for fish). If there is any scum, skim this off periodically with a spoon. Strain through a sieve. To get the extra goodness out, return the debris to the pan with a little fresh water, swirl it around and add this to the stock through the sieve. Most butchers and fishmongers are happy to give you bones. I don't make vegetable stocks specifically, but always keep or freeze any water from cooking them.

Soup base (per person)   *2+8 mins.*

1 slug of olive oil and a knob of butter

Half an onion and a clove of garlic, roughly diced

1 medium potato (unpeeled), roughly sliced

Stir-fry for 2 minutes then turn down the heat while you prepare your other ingredients.

Chuck 'em in, cover if they are roots, don't if they are green. Add stock and as soon as they are tender, liquidize. (NB don't ever liquidize anything very hot or it will end up on your ceiling - use less liquid when cooking and add this cold to bring the temperature down to safe limits.)

If you only have a food processor and want a smooth soup, strain off the liquid through a sieve, whizz the solids thoroughly and add the liquid back in afterwards.

If you don't have either machine, you'll have to chop the vegetables more finely and cook them for slightly longer, but you'll end up with a lovely wholesome texture.

Lots of ideas (start with the base unless stated) *These will take 3-10 more mins*
to cook + 1 to liquidize.
Nettle soup - free from March to July and *full* of goodies. Don't forget to take the
rubber gloves to the nettle patch. It tastes rather like spinach soup. Yum.
Courgette and spinach (add a pinch of nutmeg)
Celery, cashew nut and bramley apple
Carrot and cashew or hazelnut (roast the nuts first if time)
Parsnip and curry (and cashews again)
Leek and lettuce
Lettuce and pea (use peas straight from the freezer)
Cock a Leekie - leeks, free range chicken, stock and potatoes. Leave as chunks.
If you leave out the chicken and liquidize it, this becomes *vichyssoise.*.
Beetroot and ginger. Don't use the base here, just an onion and carrot, cook
lightly with olive oil, water and stock powder only - it should be a thin, clear
consistency. Garnish with a swirl of diluted sheep's yoghurt and fresh *finely*
chopped chives.

Adding lentils, chick peas and beans to soups - making a meal of it
Pulses need soaking overnight, rinsing and pre-cooking until they are tender (35-
60 minutes) - use the cooking water, or use tins if you are in a hurry, but rinse the
salt out of them.
There is such a wonderful variety of pulses around in the health food shops. They
store well and it is easy to buy organic ones. All the different colours are great!
Experiment with leaving them lumpy rather than liquidizing them. Grating the
vegetables works very well here and they cook more quickly. A bowl of pulse
soup makes a whole meal especially if you add some cooked brown rice and a few
seeds as well - and they are surprisingly delicious cold.

Some ideas are:
Red lentil, fresh ginger, parsley and carrot
Puy lentil, with roasted aubergine, onion, garlic, carrots and parsnips.
Roast the chunks of vegetables for 40 minutes until getting brown, liquidize
them with a rich stock and add the lentils. Cook, covered for a further
10 minutes. Serve with fresh chopped parsley.
Aduki bean and leek (brown the onion well for this one)
Chick pea, cumin and carrot (a dollop of sheep yoghurt on top is good here)
Chickpea and coconut milk and Thai spices (as in the Thai stir fry recipe)
Flagolet bean and fresh tomato and basil (good with brown/wild rice)
Green lima bean, grated courgette and watercress (only cook this for 5 minutes)

Quick, Cold Summer Soup   *2 mins+2 hrs standing time*
(affectionately known as Pink Soup).
Everyone will think you've been slaving for hours over this one. For 4 people

3/4 pint of sheep's yoghurt
3/4 pint of V8 vegetable juice, or better still, juice your own tomatoes, celery,
carrots, parsley etc.
about 1/2 pint of filtered water, add until you get the right consistency
2-3 fat cloves of garlic, finely squeezed (don't add the fibrous bits)
juice of 1 lemon (or lime)

Whisk all the ingredients together, leave to stand for at least 2 hours in the fridge.
Chill the bowls too. Serve with a swirl of yoghurt on top and float an ice cube and
some finely chopped chives or basil on top of that.

Chilled Avocado and Lime Soup   *3 minutes flat!*
*This is another knockout for a dinner or lunch party. You must do this at the last
minute.* Chill the bowls beforehand.

For 4 people
Put the following ingredients straight into the liquidiser:

some cold potato and onion base if you have it - optional
flesh of 2 avocados
juice of 2 limes (lemon will do but it is not nearly so special)
3/4 pint of sheep yoghurt
2 heaped teaspoons yeast-free stock powder
a pinch of sea salt and a few twists of black pepper
6 ice cubes (made with filtered water)

liquidize and add filtered water if it is too thick.
Garnish each bowl with a little swirl of yoghurt, a tiny mint sprig and 5 red
pepper-berries.

Stir Frying   *8-15 minutes*
Why people insist on paying a fortune for pre-prepared meals when you can knock
up something as delicious as this in 10 minutes flat, that is fresh and far better for
you, beats me. Once you have got the hang of instant stir fries you'll never go
back to a microwave supper! All you need for stir frying is a good sharp knife, a
large chopping board and either a wok (preferably) or a large frying pan, and a
wooden spatula to stir things. All you do is heat some olive oil in your wok and

114

chop whatever mixture of vegetables you feel like, adding them to the wok as you go. If some of your chosen ingredients are a bit difficult to peel or you are not very quick at chopping yet, do them before you start cooking as you might not be able to keep up with the cooking. Chop and add them in the order of those that take the longest to cook first. This could be any combination of the following (in order of cooking):

Onions (red onions are sweeter and more subtle but more expensive)
garlic
nuts and seeds
parsnips/carrots
aubergines
fennel
cauliflower or broccoli
courgettes
mange tout or sugar snap peas
asparagus
frozen peas (it's fine to cook these straight from frozen)
spinach or lettuce leaves (lettuce is surprisingly good hot!)
herbs (put dried herbs in close to the beginning and fresh ones in at the end)
sea weed flakes are good. They'll need soaking in boiling water first
wet food such as tomatoes are best left to the very end

Sauces - stir fry is delicious just with olive oil but if you prefer a saucier finish add some soya milk or rice cream or stock at the end. If you want a thicker sauce (which will turn it into a fricassee rather than a stir fry), sprinkle in some rice, potato or buckwheat flour before any "wet" ingredients go in. Cook through for a minute or two and then add the liquid.

Adding protein - whether you are using beans or lentils that you have cooked yourself or are opening a tin, these can be warmed up in the wok.

Chunks of organic chicken, tuna fish (mercury free) salmon, lamb or chunks of goats or sheep's cheese or tofu are all delicious (not all at once!) So experiment to your heart's content.

Serve with brown rice, non-wheat pasta, millet or couscous.

To cook *millet* (for savoury dishes, as it is very good as a porridge for breakfast too and very good for us), simply steam it in some stock and olive oil, stirring occasionally for 45 minutes.

Couscous is very exotic but dead easy. The Kamut brand is excellent. Cover the grains with boiling water and soak for 10 minutes, separating the grains with a fork. Then either cook it in some stock with a spoonful of olive oil, or (and this is the proper way), steam it. What works very well if you have a big pan is to sit your vegetable steamer on top of a vegetable stew. or on the Thai stir-fry (see below). Line it with two squares of kitchen roll and cook the couscous for 10 minutes with the lid on (i.e. add 10 minutes before the stir-fry is ready).

Thai Stir Fry   *15 minutes*

Using the same principles as above, choose the following ingredients and add them in the order in which they are listed. In the Far East they often cut their vegetables on the slant which looks rather exotic and much more delicate.

For 4 people
Hot red chilli (deseeded very carefully. Don't wipe your eyes while doing this!)
1 inch chunk of fresh ginger
2 cloves of garlic
2 stalks of lemon grass chopped finely
a small bunch of fresh parsley (de-stalked)
Whizz all these ingredients in a mini food processor or coffee grinder if you have one. If not, just chop them up finely.
1 large onion, chopped
1 aubergine, cubed
1/2 cauliflower, broken into bite sized bits
1 tin of chick peas, drained

Once all the ingredients are cooked through but still *al dente* add 1 tin of coconut milk. And finally a good handful of chopped fresh coriander.

Variation
Instead of using the lemon grass and Thai spices, curry powder also works very well with this combination - but make sure it is fresh. Better still grind your own.

Steaming vegetables

Steaming is quicker than boiling vegetables (because you are cooking at a higher temperature) and much better for you because all the nutrients are not boiled away in the water. All you need is a stainless steel steamer which expands and contracts to fit the size of your saucepan (this costs under a fiver - see kit list). You can also use a sieve or colander though you will not get such a good fit with your saucepan lid. There are also steamers on the market that stack on top of other saucepans which is good if you want to keep things separated - and it saves on fuel. Use only an inch of water for green, quick cooking vegetables and two for root vegetables.
The general rule for cooking vegetables (whether you are steaming or boiling them) is that root vegetables are best started in cold water and cooked with the lid on and green vegetables should not be put in until the water is boiling, and cooked

without a lid. Otherwise they will tend to go grey. When you are steaming them, you can cover them, but take the lid off several times during the cooking to let the greying gases escape.

If there is any water left over, don't chuck it down the drain! It will be full of nutrients so always drink it as soon as it has cooled off a bit, or save it for stock, or put it in whatever else you are cooking

Sweating vegetables *8-12 minutes*

This is ideal if you are cooking for one or two. All you need is an ordinary saucepan and you add things on the same principle as for stir frying in a wok One of my favourite mixtures is (for two people) one leek, one parsnip finely sliced, one large courgette, a handful of frozen peas/mange tout/sugar snap peas/sliced runner beans, shredded lettuce or spinach also go very well with this. Once everything is going, give it a stir, add some more olive oil or butter if necessary and put the lid on for another minutes cooking. This is delicious with rice or pasta. You can mix in a beaten raw egg or two with the juice of half a lemon, plenty of black pepper and fresh herbs. Heat the vegetables, pasta and egg and lemon, turning them over and scraping the bottom of the pan until the egg is *just* cooked through and you will have a perfect sauce.

Hummus *5 minutes + 45 minutes cooking time for the chick peas*

This is the absolute stand by for us all. You really need a food processor to make this easily. If using a liquidizer put the liquid ingredients in first and you will probably find you will have to keep stopping to scrape them down the bowl. Mashing it with a fork works but takes a bit longer and gives you a different consistency.

1 bowl of chick peas (either soaked overnight and cooked until soft, or a tin, drained) Reserve the juice unless it is full of salt.
2-4 cloves of fresh garlic
up to 1/4 pint of olive oil
juice of 1 lemon
a handful of fresh parsley with stalks removed
plenty of black pepper, freshly ground.
2 big tablespoons of tahini
N.B. Your hummus will not keep as long if you add parsley

Keep switching on the machine between each new ingredient and add some of the chick pea juice until you get the right creamy consistency. Finally add the tahini (ground sesame seeds). Check the taste. The final consistency may need adjusting with more oil or filtered water.

Variations
Omit the tahini and put in a heaped teaspoon of cumin powder. You can also use lime instead of lemon and experiment with other fresh herbs, eg coriander.

Kedgeree   *10+25 minutes*
(This is not ideal if you are food combining but I am including it all the same as it is such a firm favourite and so easy)

Simultaneously cook the following three ingredients (in three separate pans) starting with the rice as that will take the longest:
For 4 people
4oz organic brown rice in double its volume of water
6-8 free range eggs - hard boiled
12 oz - 1lb *undyed* smoked haddock /cod or salmon.
Poach the fish in some melted butter and a little water in a large frying pan with a
    lid on until just cooked - 5 minutes maximum.
Lift it on to a cold plate and once cool, flake it, picking out any bones.
Peel and chop the eggs - by which time your rice should be cooked.

Mix all the ingredients together with some black pepper, extra butter if you wish and the juice of half a lemon.

Variations
Prawns (frozen's fine. Add towards the end of cooking and cook through)
Chopped parsley
Chopped tomatoes
Curry powder

Serve with plain frozen peas or your favourite sweated vegetables (see above.)

Salads and dressings
It is very important to find sources of good salads and a wide variety of different types - there is nothing more tasteless or boring than iceberg lettuce and I hate to think how few nutrients there are in it. If you have a garden or a window box, fresh herbs, radishes, lettuces, spinach and sorrel all grow easily and quickly and there is nothing to beat picking your own.
Keep your mixtures simple and fresh. Make a bowl of mixed leaves and add a few cherry tomatoes or some finely sliced fennel or some peeled and sliced cucumber, then you can appreciate all the flavours rather than having a muddle.

Black olives are particularly good with oregano and basil and tomatoes. Add chunks of feta or goats cheese for a whole meal. (I marrinate olives in garlic, herbs, more oil and a couple of strips of lemon rind and keep them in the fridge.)
I love adding hot vegetables to cold salads, for instance, hot asparagus, courgettes, sugar snap peas or mange tout. Dress these immediately afterwards so they soak up the lovely flavours of the dressing and eat while still warm.

Dressings
I find a jam jar with a screw top the easiest way of making dressings, and you can make double or triple quanities and keep the rest in the fridge. Just throw in the ingredients and shake hard:

Basic French Dressing
juice of 1 lemon
double its quantity of olive oil
1 clove of garlic
plenty of freshly ground pepper
1/2 tsp of mustard (as long as you are not sensitive to the small amount of vinegar that will be in it - better to leave it out for the first month or so)
Variations
1 tsp of pesto
lime juice is a delicious change
leave three fresh or frozen rasberries in your jam jar - people will think you have used rasberry vinegar
1 tsp of tahini - more if you want a thicker dressing
lots of fresh herbs but add these fresh rather than leaving them to go soggy in your
    jam jar
experiment with different oils. Walnut and hazelnut and sesame seed oil are all
    delicious
Live yoghurt dressing - just add a tablespoon per person to the basic French dressing, omitting the oil if you'd rather.

Vegetables as salads
It is miles easier if you have a food processor to do the grating here but it does not take long to do it by hand.
Grated organic carrots with poppy seeds - moisten with some French dressing and some apple juice. Grated *fresh beetroot* makes this a glorious colour or fresh apricots go very well with this as do roasted nuts and seeds
Grated celariac 'remoulade' with either homemade mayonnaise (made with lemon juice rather than vinegar) or tofu dressing (see below)

Tomato salad with very finely chopped red onion and lots of fresh basil with French dressing made with really good mediterranean oil and plenty of black olives - add chunks of goats cheese or feta cheese if you wish for a really brightly coloured salad-cum-meal.

Cold pasta salads such as broccoli, fennel or fresh rosemary and black olives are good with a french dressing.

Potato salad with masses of fresh chives and tofu dressing (below) or homemade mayonnaise. Hard boiled eggs go very well with this if you are not food combining.

Tofu dressing *2 minutes*

(If you do not have a food processor this can be mashed with a fork but it will take a bit longer). It can also be used as a sauce for pasta, baked spuds, fish or chicken.

1 packet of silken tofu
juice of 1 lemon
plenty of freshly ground black pepper
switch on the machine and dribble in 1/4 cup of good olive oil until you reach the right consistency.
Variations
fresh herbs
curry powder
toasted sesame seeds

Avocado dip, dressing or sauce *2 minutes*
It needs to be eaten straight away as it oxidises.

Put everything into a food processor:
juice of a lemon or lime
pinch of Celtic salt and some black pepper
flesh of a large avocado, scooped out with a spoon
add olive oil and/or soya milk until you get the consistency you want.
Variations
Good with cumin or curry powder
For Mexican guacalmole add garlic, half a chilli pepper and lots of fresh coriander, stir in some chopped tomato by hand and eat with corn or tortilla chips.
(in which case don't add any extra salt)

Try using it as a sauce over pasta and green vegetables (hot) with some toasted pine nuts or on jacket spuds with chives or coriander, with salmon, trout or plaice, or chicken.

Home made mayonnaise   *10 minutes*
People make a big song and dance about how tricky this is to make, but if you have a liquidizer it is a doddle once you have got the hang of it. It is worth mastering because of course you can't have bought mayonnaise because of all the vinegar in it. Using really good olive oil make this a real treat. Yum! The trick is to chill the ingredients beforehand and patience! Otherwise, if you put the oil in too fast, the whole lot will curdle. If you only have a big food processor, you'll need to use 3 egg yolks and 3/4 pint of oil.

For 3/4 of a pint:
Start with 2 egg yolks a drop from the juice of a whole lemon,.and a little salt and pepper. Depending on how strict you need to be, add 2 tsp of mustard and a small dollop of Hellmans (this just gets it going better, but is by no means essential.) Whizz until it goes pale.
Measure out 1/2 a pint of good olive oil into a jug that pours well.
With the machine running, dribble the oil in *very* slowly. Don't add more until it is all emulsified. As it gets thicker, add the rest of the lemon and some water until you get to the consistency you prefer. In case it does curdle, don't panic. Empty the liquidizer, start with another egg yolk and add the curdled maionnaise bit by bit (only slower) and it should be fine.
Add some fresh herbs if you like. Lots of garlic, a hot pepper and 2 tsp of tomato paste makes aioli (to go with fish or on toast). Always store it in the fridge.

In case you are not sure how to separate eggs, again it's a knack that doesn't take more than a few goes to get. Crack one egg smartly on the edge of a bowl. Separate it into two equal halves with your thumb nails. Holding the yolk in one half, let the white fall into the bowl and empty the other shell. Then without catching the yolk skin (or it will break) transfer it into the other shell, letting the rest of the white fall into the bowl as you go. You may have to do this a couple more times. The point of being so careful about this is that egg whites won't whip if there is any fat or yolk with them. If some yolk does go in, scoop it out immediately with a clean shell. So once you have your clean whites you can give them to someone else to make merringues (they'll freeze) or make fruit snows, by whipping them into a firm snow and folding them gently into fruit purees.

Comforting stews
Whether you like bean, lentil, root vegetable, meat or fish stews, there is nothing so comforting and they are suprisingly delicious cold for a packed lunch next day, so make extra.
If you are making meat stew, don't cook the vegetables to death. Sweat them in a separate pan and add them to the meat and sauce with less than 10 minutes to go.

It is easy to adapt your old favourite recipes: Replace any alcohol with fresh stock or Marigold stock power and water (or preferably vegetable or bean water), use potato or rice flour instead of wheat flour, and use extra onions and garlic.

If you find you are wanting to cut down on meat, replace it with lentils or beans. Remember pulses with rice make a complete protein. See under stir-frys for steaming Kamut couscous over your stews.

Pates & terrines   *10 minutes cooking + 3 minutes*

With a food processor, one can knock up any pate in a few minutes flat. The basic idea is to use a main ingredient plus some type of oil or fat. Many recipes involve baking the pate, but I find cooking the main ingredient first (if necessary), letting it cool, then processing it with the fat is quick and simple. Serve with oat cakes, rice cakes, rye toast or kettle chips or if food combining, just in a bowl with salad.

Some ideas include:

- Undyed smoked haddock, hard boiled eggs and either butter or mayonnaise
- Layered vegetable terrine - grate and simmer three vegetables with contrasting colours (e.g. carrot and nutmeg, cauliflower and courgette) into three thick purees. Season, beat an egg into each vegetable and take straight off the heat. Scoop into a loaf tin in three layers and cool. Turn out and serve in slices.

Monika's Walnut and Lentil Pate   *5 + 15/45 minutes*

This is dead easy to make, tastes, looks very 'meaty' and freezes well.

2oz (dry weight) of red or brown lentils, washed and soaked over night
1 onion, finely chopped
1 clove garlic, crushed
1 tsp. thyme, 2 tsp. Marigold stock powder and water or stock, black pepper

Fry the onion and garlic in a generous slurp of olive oil. Add the lentils and thyme and enough stock to cover them. Bring to the boil and skim off any scum. Simmer for 15 minutes for red lentils and 45 minutes for brown ones. You may need to add more water, but don't make it too sloppy. When the lentils are soft, add black pepper and cool the mixture in a serving bowl. Garnish with parsley and serve with toasted pumpernickel, Ryvita or oat cakes. For a more formal meal, cool it in a loaf tin and serve in slices with salad with a tomato or tofu and herb sauce.

FISH

The essential fatty acids in round/fatty fish (herring, mackerel, trout and salmon) are what they say they are - essential for your health, particularly for healing your gut and immune system.

Herring or mackerel in oatmeal.   *1 + 8 minutes*

This is how the Scots cook their herring, but it works just as well for mackerel. It is not kosher food combining, but so little oatmeal is needed you can get away with it.

Gut and clean the whole fish and while damp, roll in a little oatmeal. Either grill with a few dots of butter on top, or shallow fry in olive oil and butter.

PUDDINGS

Puddings are obviously rather limited on a sugar free diet. Though Sue Elliot has come up with some delicious ones. Goat and sheep yoghurt or cheeses are always an option, but as long as you have plenty to eat for your first and second courses, you'll soon not mind not having puddings every day.

Fruit crumble   *15+30 minutes*

1 cup of rolled oats   ½ cup of Spelt flour, rye, barley or buckwheat
4oz melted butter   ¼ cup mixed seeds and nuts (either ground or whole)
a *little* honey melted with the butter
Bramley apples, either plain or with cranberries or apricots or brambles.
unsweetened apple juice

Mix all the crumble ingredients in a bowl with your fingertips, cover the uncooked fruit and juice with the mixture and bake in a medium oven for 30 minutes.

Variations

Experiment with chopped fresh ginger, cinnamon, ground cloves or coconut.
Grating the apple is quicker if you have a food processor and it cooks more quickly. You can leave the skins on if you like.

Sue Elliot's Lemon and Coconut Pancakes.

Sue is an ex-sufferer who has very kindly said we could have this recipe from her very imaginative cookery book Coping with Candida. The pancakes can be frozen (interleaved with freezer tissue) and reheated.

Pancakes:

4oz barley or rye flour
2 eggs beaten
2 tbs. olive oil
7 fl oz soya milk

Sift the flour into a bowl, make a 'well' in the middle and gradually beat in the eggs, milk and oil. (If you have a liquidiser, just chuck 'em all in together) When smooth, leave to stand for 30 minutes. Heat a small frying pan, brush with oil and/or butter. Drop in 2 tbs. of the batter, swill around and cook until bubbles rise and the underside is golden brown. Toss the pancake over and cook the other side.

Lemon and coconut sauce
Put the juice of 3 lemons in a liquidiser with 3 tbs. of desiccated coconut.
If you don't have a liquidiser, you can grate a block of coconut (available from Indian shops) into the lemon juice and end up with a smoother sauce.
Roll up each pancake with some sauce in the middle and pour some more sauce over the top of the pile.

BREADS

Lynette Coffey has some excellent recipes. She wrote her book for her son who has coeliacs disease and can't eat any wheat at all. Several include yeast which you'll have to skip, but she gives many sugar free recipes as well.

Rice and oat muffins (bread rolls substitute) Makes 12   *5+25 minutes*

1 cup oatmeal	½ teaspoon salt
½-¾ cup rice flour (sifted)	¾ cup milk
3 teaspoons baking powder	1 egg

Preheat oven to 175°C (350°F). Grease muffin tray. Sift flours, baking powder and salt and mix in remaining ingredients. Pour into tray and bake for approximately 25 minutes. Cut muffins in half, butter and spread with nut butter.
Variations
For a multi-grain variation add 2 tablespoons of each of the following: unroasted buckwheat; unhulled millet; chopped sunflower seeds; flax seed.
For cheese, herb and onion muffins, mix herbs into mixture, place an onion ring on each muffin, sprinkle generously with grated cheese. Bake as above.

Corn Bread   *10+30 minutes*

1 cup corn meal (polenta)	½ teaspoon salt
¼ cup of soya flour	1 egg
¼ cup oatmeal	1-1¼ cup soya milk
3 teaspoons baking powder	

Preheat oven to 190° (375°F). Grease 20 cm x 10 cm (8" x 4") loaf tin. Mix dry ingredients. Add milk and egg and mix until smooth. Pour into prepared tin and bake for approximately 30 minutes. Can be eaten hot, cold or toasted.

Variations

For a lighter texture fold in two stiffly beaten egg whites just before baking (use the 2 yolks in place of the egg in the recipe).

Savoury Millet Muffins (bread rolls substitute) Makes 12   *10+20-30 minutes*

1 ½ cups millet flour	1 cup soya milk
1 ½ cups barley flour or oatmeal	2 eggs
1 ¼ tablespoons baking powder	1 ½ tablespoons melted butter

Preheat oven to 175°C (350°F). Grease muffin tray. Mix flours and baking powder thoroughly. Lightly beat eggs and milk and add to flour mixture. Beat in butter. Bake for 20-30 minutes.

Yeastless Barley Bread   *5+65 minutes*

1 ½ cups barley flour
½ cups water
1 ½ cups rice flour   6 teaspoons baking powder
2 teaspoons oil

Oil a 20 cm x 10 cm (8" x 4") loaf tin. Preheat oven to 175°C (350°F). Combine sifted flours and baking powder. Add water and oil. Mix well until combined. Place dough into oiled loaf tin. Bake, covered with Bakewell paper and foil for 65 minutes. Remove foil and bake for a further 10 minutes if you want a crisper crust.

Variation

Yeastless Rye Bread.   *5+70 minutes*

Replace the two flours with one cup of rye flour. 1 ½ cups of rice flour and 1 cup of soya flour. Leave plenty of room for expansion under the Bakewell paper and foil and bake for 70 minutes.

Variations for Breads

Experiment with adding the following either in the dough or as toppings:

Seeds (either ground or whole), poppy seeds, caraway seeds and spices such as nutmeg and cinnamon, fresh grated ginger.

For savoury breads add garlic, herbs and gently fried onions, olives, goats cheese, small lumps of tofu - really anything you like that will make a change.

Remember that homemade bread never keeps as long as shop bought bread so after you have eaten the first few slices fresh out of the oven, keep it in the fridge.

PASTRY

Barley or Rye Pastry   *5 minutes with a food processor, 10 without*
Makes enough to line and cover a 20cm (8") to 23 cm (9") pie plate.

1 cup barley or rye flour	125g/4 ounces butter
½ cup soy flour	2 eggs beaten
½ cup rye flour	salt (optional)

Sift flours together. Rub butter into flour. Add eggs to mixture and mix to a firm dough. Knead lightly and use as required. This is suitable for savoury pies, quiche, sweet pies and tarts.
Note: When rolling do not use flour. Place ball of dough between two sheets of plastic wrap and roll with a rolling pin.

TAKING YOUR OWN FOOD TO WORK

If you work, and have been taking sandwiches for lunch for as long as you can remember, you may think that lunch is going to be a major problem. It is true that most of our patients look horrified when it dawns on them that this diet means that they *can't eat sandwiches!* But with a little bit of forethought and imagination it is quite easy, a lot cheaper and far more interesting, to take in your own.

Containers:
Rather than using empty yoghurt pots which may crack and leak in your bag, buy one or two small square Tupperware containers and a plastic beaker with a screw lid (i.e. one you can drink out of). Zippable plastic bags are also useful for salads, and a small jam jar with a screw top is good for carrying lemon & oil dressing. It is also useful to keep a sharp knife, fork and spoon at work, as well as a mug and small electric kettle for making your own herb teas.

Find out if you have a fridge you may use: if so you can shop for the week, but do keep your things hidden in a bag, or your colleagues may be tempted to try them!

Things that will keep. Keep a stock of some of the following in your desk drawer:
- Oatcakes (Patersons are good - avoid Sainsbury's own brand, they taste like cardboard and actually contain wheat and sugar) and rice cakes
- Rye bread (check it is wheat- and yeast-free)
- Ryvita (the sesame seed one is delicious) - not the dark type, it contains malt.

- Fresh almonds or hazelnuts, pumpkin and sunflower seeds
- Fresh fruit
- Carrots (organic taste so much better)
- Kettle chips
- Nut butters: almond, cashew and hazelnut are all good - ideally they should be kept in the fridge

All of these can be eaten with:
- Dips: Humous, Tzatziki, aubergine, goats cheese/tofu, and herb dips (see recipe)
- Avocado (mashed or eaten straight out of the skin with a lemon and olive oil dressing - or just a tiny pinch of salt)
- Mashed banana
- Goats or sheep cheese

Salads:
- Bring washed mixed leaves and herbs and add a lemon and olive oil dressing. Add bean sprouts or seeds for a change.
- Raw vegetables are great to dunk into dips, either whole raw carrots or celery sticks or a bag full of mixed vegetables. though ideally it is better not to cut them until you eat them

Last night's supper. Simply make extra and put some straight into your Tupperware. E.g. Stir fried vegetables and rice, Bean/lentil stew with potatoes (very good cold)

Hot food:
- New Covent Garden Market Soups (some of these are actually delicious cold too)
- Jacket potatoes with butter and some of the above
- Last night's supper
- *If you have no means of heating things except a kettle:*
- Thermoses are great for soups and wide-necked thermoses are good for stews, but it not do wonders for your *al dente* vegetables to keep them hot all morning.
- Bring in very concentrated home-made soup and add boiling water
- Sit your Tupperware (with lid on) in a bigger bowl full of hot water for 10 minutes

Puddings

- Home-made muesli is delicious soaked in some sheeps' yoghurt, soya milk or a little apple juice and water.
- Pots of sheep's or goats yoghurt, plain or with ground nuts and seeds.

General guidelines

Try not to carry on working when you eat. Before you eat, stop and get some fresh air and sunlight (even if it is raining, and only for 10 minutes). If you chew thoroughly and think about, i.e. appreciate, what you are eating, you will digest it far better - try it! Robert MacCarrison, the modern father of nutrition, used to say "chew your drink and drink your food!"

Check out your local lunch take-away places. Jacket potato places are becoming more popular, as are vegetarian take-aways (have a look in vegetarian magazines). Many places do plain salads these days.

MENU IDEAS INCORPORATING FOOD COMBINING

Food combining (i.e. not mixing proteins and starches in the same meal) will speed your recovery from candida considerably because it improves absorbtion and takes a load off your digestive system, leaving it more energy to heal.
But do not feel you have to achieve this immediately on top of all the other changes you will be making. We emphasise again, that both for your body's sake and for your sanity, changes must be made gradually, and this is what you should be aiming for. So take your time, one step at a time, ask for help if you need it and you **will** get there!

General Guidelines

- Keep protein foods and starch foods separate.
- Drink between 1-2 litres of filtered or bottled water a day.
- Never eat fruit with a meal (except for banana with starch).
- Avoid the foods to which you personally are intolerant or allergic, as well as all of the foods on the candida list.
- Lunch and dinner can be swapped around.
- Never eat in a rush or when you are angry. Try to go for a walk in the fresh air for a few minutes before you eat, breathing deeply and evenly, and you will find that you will digest your food much better and not be so tired. Do not eat less than 1-2 hours before you go to bed.
- If your stomach is very sensitive, try eating several smaller meals. It is important that you eat enough.

BREAKFAST
- Porridge made with filtered water. You can add banana/cinnamon/some seeds plus a little butter or cream if you wish.
- Wheat and malt-free muesli. Wild Oats do a delicious mixture for anti-candida, (available by mail order see appendix 2) or mix your own. Soak it, preferably overnight, in a little apple juice and water or sheep's yoghurt.
- Homemade crunch, i.e. the muesli above, roasted in a little butter and sunflower oil and stored in an air tight jar. Try with some diluted apple juice, or soya milk.
- Sheep's/goats' yoghurt with seeds, e.g. linseeds, sesame, sunflower, pumpkin. Keep these ready mixed in an airtight jar. Grind 2 days supply at a time and keep in the fridge.
- Ryvita, oatcakes (check they are wheat free), rice cakes with butter. 100% Rye bread (i.e. wheat and yeast free) is very good - especially toasted.
- Eggs - boiled, poached or scrambled. You could add chives, parsley, haddock or salmon to it but do not eat any toast or biscuits with it.

LUNCH   STARCH + SALAD

- Soup (not meat or fish). The New Covent Garden soups are very good (but a few of them have dairy and wheat in them, so check the label), with oatcakes/rice cakes/ryvita/100% rye bread toast.
- Buttered jacket potato with a large salad with an olive oil and lemon dressing.
- Avocado and salad with dressing.
- Hummus and salad with Ryvita, oatcakes, rice cakes and butter. Raw carrots are particularly good for dipping into hummus.
- Brown rice/rice noodles/rice pasta with herbs, olive oil and vegetables and/or salad.
- Pasta (Corn, Spelt or Kamut, Buckwheat, Rice, all available from good healthfood shops or Wild Oats mail-order) with mixed vegetables cooked in olive oil.
- Salads of any kind as long as they do not include tuna, eggs, cheese, etc.
- Any pea, bean, lentil dish with salad. Try sprouting seeds, peas and lentils to go on salads.

PUDDING
- Mashed banana with homemade breakfast crunch.

SUPPER - PROTEIN + VEGETABLES OR SALAD
(NO RICE, PASTA, POTATO, BREAD, BISCUITS OR PASTA).

Starters
- Home-made fish or meat soup. (most bought ones will have starch thickeners). Egg and lemon soup is also delicious. See recipe for avocado & lime soup.
- Avocado with a dressing, or with prawns in lime and yoghurt. Add fresh ginger and fresh coriander if you like.
- Crudités with a herb and Greek yoghurt dip, or Tzatziki.
- Salad with warm roasted peppers or aubergines with parmesan or with avocado and roasted seeds.

Main Courses
- Organic chicken/turkey or game
- Organic lamb
- Fish or seafood - herring, mackerel, trout and salmon for your essential fatty acids.
- Omelettes (don't forget fresh herbs) or make a fish or vegetable terrine.
- Tofu - see books on Japanese cooking and macrobiotic cooking.

Pudding
- Yoghurt with ground nuts and seeds
- Cheese board à la française i.e. with no biscuits or bread

SNACKS
- Fresh nuts and seeds
- Kettle chips
- Ryvita, oatcakes, rice cakes with butter and/or Hummus/nut butters (almond, hazelnut, cashew)
- Crudités with hummus
- Olives - marinate in olive oil, garlic, parsley and a piece of lemon rind.
- Some fruit - always eat by itself

COOKING FOR THE FAMILY
If the changes you need to make from your old diet are pretty major, then presumably they would be as great for your family if they were to make them with you. It depends on how much they help in the kitchen already - though now is the perfect opportunity to start to include them on the food front if you have traditionally been the 'sole provider' there.

Many families are fantastic and enter into the spirit of adventure, coming up with ideas for you, learning about the new foods and special ways of cooking them and trying whatever is on your menu themselves. Many sufferers report back after a few weeks that their husbands confessed that they actually feel better and prefer their new diet!

In other families, whether particular members or the whole gang, they simply won't budge and inch from their sausages and ketchup, takeaway pizzas and beer and the latest triple chocolate-chip ice cream that has just been advertised on the TV. Obviously your ending up with twice as much cooking and shopping as before is going to defeat the object entirely, so you must find a compromise. There might be some helpful ideas in chapter 8.

If your family is co-operative, but conservative in their tastes, the recipes in Erica White's cook book may well be the solution. It is full of great looking recipes for pizzas, cakes, turkey burgers, sauces and stuffings and pastries and puddings that children, teenagers and husbands will love. All of which you can eat as well! (See appendix 2 for where to get a copy). If they are more cosmopolitan in their tastes, I highly recommend Sue Elliot's book.

Adapting recipes
Often it is simplest to have the same food as the family, but add the sugar or whatever last and making a special little bowl for yourself without it. It is worth buying an individual ovenproof dish and a small pan for yourself if this is going to be your solution. If you enjoy cooking (and I hope you are beginning to do so having read this chapter), you will equally enjoy the fun of adapting recipes.

Really the only things that tend not to work on a straight swap basis are breads, cakes and pastries because wheat flour behaves differently to rye, barley or corn flours and sugar works as a binding agent. If you enjoy baking, order a copy of Lynette Coffey's lovely book. She goes into the science and behavioural idiosyncrasies of the various grains in clear and charming detail - and it is full of delicious recipes. Otherwise, the chart at the end of this chapter giving you the foods to avoid and their alternatives should be self explanatory and give you some ideas.

Here are a few extra thoughts:
Eggs and yoghurt both thicken sauces beautifully, but don't overheat them or they will curdle and separate.

Don't use artificial sweeteners in place of sugar! They are chemicals that we can well do without and much more to the point, seem to perpetuate or bring back any sugar cravings

Stock cubes, gravy brownings, cook-in sauces, MSG, sugar and salt are called "flavour enhancers" but they are usually used when there is nothing to enhance! If you use really good, fresh ingredients and herbs, you won't need any of them, so just leave them out altogether. (Though a teaspoon of yeast-and-everything-else-free stock powder such as Marigold, doesn't go amiss occasionally.)

Christmas without candida!

A special sheet of recipes and ideas for a Happy Candida-free Christmas, will be available from mid-November. If you would like one, please send a C5 s.a.e. plus two extra first class stamps to: Christmas without candida, All Hallows House, Idol Lane, London EC3R 5DD

FINDING A GOOD HEALTH FOOD SHOP

The very first thing you need to do when you have had candidiasis diagnosed is to find your nearest, good, i.e. independent health food shop. First, because you'll discover masses of delicious foods that you can eat, that are probably quite new to you, and second, because their staff are usually very well trained and knowledgeable about candida (many of them are ex-sufferers themselves). Particularly if you catch them at a time when the shop is not too busy, they are usually terribly helpful and will spend quite some time with you introducing you to all the sugar, yeast and wheat-free goodies, how to cook them and the latest tip they have picked up for bloating or thrush, or whatever. If they don't stock something, they will usually be only too delighted to order it for you, especially if it is something they haven't come across yet.

The big health food chains tend not to be so good, either in the range or quality of their stock nor in the experience of their staff. But there are always exceptions so check them out, ask your questions and don't be afraid to ask where the staff trained.

SUPERMARKETS

Happily the variety of foods we can eat on a sugar and yeast free diet is improving all the time. I have listed specific foods normally stocked by the big supermarket chains in the notes by your checklist of foods to avoid and their alternatives at the end of this chapter.

That said, you still have to *check every label* as they can and do change the ingredients without warning and you'll find sugar, yeast, vinegar, flours and of course flavourings and additives in the most surprising places.

If your supermarket does not stock certain things *speak to the manager about it,* otherwise he won't know there is the demand for it. Keep pestering - it'll pay off in the end.

Fruit and Vegetables leave a lot to be desired. They might look perfect, but you compare them with their organic equivalents for taste and vitality and you will see what I mean. Supermarkets are experimenting with stocking organic foods, usually carrots, onions, potatoes and lettuces. Do give the staff your feedback and keep encouraging them, or they might stop stocking them - and encourage your friends to buy them.

KITTING OUT YOUR HEALTHY KITCHEN

- water filter - Waymaster or Brita £13-£19 plus cartridges
- sharp knives, a sharpener and a large wooden chopping board
- wok with a lid
- stainless steel collapsible steamer £4
- stainless steel or enamel pan. Le Creuset are wonderful to cook with but may be too heavy for some people.
- salad spinner
- rubber spatula for scraping out bowls without wasting anything
- Tupperware containers to take food to work
- food processor and/or liquidizer. Braun and Kenwood are both good.
- mini grinder (Tefal Foodmaster)
- juicer. Kenwood, Braun and Moulinex range from £38-£45
- pressure cooker (useful, but don't buy one specially)
- pegs or freezer clips to keep things in cellophane bags fresh
- air tight, dark glass jars for general storage
- individual sized oven-proof dish and pan etc if you are keeping your food separate from the family's
- a freezer, so you can cook several meals for yourself in one go
- AVOID microwaves - they don't do anything for the nutrients in your food.

CHAPTER 7

NUTRITIONAL SUPPLEMENTS
Some good brands and products and where to find them

Many of the books, and I'm afraid a few practitioners recommend a whole shopping list of supplements that can cost into three figures. I have met so many sufferers who say they could open a shop with all the bottles and pills they have been advised to take over the years.

Particularly if you have several associated symptoms and read up on each piecemeal, it can seem as if you do need a whole list, but remember that candidiasis is a "syndrome" and that we are aiming to help your body-mind heal itself as a whole. Once you start getting the general environment in your gut into better shape, most of the associated problems will clear up as your body-mind gets itself back into balance. Most people should only need the baseline treatment to start this happening. The next stage, after 4 to 12 weeks is to review things with your practitioner, as now you will be able to see the wood for the trees, and any distinct problems that are still troublesome can be treated. This process may have to be repeated several times if you have been ill for a long time, but at least this will be a more focused and specific approach.

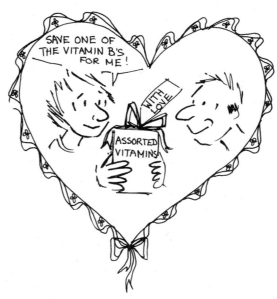

Of course you can take a whole list of supplements from the outset if you wish. As long as your constitution and absorption has not been too damaged, you may get better more quickly. But do not think of buying more supplements as a short cut to doing the diet properly! If however your job and lifestyle makes it genuinely difficult to stick to the diet as closely as you would like - as with many of our clients who work in the City of London, then it is a good idea to take more. Your nutritionist will suggest which.

If you are very ill and your absorption and energy levels are poor, there will be a limit as to how many goodies your system can actually utilise - or you really will be producing 'expensive urine'. Sustaining herbs, Celloid minerals, Replete and a *very* gentle detoxification and *very* pure, fresh foods are what you need to start with - and expert professional care.

I had an interesting conversation last year (1994) with Leon Chaitow on the subject of the number of nutritional supplements one needs to take. I recommend his book *Could Yeast be Your Problem?* to everyone, as I think it is still one of the best, most concise and most practical available. However, I do this with the major proviso that in our experience, it is not necessary to take anything like the number of supplements he recommends. He had been working in a GP's surgery for a year, where of course most of the patients simply couldn't afford, or were not expecting to pay for, as many supplements as his private clients. (Very few supplements are available on the NHS.) So he had to keep to the barest essentials: a probiotic, an anti-fungal, something for a leaky gut (or this came in phase two if necessary) and perhaps one or two other things - and they got better, perhaps a little more slowly, but with the same end result! Very good news is that Leon is bringing out a new edition of his book early next year (1996). I for one very much look forward to seeing it.

Self help and self-treating

Helping yourself and your family through minor ailments by learning about the natural remedies and supplements is certainly to be encouraged, and you will find that by using the brands mentioned here, you will get good results. See chapter 7 for more specific suggestions.

I have already warned of the hazards of trying to self-treat more serious conditions in chapter 3, so please read that section if you haven't already done so. Some of you will only have candidiasis mildly and others will think you can do it yourself whatever someone like me says, but I'd much rather you used good brands and products than wasted your money on inappropriate ones. This chapter will give you that information - but I'll say it once more, don't forget that natural remedies are not meant to be "this pill for that ill" like the over the counter drugs. So the information here can never be more that broad generalisations, with none of the subtleties of the individual attention you will get if you see a practitioner. If you are seeing a practitioner, then this chapter will hopefully be a helpful reference.

Which brands?
The brands mentioned here are those that are backed up by excellent research. We have used them ourselves and get consistently good results - and they are used by practitioners we know and trust. I do not have shares in any of their companies and they are not buying huge blocks of advertising space - we just listen to our clients and to their researchers. But we can't know everything on the market, so if you find any good products that are not mentioned here, please write and tell us.

Generally, those recommended by trained practitioners, such as those below, are far better researched; more effective for therapeutic purposes than those freely available to the general public; and do not contain any of the allergenic substances known as "fillers", nor the flavourings and preservatives such as yeast, sugar, talc, lactose, whey, gluten, corn, soy - all of which are commonly found in other products. Check the labels. But perhaps the most important factor is that they are more synergistic. That is, all the compounds needed for the main ones to be utilised are included, such that the whole effect seems to be greater than the sum of the constituent parts.

The supplement manufacturers we rate include **BioCare, Blackmores, Higher Nature and Lamberts**. All of these have pretty comprehensive ranges, some have over 200 different products, but here, I am only mentioning the essentials for candidiasis and its associated problems.

As far as treating candidiasis is concerned, one must remember that it is a relatively newly recognised condition, so only those companies backed by the most innovative research teams who have focused specifically on candida will be at the leading edge in terms of new product research and development and effectiveness. BioCare leads the field here with some of Britain's top bacteriologists, biochemists and practitioners, as well as new biotechnology from the United States. Brian and Celia Wright who set up Higher Nature were among the first in the UK to write about and encourage the natural treatment of candidiasis and ME. They have also developed their range well and have brought over some new products and protocols from the States.

Prices
Those quoted here are the recommended retail prices, including VAT and are correct at the time of going to press (September 1995).

136

If you compare them with other brands which may seem cheaper, remember that most of these come in larger packs and that because of their quality and higher strengths, they will end up being much more cost effective. So as ever, "you gets what you pays for". That said, do make sure you are clear about the appropriate dose, as people often take more than they need and "more" is not necessarily "better" - and can cause problems. And before anyone starts whinging about how expensive they all are..... remember to include in your calculations the fact that you are not drinking coffee and alcohol nor fizzy drinks, nor eating so much meat, processed foods and bars of chocolate, though hopefully you will be investing a bit more in organic vegetables, good olive oil and so on. Your daily needs for supplements should come to between £1.10 and £2.00. so with the savings above, we reckon you'll actually come out quits financially - but you are bound to gain overall, since your health is priceless. If you really can't manage financially, speak to your GP or practitioner.

STORAGE: Store all supplements in a cool, dark, dry place.

DOSAGES: These are very individual and depend on what other combinations you might be taking. To avoid die-off symptoms, the anti-fungals and in some cases the probiotics must be built up gradually. Your practitioner will advise.

If you have trouble taking pills
There are many multiminerals and vitamins in liquid form (often formulated for children) but you could also try Cantassium's pill crusher which turns a pill into a powder in one twist. But do check that this will not affect any necessary slow release capability intended for that supplement.

PROBIOTICS

Everyone knows that antibiotics kill bacteria, but perhaps you hadn't come across probiotics. They encourage bacteria - but unlike antibiotics which affect all bacteria, good and bad indiscriminately, probiotics only encourage the friendly bugs that are essential to our well-being to recolonise our gut lining.
Thanks to great technological advances in bacteriology over the last ten years, we now understand more exactly how lactic bacteria work and how they can be supplemented effectively. However, they are very fragile things. They cannot live in air, and are highly specific to the human gut, so strains cultivated on bovine (cows) substrate for instance will not recolonise the human gut. Therefore it is essential that you look for good quality products. (Beware as there are some rather dodgy ones around - though the situation is better than it was. Penny

Woolley's independent register of nutritionists have investigated and recommend those below plus Naturdophilus from Larkhall.)

Checklist for good quality probiotics:
- Must include both *Lactobacillus acidophilus and Bifidobacterium* whether separately or together.
- Number of viable micro-organisms should be guaranteed. (Dose should be at least 1 billion.)
- Must be able to survive through the stomach acid
- Must be shown to be able to colonise the human gut lining, i.e. be of human origin.
- Must not include other bacteria, sometimes used because they have a longer shelf-life, such as *streptococcus faecum or S. faecalis.* These, while found in the human gut, are opportunistic pathogens and can and do cause secondary infections in vulnerable guts.
- Strict product quality control. Check the capsules are microencapsulated and vacuum sealed and that it is recommended that they are refrigerated after opening. Check the sell-by date.
- *Avoid* Powders as they will not survive the stomach acid and will quickly deteriorate on contact with oxygen.

The only independent analysis of commercially available products carried out to date showed NaturChem Ltd's supplement is of the highest quality (**available from BioCare and Blackmores),** with the Life Start preparation by Natren Inc. having a "satisfactory" specification.

NB Yoghurt is NOT a substitute for these supplements. The bugs in yoghurt, i.e. *Lactobacillus bulgaricus and Streptococcus thermiphilus* are not normal residents of human guts and therefore will not help with the job of re-establishing the healthy flora. However, to a certain extent eating natural, live yoghurt will make it easier for the right strains of our own bugs to re-establish by improving the environment in the gut and is a good general food source.

Other occasions on which to take probiotics As recommended by Dr Nigel Plummer of BioMed.
- Post-antibiotics, when you will need a hefty dose immediately after the course, (e.g. Replete). See also alternatives to antibiotics in chapter 4.
- after illness (including colds or flu)
- before and during long distance travel, and when abroad
- after stressful times
- following digestive or bowel upsets (great for hangovers!)

- after several days' eating too much meat and dairy foods.
- after an intensive diet or fast.
- if having colonic therapy, double check the therapist is replacing your bowel flora with a probiotic supplement.

The following products are listed under each supplier:
BioCare
Bio-Acidophilus *providing 4 billion organisms of Acidophilus and Bifidus per capsule fulfils all the criteria above. Only one capsule a day needed.*
60 capsules £15.25
Vegi-dophilus *the vegetarian equivalent, in a base of Bifido Growth Factor*
60 capsules £15.95
Replete *7 day intensive post-antibiotic recolonisation regime 30 billion organisms per sachet and specific fructooligosaccharides to selectively stimulate the regrowth of the three strains of Lactic acid bacteria.*
7 sachets x 20g £29.95
Follow with Bio-acidophilus.
Strawberry Acidophilus for Children *chewable tablets that they love!*
60 tablets £10.65
Cervagyn cream *for vaginal thrush, can also be used on the skin. Applicator included.*
55g £11.70

Blackmores
Acidophilus Bifidus capsules *(identical to the BioCare product above)*
30 capsules £7.99

Higher Nature
Entero-dophilus *90mg of lactobacillus acidophilus and 360 mg fructooligosaccharides.*
30 capsules £8.65, 60 capsules £16.95
Acidobifidus *Acidophilus and Bifido bacteria in a powder form. More economical when a lower concentration is needed later.*
90g £3.50, 180g £6.70
Probiogest *A probiotic formula containing Lactobacillus salvarius and F.O.S.*
30 Capsules £8.75 60 Capsules £17.25

Lamberts
Acidophilus Extra
30 capsules £6.50, 60 capsules £12.50

ANTI-FUNGALS

The case against pharmaceutical anti-fungals
Most doctors will tell you that fungal conditions aren't a problem except in the severely ill, because we have such effective anti-fungal drugs that wipe out fungi on contact. Then they will add that Nystatin is cheap, well tried over years and very 'well tolerated' (i.e. it is non-toxic) because it is not absorbed by the gut. (Some of the others such as Amphotericin or Fluconazole (Diflucan) do affect the liver and kidneys so have to be carefully monitored). Yet we frequently see patients who have been on Nystatin, and sometimes repeated courses of the others, for a year and more - and they are not better. Many people say that when they come off the drug they actually feel worse than they were before. First, it only seems to kill on contact but do not reach the roots of the fungal overgrowth (the "lawn mower effect") and secondly, though it is not fully understood why, the drugs seem to make the colonies of yeasts and fungi *better* able to establish themselves than before.

As I emphasised at the beginning of chapter 4, with any conditions like candidiasis, gut dysbiosis or food sensitivities, the liver will be under pressure, if not actually damaged, so it is important to avoid pharmaceutical drugs where possible because they only add to that overload. While there is a time and place for pharmaceuticals occasionally if used judiciously, we believe the natural anti-fungals should be tried first (in conjunction with the whole programme). This is, as ever, because natural remedies work in synergy and support the body's healing processes.

The natural anti-fungals
These are based on either caprylic acid which comes from coconut oil and is found in human breast milk, or on grapefruit seed oil. Garlic is another good one. Herbalists have many others and there are several essential oils such as Tea Tree.

Depending on where your candidiasis is, i.e. just in the gut, or whether it has spread to the throat, mouth, nose and ears - or is in the vagina, it is important to choose the most appropriate product. For instance, it has to survive the stomach acid and be 'time released' to get right down into the lower, large intestine and colon to do any good for the gut. The liquids below can all be used as gargles, nasal sprays, ear drops and vaginal rinses, for skin and nails, even to clean toothbrushes and food.
NB If you have not been well for some time, don't start taking anti-fungals until you have started to detoxify for 1-3 weeks, build up dose gradually (see 'coping with die-off' in chapter 5) as prescribed and take with food.

NB Most of the anti fungals below should not be taken during pregnancy. Check with your practitioner.

BioCare
Mycopryl *for candidiasis in the lower gut*
680 90 capsules, £17.65
400 100 capsules £15.25
250 (for children) 60 capsules £10.95
Magnesium Caprylate which is non-irritating, though not suitable if you have gastritis or ulcers. Provide 680, 400 and 250 mg per capsule respectively.
Caprycillin *the vegetarian equivalent of Mycopryl*
400 90 capsules £15.25
Candicidin *for systemic candidiasis i.e. in the gut, upper respiratory tract and for parasites*
60 capsules, £15.95
A relatively new product including plant oils and Artemisia absynthium extract with a broad spectrum anti-bacterial, anti-fungal and anti-parasitic action which has been extensively tested with very good results.
Oxypro *for the upper respiratory tract.*
Liquid, 15ml £6.55
Garlicin *Garlic is one of the oldest known antifungals. Freeze dried fresh garlic, to make an active concentrate. With Biotin.*
400mg 90 capsules £8.50

Blackmores
Garlix
30 capsules £4.99, 90 capsules £11.50

Higher Nature
Citricidal *Grapefruit seed extract in liquid form. Broad spectrum, hypo-allergenic and non-toxic even over long periods.*
Liquid, 15 ml £3.20 (travel size)
Liquid, 50ml £8.50
Liquid, 120 ml £19.50
Candiclear *Buffered Caprylic acid with antifungal herbs.*
30 tablets £
90 tablets£
Paraclear *Citricidal and Chinese Artemisia plus 7 other herbs in capsule form.*
30 capsules £5.25
90 capsules £15.00

Lamberts
Caprylic Acid
90 tablets £14.95
Pure-Gar *(garlic)*
90 capsules £7.95

LEAKY GUT
F.O.S. or Fructooligosaccharide
This enables the friendly bugs in the small intestine to make butyrate which is essential for the a healthy gut lining (mucosa) in both the small intestine and the colon. It also provides the Bifido Growth Factors that encourage the growth of bifido bacteria in the gut, without feeding the yeasts.

It is a natural food substance with the properties of a natural fibre, which occurs in fruit and vegetables (It is particularly rich in Jerusalem artichokes - the "fartychoke" type and dandelion leaves.)

F.O.S also tastes sweet, though it doesn't encourage the yeasts, so it makes a welcome addition to sugar-free diets.

All the following are available from most of the manufacturers mentioned above.

Butyrates have a key role in restoring a leaky gut, as it supplies the food necessary for the epithelial tissue to regrow and helps maintaim the natural barrier. (NB Butyric acid is what we bring up when we are sick, so will have that familiar unpleasant smell!) For more information, see BioMed 1989 by Dr Torben Neesby.

N.A.G (N. Acetyl Glucosamine) is an integral part of the "glue" which holds our cells together, especially for the mucous membranes lining the gut.

Zinc ascorbate is needed to maintain the defences of the gut barrier and for healthy tissue repair.

Magnesium ascorbate (Vitamin C and Magnesuim) strengthens and heals connective tissue and the magnesuim maintains the muscles and nerves.

Vitamin A protects against infection and helps the healing process.

Replenishing the friendly bugs with probiotics also directly helps the gut lining to heal by helping the nutrients it needs on site.

NB Allow a leaky gut at least 3 months to heal.

Avoid herbs that will irritate such as cayenne, pau d'arco and sometimes even goldenseal. Even aloe vera can gripe sensitive tissues when taken in a concentrated form.

BioCare
Enteroguard. A synergistic combination of all the nutrients mentioned above to heal a leaky gut. Best taken with Mega GLA and Bio-Acidophilus
150g powder £24.95

142

This is highly effective, but smells pretty nasty - a mixture of silage (fermenting cellulose) and sick (the Butyric acid). However, don't worry, this is entirely contained in the gut so it will not smell on your breath or your skin. If you really can't stand it, try

Permatrol
90 capsules £13.95

Mega GLA Emulsified Gamma Linolenic Acid. (rich in Omega 6 fatty acids.)
30, 60, 90 and 180 capsules £5.10, £9.05, £ 12.60, £ 21.15
It works as an anti-inflammatory and helps the action of other nutrients163mg per capsule - i.e. 4 times as much GLA as a 500mg capsule of Evening Primrose Oil. Good shelf life. You only need take 1 per day so it is far more economical.

Lamberts
Biotin *500iu*
90 capsules £6.25

MULTIMINERAL-VITAMINS

It is certainly a good idea to take one multimin-vit a day particularly in the early stages of your recovery. But it is particularly important to go for quality at this stage, so avoid shiny tablets (you may not be able to digest the coating) and stick to the manufacturers mentioned here.

BioCare
Multivitamin/mineral Complex *very well formulated, time released*
30 capsules £6.75
60 capsules £12.15
90 capsules £16.65

Femforte *a specially formulated mulitmin-vit for women. Some women find these difficult to swallow, but a pill crusher solves this.*
90 tablets £15.45

Children's multivitamin & mineral *formulated especially for the Hyperactive Children's Support Group. One capsule suitable for 2 year olds. Break capsule and sprinkle on food for younger children. Made from freeze dried fruit.*
30 capsules £3.85, 60 capsules £6.75, 90 capsules £9.70

Vitaforte Banana for children *in powder form if they won't take capsules. Made from freeze dried fruit.*
Powder 150g £7.45

Blackmores
Naturetime sustained release vitamins *with anti-oxidants, very well formulated*
31 capsules £5.85, 75 capsules £10.50., 200 capsules £22.85
Their **Executive B Formula and B plus C** are also good.

Higher Nature
Optimum Nutrition,
90 capsules £10.45
Maxi Multi
90 capsules £19.95
Get Up & Go
300g powder £9.95
Dinochews *for children*
90 tablets £9.95

Lamberts
Vitamin/Mineral complex
60 tablets £6.95,   180 tablets £18.95

LIVER SUPPORT
Essential for detoxification (though can be stage 2), known liver infections, heavy drinking (alcohol) or exposure to pollutants in the past or present, or if multiple allergies, aches, or dark rings under the eyes indicate general toxicity. NB take with anti-oxidant vitamins to "quench" the free radical activity.

BioCare
HEP 194 Hepaguard *high potency to build up the liver and blood, enzyme activated.*
60 capsules £5.75
90 capsules £10.50

Blackmores
Dandelion Complex 75 tablets £3.99

DIGESTIVE ENZYMES
Until your gut is back in balance, digestive enzymes can be invaluable, especially in the early stages when you may be sensitive or intolerant to many foods. Particularly useful when eating out.

BioCare - do a whole range of specific enzymes that can be a lifeline for people with food intolerances
Digest Aid *a combination to help you digest proteins, fats and carbohydrates. Take one capsule with each meal and a little water.*
30,60 and 90 capsules £6.30, £11.35 and £15.55
Carbozyme *providing Amylase to digest starch and carbohydrates*
90 capsules £10.70

Lipozyme *helps breakdown fats so they can be assimilated (not if you have ulcers or gastritis)*
90 capsules £12.30

Prolactazyme Forte *for milk intolerance plus Acidophilus. Most people can't digest the lactose (milk sugar), but some can't deal with the fats or proteins. This product deals with all three (not if you have ulcers or gastritis)*
30, 60, and 90 capsules £5.30, £10.25 and £15.25

Liquid Lactase Enzyme *to put straight into milk so you can take it normally. (4 drops to one pint) One bottle does 68 pints.*
15ml liquid £7.75

Glutenzyme Forte *to take with gluten cereals*
42 capsules £8.55

Blackmores
Digestive Aid Tablets 84 tablets £8.99
Digestive Bitters Fluid Extract 220ml £11.75

Higher Nature
Easigest 30 capsultes £4.15, 90 capsules £11.85

PARASITES
Biocare
Eradicidin Forte for gut parasites
90 capsules £13.75
Alan Hibberd finds that this will shift even *Helicobacter pyloris,* so always try it before resorting to antibiotics.
Candicidin
An anti-fungal for all strains of *candida* which also has also been shown to be effective against against *E coli, salmonella,Camplylo Bacter and Helicobacter Pylori.*

Higher Nature
Paraclear *a complete herbal formula for many parasites.*
30 capsules £5.25
90 capsules £15.00

LOW BLOOD SUGAR
BioCare
Chromium Polynicotinate
15ml £11.70

WHERE TO FIND SUPPLEMENTS AND REMEDIES.

Many of the brands of nutritional supplements recommended here are not readily available to the public unless they go through a trained practitioner who order them by mail. However many specialist health food shops are now stocking their retail (as opposed to professional) ranges. This is not to maintain a monopoly for alternative practitioners - it is because there are no prescription controls as for orthodox drugs and you do need to know what you are up to, to know which ones are the most appropriate to take, what dose and for how long. Otherwise, they won't be so effective, or may trigger some reactions, and they, and all alternative medicines with them will (and do) get a bad name!

Herbal and Homoeopathic Remedies and Essential Oils

Most health food shops have a good stock of all of these and will advise you on the best brands and products. The ones we have found to be good are:
Herbals: Blackmores, Gerrards, Bioforce, Potters, Weleda,
Homoeopathic: Weleda, Nelsons (now also available in Boots),
Essential Oils: Neal's Yard, Tisserand, Shirley Price,

If you have any difficulty in getting something, **The Nutricentre** offers an amazing *mail order service.* They have one of the most comprehensive selections of nutritional supplements in the UK in their treasure trove shop at the Hale Clinic. They certainly stock everything mentioned in this guide - and more, and will do their best to locate anything else you want, or a suitable alternative. They also stock books, aromatherapy oils and a small range of health foods for special regimes. Their staff are well qualified and very helpful if you want advice on products. Orders received before midday are sent by first class post to reach you next day.

Payment can be made on either a prepayment basis by cheque, or by credit card. If you know exactly what you want then an order by fax with your credit card number is easiest. They need your name and mailing address, the exact details of the things you want (name of product, brand, number of capsules, title of book and publisher etc.) Don't forget to include your credit card's expiry date and your phone number in case anything is illegible. Otherwise they are happy to speak to you on the phone.

The Nutricentre, 7 Park Crescent, London W1N 3HE Tel 0171 436 5122
Fax 0171 436 5171

What can I get on the NHS?

The list of both drugs and supplements that can be prescribed on the NHS has been honed down considerably over the last 3 years, and it seems as if this trend will continue. Unless you are under 16 and over 55 (women) and 60 (men), or pregnant, you have to pay £5.25 per item anyway, so we are not often talking about a great saving for you. If however you are entitled to free prescriptions, then obviously it is worth finding out what is available. The Drug Tariff (the list of prescribable drugs) is changing all the time so it is best to ask your pharmacist. Many vitamins and minerals are marketed at below the £5.25 threshold, particularly the mass-marketed - but these are the ones that while they are fine for healthy people, they do not generally have as good results as the brands recommended above for people who need to take them therapeutically.

Hills and other pharmacies will be stocking the *BioCare* range from this autumn (1995). This very welcome new initiative will be backed up by local nutritionists on site and well trained staff who'll be able to give you a candida questionnaire, written information (or a copy of this directory and guide) and some personal advice. New pharmacies will be added to the list of stockists all the time, so to find out if there is one near you, *phone BioCare Pharmacy Ltd on 01276 36638*

CHAPTER 8

FINDING MORAL SUPPORT,
asking for help and joining a self- help support group
Breaking out of the low self-esteem spiral

No one is pretending that sticking to this programme is easy - particularly as the months go on. As I've said all along, asking for moral support and practical help is an essential part of beating your candida. The trouble is that many candida sufferers (particularly women) are the 'don't worry about me, I can manage' types who find it very difficult indeed to ask for help. Either they think they are not worth it or they don't need it. This has a great deal to do with low self-esteem and our tendency to put our own needs at the bottom of the list. (I'm speaking from personal experience here.)

Here we have yet another vicious circle that you need to recognise and break. While candida sufferers seem to have a pattern of low self-esteem in the first place, (though this is often very well disguised) *it seems as if the candidiasis makes this tendency worse.* After all, how can anyone feel like taking charge and convincing an entire support team of people that they are worth helping, when one is feeling lousy, depressed, anxious, fat, a failure because one doesn't even have the will power to lose weight, puffy, spotty, a party pooper, premenstrual, a hypochondriac and a general downer to be around? (I hope not *all* these things apply to you, by the way!)

One of the problems is that you only have 'vertical disease' (another of Jeffrey Bland's lovely expressions). In other words since you are still upright as opposed to prostrate in some hospital ward and don't have an official label, you think nobody will take your illness - which is exactly what it is - seriously. Well, starting with yourself, you are just going to have to do some convincing. Easier said than done I know, but you need to start accepting that you have as much right to be bursting with health and go as the next person - probably more so as most candida sufferers are very special, giving people. (Go to a candida support group and you'll see what I mean). Until you really recognise this, you will continue to drag yourself through your days, making compromises with yourself and your family and friends, and life will carry on passing you by because this thing ain't going to go away by itself!

Getting your GP on your side.

If you are one of the many sufferers whose GP can't put his finger on how to help you, you may have been told you something like 'it's what women of your age must expect' or 'you'll have to learn to live with it,' or worse (having done umpteen tests), 'there is nothing wrong with you physically, it is obviously psychosomatic, so I'm going to refer you to a psychiatrist'. Far from backing you up and giving you the moral support you need, this negativity, denial and abandonment by your doctor, is probably acting as a powerful *nocebo* effect. This is the opposite of the placebo effect and means that negative feelings and beliefs that you have accepted are directly hindering your ability to get better. (See *The Healing Brain,* Ornstein & Sobel 1987)

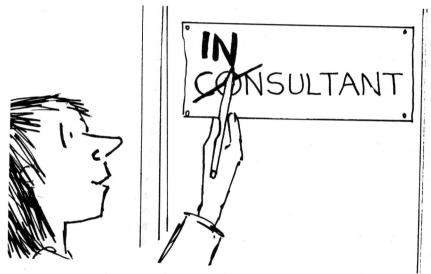

You need your GP's support even if it is only to get a medical certificate - but you'll have to try another tack. Put yourself in his or her's shoes. How would you like to have a baffling problem to solve in 8 minutes flat? Many of our clients who have had this experience find that if they do their homework, then go back and say clearly and briefly, 'I have read these books and am pretty sure that candida could be my problem. I think Mrs X a nutritionist might be able to help me/I think this test will confirm it, but I'd like your approval. I have high-lit the important parts, would you have time to read them and let me know what you think? I could come back next week.' Then give your GP whatever literature you have found most helpful, or a photocopy - but make sure it is *brief and to the point.* You will probably be pleasantly surprised. If not, and your GP still doesn't want to know, remember you have the right to change GPs.

It may also help you to know how many other people are out there having as rough a time as you - or even worse. Gill Jacobs has included several amazing case histories in her book, that she documents with such perception - I highly recommend you read it.

Next, start asking for support generally. Begin with the people you know will be positive and helpful: your healthfood shop manager; friends who have or have had candida; those who love you.   Tell yourself, and your family, friends and colleagues that you are ill, that the only way to get better is to make some changes to your diet and lifestyle for several months, but that you are determined to do it. Treat it as a big adventure *and ask for their help, love and support*. Then remind them that within a few weeks, you will be *much* more fun to be around and will be beginning to get your old energy back and be your old self again. (Though warn them that there may be some downs as well as ups on the way.) *You will be amazed at how positively they respond!*

Make a list of the areas that you anticipate will be particularly difficult for you. For example, cooking for yourself *and* the family - or cooking at all; getting transport to the healthfood shop for your monthly stock-up; not drinking at parties; just finding the energy to learn about the alternative foods and so on. Then put the name of the people who will be able to help you most next to each challenge (they are not problems, they are challenges....) and discuss it with them. Within a week or two they won't even be challenges, let alone problems.

Cooking for the Family
Many women think they will find this one of the most difficult things about managing their new diet. It certainly is much easier for single folk who only have themselves to worry about.   But as with anything in life, if you look for the positive potential in a challenge like this one, you might be pleasantly suprised at the solution.

Obviously your ending up with twice as much cooking as before is going to defeat the object entirely. Depending on the ages and tastes of your children and the culinary skills and schedule of your partner, you have several options. If you are not already, it is an opportunity to start to share the family cooking for a start. I have heard of many partners who offer to step in and look after the children's meals (largely, I suspect so they'd not find themselves eating your 'funny' food.) If we handle it right, are patient and state our own needs clearly, most of us can get the family on our side.

Some of the greatest support of all comes from others knowing what you are going through because they have been there themselves. You will find a whole room full of them if you join a support group.

The Story of One Candida Support Group

The group we set up at All Hallows House in 1994 arose simply out of one of our star clients, Anya Harris, insisting that there was such a need for it - and she was absolutely right. No sooner had we mentioned the idea to other clients, we had a core group of about eight with others making it up to 10-18. We met every three weeks after work and had supper together.

At each meeting, we started by going round the circle, introducing ourselves and telling our story, just for a few minutes each, the new ones going last if they were shy - though nobody was ever shy for long. You would not believe how 15 people all supposedly with the same 'problem' could have such *totally* different stories to tell - different symptoms, different experiences with the medical profession, different rates of getting better - and often getting worse again - and the lessons they had learned from this. This is where a support group really comes into its own. They all had their theories and philosophies, and tips, triumphs and sorrows. Many people's lives, or at least their attitudes towards them, had changed track completely and they were even grateful to their candida for it.

Everyone got different things from coming to the group, but virtually everyone said how much they valued seeing that they were *not alone*. However sorry for themselves they were feeling, there was always one who sounded even worse - and others who used to be, but had persevered and pulled through to their vibrant and enthusiastic new selves, giving masses of encouragement to the others who still had a way to go. We also made such good friends. Virtually every meeting

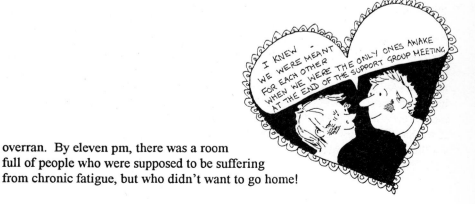

overran. By eleven pm, there was a room full of people who were supposed to be suffering from chronic fatigue, but who didn't want to go home!

We always had something to eat together. I used to cook professionally, so sometimes I would start by demonstrating how easy it was to conjure up various delicious things that everyone could eat with abandon. Many sufferers had been feeling very 'deprived' and found this very reassuring. Or we would take it in turns to do the food. On one unforgettable evening, a sufferer's husband made us a scrumptious Thai coconut and chickpea stew with rice, but unfortunately he made it up as he went along, so was unable to give us the recipe, although there is something similar in chapter 6. Then either one of the practitioners from All Hallows spoke about how their particular therapy can help candida or its related symptoms, or we invited in people from outside. One of the most popular was when Angela Holden a long term sufferer who worked at Wild Oats, a fantastic health food shop in London NW2, brought in a whole lot of examples of the wheat-, yeast- and sugar-free goodies they sell there and told us all about them. Then we had a feast! Other speakers we had that went down especially well were a talk from Sydney Chang, an ex-ME and candida sufferer, about spiritual healing and the key role it had played in his recovery. Also one on creative visualisation by Dr Richard James, our holistic physician and acupuncturist.

If you want to join a Support Group locally...

Of course the level of involvement on your part can be anything from having someone to talk to on the phone occasionally, to going to a few groups and meeting fellow sufferers, to running the whole show.

Thirty practitioners have agreed to host or co-ordinate groups all over the UK, so first look in the directory and see if there is a one in your area and ring them up. The 'co-ordinators' will organise their group. If they are listed as an 'initial contact', this means that they will support and/or provide a venue for a group, but won't actually have the time to run it. In this case, they or their receptionist will take your name and number and to what extent you would like to play an active part in the group (if any). They will either give you a time and place for the first meeting or ring you back once they have got enough people to start the group. Then at the first meeting, after you have all met each other, it will be up to you and whoever turns up, to decide how your group will happen.

If there is not a group mentioned in the directory that is close enough for you to get to, send a medium sized s.a.e. and either a cheque for £2 made out to AHHF Candida Support Groups, or postage stamps to the value of £2 to:

(Candida Support Groups), All Hallows House, Idol Lane, London EC3R 5DD

Please mention whether you can offer anything such as a venue, administrative support (though we recommend keeping this simple), a bit of time occasionally or that you would like to co-ordinate the whole thing (with help of course).

By October 1995, we will have the database up and running, so by then you will receive a list of any other people in your area who have already contacted us - or a phone call from one of them. Please allow 2-3 weeks for a response. You will also receive a 'tip sheet' giving you ideas or your group and passing some of the successes and pitfalls that other groups have had. There will also be a few notes on how to contact other candida sufferers in you area.

We have heard of several 'candida support groups' with quite substantial membership fees, which were not run to bring fellow sufferers together, but to sell products. Please make sure you are paying for what you think you are.

A Candida Newsletter

We will also send you details of the newsletter we are planning with leading writer on candida, Gill Jacobs. Of course you can ask for this separately if you're not interested in a group at the same address. The first issue will be out before the end of 1995. It will be for practitioners, so it will be more technical than this guide, but sufferers are welcome to subscribe as well. The more you can inform yourself the better. It will include sections for news from support groups, new products, new research, case histories, letters - and whatever else you and your practitioners want in it

L.E.T.S. Local Exchange Trading Systems

You might not have come across LETS, but it is a brilliant idea that has been flourishing in several parts of the country since the end of the eighties. Briefly it is a group of people who live near to each other and want to exchange their services, skills or advice by barter rather than for money. When they give their skills they build up credit and vice versa. The reason that this is such a good system for candida sufferers is that there are usually lots of natural therapists offering their skills and a few organic gardeners and it might be way for you to get some regular treatment and help without blowing the budget. You can also get help mowing the lawn, baby sitting, shopping - whatever will take some of the strain off you and give you some time for yourself. It is also rebuilds that valuable sense of community that we are losing so sadly in our modern society. See Appendix 2 for for a contact.

Other Support and Self Help Groups

There are numerous national support groups, each for a different problem such as Action for ME, The Hyperactive Children's' Society, The Soil Association (who'll put you in touch with your nearest supplier of organic vegetables.) There is a list of several of them in appendix 2. *WHEN CONTACTING THEM FOR INFORMATION, PLEASE REMEMBER THAT MOST OF THEM ARE CHARITIES AND WOULD APPRECIATE AN S.A.E.*

Be well informed

Books, both about candida and other aspects of health and healing that will help you to understand what you can do for yourself more clearly, are listed in *Appendix 1*.

Laughter is powerful medicine!

Whether it is through fellow sufferers, some of the Arbers' cartoons, books such as Kathryn Mrsden's *All Day Energy*, which is a hoot, or your favourite videos, do make a point of finding things to have a good laugh about. Find out when Patch Adams is next performing from the BHMA, (see Appendix 2.) He is doctor and a clown - and you'll be laughing for weeks.

...but you can have too MUCH support

There is one aspect of moral support that might take you by surprise - and could be a real problem. It is that some people 'need to be needed' to such an extent that they find someone who is needy (you perhaps), whether emotionally or physically, and form an almost parasitic or symbiotic relationship with them. It sounds dreadfully harsh to say so, as everyone will be saying how amazingly kind and selfless they are. But this is a well recognised phenomenon amongst psychotherapists, who call it *co-dependency*. This might be exactly what you need to start with, an absolute godsend in fact, but later on, when you are well on the way to recovery, you may find re-establishing your own individuality and independence again is blocked. This is usually completely unconscious on the part of your valiant rescuer-carer-protector, which makes it all the more difficult. On the other hand you may prefer to comply with the situation and continue to play the needy role long after you are better. If you find yourself with a genuine case of co-dependency on your hands, you both may need help. Recognising it is the first step to getting things back into proportion. A psychotherapist will probably be the best person to go to.

ACTUALLY I RECOVERED TWO YEARS
AGO - BUT HE'S HEAVILY INTO
COMPULSIVE CARING

CHAPTER 9

I AM STILL NOT BETTER. WHAT ELSE COULD BE WRONG?

When clients have been doing the programme faithfully for over six months and have seem to have 'got stuck', there are three things we ask them to look at (if they haven't already done so), which in our experience are the most common blocks to full recovery. Are you being poisoned by their mercury fillings? Are you sleeping in a safe place? And do you need to look at your spiritual life?

COULD YOUR MERCURY FILLINGS BE AFFECTING YOU?

Mercury-silver amalgam fillings have been used since the turn of the century and at least 90% of adults in the Western world have at least one. We all know from our chemistry lessons that pure mercury vaporises very easily and is extremely poisonous, yet it has always been said that amalgams are stable i.e. they don't affect us at all because they are bonded with other metals. It is true that any mercury that is breathed in, unlike other heavy metals such as lead and cadmium, leaves the body pretty quickly (half goes within 5 days). However over the last ten years, more evidence is coming in, which suggests that in low doses, over time, the mercury in our fillings may be affecting our health. As ever, this seems to be true for some individuals and not others. But as Alan Hibberd points out, something to bear in mind is that since mercury fillings are so universal, any effects will be considered the 'normal' baseline for health for the entire population. It is also highly unlikely that any official statement will be made questioning its safety, given the scale of its use and presence in our mouths already.

Two other points must be made. One is that its effect is not just biochemical. Like all metals, mercury conducts electricity and when you have a mixture of metals in your mouth (say a gold bridge or crown or a steel screw as well as a filling or six) the electrical potential will be higher and therefore there will be a current or exchange of ions in your mouth (galvanism). In other words, mercury vapour will be released.
The second is that when mercury is turned into compounds such as methyl or ethyl mercury by bacteria in the mouth, these are far more toxic to humans than plain mercury.

How can I tell whether I am sensitive to mercury?

Many symptoms are shared with candidiasis, so this will not be obvious.

- You are likely to also be sensitive to nickel i.e. costume jewellery.
- Migraine, multiple nutritional deficiencies, allergies and sensitivities are common.
- Methyl mercury primarily affects the nervous system, causing mental and neurological problems e.g. foggy brain, poor memory, fatigue, depression and anxiety. Severe cases have muscular and visual disturbances that have been mistaken for multiple sclerosis. On many occasions, patients' symptoms have cleared completely once their fillings were changed and they were treated for the mercury in their tissues.
- Methyl mercury in the gut also favours candidiasis and may well be a factor if you feel you are not getting better as fast as you should be - if at all. Gut protozoa and parasites are also common.
- See the diagnostic tests in chapter 2. Hair or sweat analysis and vega tests - but start with dowsing or kinesiology if you have access to them.)
-

If so, should I have all my fillings replaced?

- If you can afford it (it will probably cost £60-£100 per filling), then definitely, yes. But make sure you go to a dentist who is experienced in doing this as it is a very specialist business. (See Appendix 2).
- If you are planning to have a baby or want one and are having any difficulty conceiving, then also yes. We know that methyl mercury is more toxic to a growing foetus that to an adult. Many babies were miscarried or were born mentally damaged after the Minimata River disaster in Japan, where methyl mercury sulphide and chloride was spilled into the river upstream by a plastics factory.
- If money is tight, get an estimate so you know what you would be in for and weigh this up against *how* bad your mercury levels are, how bad your symptoms are and the following alternatives:
- Contact the International Academy of Oral Medicine and Toxicology, or the British Society for Mercury Free Dentistry (incorporating the British Dental Society for Clinical Nutrition) - see Appendix 2 They will be able to recommend dentists who are experienced in replacing mercury fillings.
- Galvanometers can measure how much current is being generated by individual fillings, so it might be worth just having just a few replaced.
- If you are sleeping or working in a 'hot spot' of electromagnetic fields, this could be making things worse, both by adding to the overload on your system with radiation and free radical activity, and because being in a field of certain

frequencies can make any mercury more volatile. Having this checked out and corrected can cost only £60-£100. See Alf Riggs in the directory and his paper below. While this can make all the difference, you obviously still have the mercury in your head.

- There is a great deal that can be done with *chelation therapy* i.e. using specific nutritional supplements and compounds to encourage your body to rid itself of the overload of mercury in your tissues. You will need this anyway if you are thinking of having your fillings out.

How to mitigate the mercury leakage and encourage your body to detoxify.

- Cut out salt and salty foods as this increases the electrical current in your saliva.
- Keep your mouth scrupulously clean as some bacteria will methylate the mercury - but not with any of the very astringent mouth washes.
- Don't chew gum! Dr Stephen Davies who runs Biolab reports that up to seven times the amount of mercury will be released if you chew gum all day.
- Avoid hot or spicy foods as these tend to release more mercury.
- Check that you are not grinding your teeth at night (this is known as 'bruxing'). If your partner hasn't already told you, your dentist can tell. Your jaw muscles will feel hard and knotty if you do. Relaxation techniques may help, and/or a rubber guard from your dentist.
- Anti-oxidant vitamins have been shown to encourage the body tissues to rid themselves of mercury. Special chelators and activated charcoal are available through specialists.
- The management of a pre- and post-replacement detoxification and chelation programme needs special expertise. Your practitioner will be able to get a copy of Alan Hibberd's very full and clear protocol from BioMed (BioCare).

ELECTROMAGNETIC FIELDS AND RADIATION. COULD THEY BE AFFECTING ME?

EMFs and Sick Building Syndrome as it is also more loosely known, is another example of a major factor causing certain diseases, that is not discussed in public. Furthermore, it seems to be increasing, due to the greater number of man-made sources of radiation. Research that has been done since the 1920's in Germany and the UK has shown again and again that EMFs can be measured very precisely and correlate to the incidence of disease in people sleeping and working in those spots - so that scientists can predict which houses will have generated most disease.

The common diseases are cancer (including leukaemia), CFS(ME), Sudden Infant Death Syndrome (Cot Death), general tiredness, migraine and depression and candidiasis. People often find it difficult or impossible to hold down a job or lose the support of partners, family and friends. Once corrected, or their bed or desk is moved, people get better in a matter of days. It is only in rare cases that it is necessary to actually move house.

Alf Riggs has been investigating and treating buildings and places for 23 years. He has particular success with people with (CFS)ME and also sees a lot of candidiasis. The following is taken from a paper he gave in Copenhagen in June 1995, that was reproduced in Cadeuceus magazine. (Issue 29). He also features regularly in *Interaction* the journal for Action for ME.

'The human body, like any living organism has a direct current (D/C) which interacts in a living relationship with the geomagnetic field of the earth...The earth's magnetic field is responsible for the motivation the bioelectric system of the body, to the extent that every cell and function in the body relies on a stable D/C frequency of the geomagnetic field. An unstable geomagnetic field can invade the body's cell structure and alter the values of the bioelectric system within [causing] malfunction and disease, physical and/or mental.'

Alf locates and identifies different types of radiation using dowsing. (See chapter 11). 'The earth radiation that I locate is confined to the so-called global grid systems created by cosmic radiation inter-acting with the earth's magnetic field, mainly the Curry Grid, Hartmann Net, geological fault lines, underground streams [whether man made or natural] and ...Ley lines.' Radon Gas may also be a component. Most hazardous is where two or more fields or lines cross. Alf observes that even low frequencies change the molecular structures of natural constituents of water, and of water-borne bacilli. Dr Mersmann has found effects to the oxidation processes in the body, resulting in damage to the hormone and immune systems. The exact point at which the lines cross your body when asleep often determines what symptoms you suffer.

Based on more than 1,600 energy-depleted cases, Alf observed that young girls can sleep on the edge of lines for years, but as soon as they reach puberty, 'at which stage, almost without exception, they go down with ME.' Men suffer in only a small percentage of cases. His contention is that 'the ultra short waves emitted from the outside edge line interacts with oestrogen, setting up a resonance which alters the messages sent along the mitochonrion electron chain, resulting in a deficiency of adenosine triphosphate (ADP), the main energy releasing agent in the cell.'

Dr Ernst Hartmann found one of the first things to be adversely affected was the immune system, and that there was a very firm link with the development of cancer. In 1989, Austrian researchers did a two year study looking at the short term consequences in a group of nearly 1000 subjects. Many biological functions were seen to alter after 10 minutes exposure. This included changes in serotonin and levels of calcium and zinc. The other findings supported Dr Hartmann's work.

How can I tell if EMFs are affecting my house?

- If your symptoms are worse in the mornings. (This could also be due to a sensitivity to house dust mites.) If you also notice symptoms such as broken sleep patterns, migraine type headaches and depression are found to be standard almost without exception. In ME cases, if you wake refreshed but get tired as the day wears on, a viral cause is more likely.
- Domestic electrical appliances are likely to breakdown more frequently, light bulbs do not last as long.
- If you have metal parts in your bed, mattress and headboard. (Cancer and SIDS is much less common in SE Asia where wooden beds and organic mattresses are the norm.) Sleeping against a radiator is a real hazard.
- Electrical kit near the head of your bed, whether in your room or the one next door. e.g. radio alarms, electric blanket, Teasmade machines, computers in the room.
- Did you start feeling ill shortly after having moved house or bedroom or having bought a new bed? It could also be after starting a new job or moving offices.
- Sick buildings syndrome is particularly common in those buildings constructed in the sixties where steel cages were used in the concrete walls.

Moving away from these harmful rays can mean that sufferers can enjoy an improved quality of life without necessarily achieving a full recovery. ME sufferers have found that healing the cell batteries is best done by a healer. Alf says 'I have found that each healer has their own characteristic frequency of emission, and therefore has an individualised suitability to heal a specific disease.' Seka Nicolic who works at the Hale Clinic in London has a particularly high degree of success with CFS(ME). Brain scans can demonstrate changes in blood flow to very specific parts of the brain known to correlate to particular functions in the body. Following healing, one woman measured had 20% greater blood flow.

For a copy of the whole paper, references or further information, either contact Alf directly (he is in the Directory) or send 4 x 25p stamps to: Cadeuceus, 38 Russell Terrace, Leamington Spa, Warwickshire CV31 1HE

WHAT DIFFERENCE CAN IT MAKE TO LOOK AT MY SPIRITUAL LIFE?

In our experience, and especially when people have got stuck, a great deal. The first thing to say is that this does not necessarily involve any kind of organised religion or sect. We all have a spiritual side to us, and ignoring or neglecting it can sometimes mean a significant imbalance in us. We all have a body, mind, emotions and spirit and it is like trying to sit on a four legged stool with one of the legs missing.

What spirituality means, varies with each individual and needs to be discovered for themselves, so I am not going to give any suggestions or explanations other than to say that once you become open to the possibility of your having a spiritual part of you that you would like to explore, help will start popping up unexpectedly. You will meet someone, have an insight about the healing process or what candidiasis means for you, or find a book that sheds some light on things for you. Your practitioner might be a good sounding board, and you probably have several friends who have been interested in developing this side of their lives for some time, but just haven't showed it to you until now. A few books are listed in the Appendix 1.

People wake up to their spiritual selves in all sorts of different ways and often at the most unexpected times: through music or Nature, meditation or prayer, Buddhism or Alcoholics Anonymous. But when they do, life takes on a greater meaning and depth, and it often results in people feeling they can tap into a greater source of power or universal Love that is available to heal them - and for them to help others too.

So be open to the possibility and wait and see....

PERHAPS IT IS NOT THE RIGHT TIME NOW?

Some people are not willing or ready to re-examine and make any changes to their habits, feelings about themselves or their relationships. Being stuck like this usually involves a lot of fear that may be deeply buried, so it is understandable they are not keen to stir things up.

You may still be overwhelmed by reasons why you can't make so many changes. That's fine. Perhaps now isn't the right time - if it isn't there is no point pretending by doing it half-heartedly, because you will only 'fail' and end up feeling even worse about yourself and your lot! If this is the case, it is much more sensible to be honest and leave it. Something will tell you when it is the right time - and this could be in a few months or a few years. But please don't put this book on the shelf just yet, until you have done three things:

- Make sure you have dated the questionnaire in chapter 2.
- Sit quietly and ask yourself 'what does having candidiasis mean to me? Are there any lessons I need to learn?' (you don't necessarily have to do anything at all for now).
- Read the guide anyway because without realising it, it will plant a seed or two that will sprout up when the time is right.

Let me leave you with a quote from Caroline Myss, one of the world's most remarkable healers who works with a physician in Massachusetts and is said to have an accuracy rate of 92% in her psychic diagnoses. This is her 'energy analysis' for candidiasis, from their book, *The Creation of Health, The Emotional, Psychological, and Spiritual Responses that Promote Health and Healing.*

'This disorder occurs mainly in people who have been psychologically, emotionally and physically over-active and are in serious need of stabilizing their lives. As in the [ME] virus, women are particularly susceptible, but for different reasons. Whereas the [ME] virus relates to issues of emotional safety, candidiasis corresponds to issues regarding the creation of a stabilized living situation, specifically what is known as the "nesting bug." The stress emerging from the unfulfilled desire to lay down roots and establish a home and family is directly connected to this virus.

Chronic candidiasis is a rather recently recognized disorder, and my opinion is that it reflects very accurately our contemporary human stresses, lifestyles and concerns'.

CHAPTER 10.

RESEARCH ON CANDIDIASIS, Past and future

Good work has been done on various aspects of candidiasis and gut dysbiosis by doctors Truss, Crook, Galland, Bland and Trowbridge in the USA, and Plummer Brostoff and Hibberd in the UK, though little notice seems to have been taken of it by mainstream medicine or general practice as yet. Full references and a synopsis of their work will be available with the practitioners' candida newsletter. In the meantime, for a very full list of references see Erica White's Healthcare Bulletin on Candidiasis, available from Lamberts Healthcare Ltd.

However, as I mentioned in the introduction, apart from the field of bacteriology and probiotics, there has been precious little research done on candida in the UK - and none as far as we know on holistic approaches to its treatment, by non-conventional therapists. The work that has been published is mostly in the United States or on anti-fungal drugs (mostly for thrush) rather than on the multi-faceted approach that alternative practitioners recommend.

Alternative practitioners know that most of their clients get better but until proper research or audits are done, we do not actually know just *how* successful the treatments are and whether some are better than others. And we certainly will not be able to convince doctors that they should be looking at any of the supplements or techniques that we use until that research has been well designed, done and published.

Why has so little research been done on holistic or alternative approaches to date?
1.   Until very recently there has been virtually no tradition of teaching research methods in the schools of alternative therapies.
2.   The sources of funding are usually from drugs companies or large charities, for research products or techniques that can be mass produced or standardised, or in an area that has already had research published on it.
3.   Again until recently, virtually the only type of trial that doctors would accept is the double blind, crossover trial. As I shall explain, a multi-faceted or holistic approach to treatment cannot be made to fit into this mould. There has been a sad history of doctors finding fault with the initial design of trials based on new approaches. They dismiss them as "flawed" without really giving due consideration to the treatment's intrinsic value. You can imagine how that feels for therapists who have probably put in months or years of dedicated work, and

out of their own pockets. I think this is the main reason why alternative therapists have been put off even attempting any research.

Obviously, for the good of the general public and so that choices of approaches to treatment are available, someone has got to start the ball rolling to break out of this situation. It is possible to come up with designs that are acceptable to the mainstream. The Research Council for Complementary Medicine has already gone a long way to getting new ideas about health and healing and new research models accepted. They are providing invaluable advice and support both on how to design and run trials - and how to get them published and how to raise the funds. They have shortlisted us for one of their awards to do a pilot study on a common symptom associated with candidiasis, starting in the Autumn of 1995, which is very exciting.

More background to orthodox research trials
So you can understand what we are dealing with, here is a very brief background to the way clinical trials are designed in the orthodox field because they still apply to trials whatever their design. They normally are designed in such a way that the drug or whatever being tested is the single factor that can have made the difference.
Other factors that are known to influence the result of the trial are eliminated or *controlled* and *randomised*. For instance:
the placebo effect: over 30% of patients get better because they think the treatment will help, so dummy pills have to be given to some of the group.
the doctor-patient relationship: some patients get better because they want to please their doctor, so any personal contact has to be standardised or eliminated.
blinding: if either the patient or the doctor knows who is receiving the real pills and who the dummies, it is known that this will influence the outcome. When a trial is designed where neither the patients nor the doctors know who is getting what, it is known as a "double blind". If just the doctors know, it is called a "single blind".
crossovers: The most common method of eliminating all these factors is to do a "double blind, crossover" trial. This means that half the group is given a dummy drug (placebo) and half the active drug, nobody knows which is which. Then the two groups are swapped over in the middle of the trial.

Why the holistic approach does not fit into the accepted models
As you have probably worked out for yourself, the type of multi-faceted treatment we suggest will not fit into the design of randomised, controlled trials (RCTs). While theoretically it would be possible to study each of the components of a treatment protocol in a series of trials, in our experience each individual needs all

the aspects of treatment simultaneously for optimum improvement. But more important is that even for an 'identical' symptom as recognised by orthodox medicine, six individuals will need six completely different blends of treatments because each will have their unique biochemical, genetic, energetic and psychological blueprints. *Holistic treatment cannot be standardised.*

Furthermore, if the placebo effect or the practitioner-patient relationship can make all that difference, far from eliminating it, let us study and maximise it! And, once you have explained how to make diet and lifestyle changes to a patient, you cannot then cross them over. But most important, when patients are participating in their treatment to a greater extent that taking a pill as instructed, we feel that it would be unethical not to treat half the patients on the trial.

The obvious difficulties in coming up with a trial design that will satisfy the arbiters, i.e. the medical and peer review journals, is why so many would-be researchers in the alternative field are put off even starting and why so little of this type of research has been done so far. But there are other designs that are becoming accepted, just in the last few years.

New models or paradigms

One is the *case study* approach where each individual patient acts as his or her own "control". In other words, if a woman has had recurrent thrush every month for the last two years, and when she starts a treatment it improves or goes away altogether, it could be "natural remission" or chance. But if you get a similar result with 70% of a group of 50 women with recurrent thrush, you can be pretty sure it was the treatment that made the difference.

The "black box" approach. This is when the actual treatment given to each individual patient is entirely at the discretion of the practitioner. The classic example of this is the comparison between (unspecified) chiropractic and hospital outpatient treatment for low back pain, which showed that chiropractic was more effective, both in the short term and after two years.

Quality of life measures are now being developed so that the patients' feelings of what effect the treatment has had on their lives in general can be taken into account. This obviously is much more appropriate to the holistic approach.

Clinical audits. Scales of improvement following treatment can be devised such that large numbers of individuals can be put together statistically. Factors such as cost effectiveness and risk:benefit can be analysed statistically in this way. It is important that where holistic treatments are concerned, that these studies are done over a long term.

Some of the research must be done by holistic practitioners

Since the establishment of the new chair of Complementary Medicine at Exeter University, Professor Ernst has been very successful in getting many trials on alternative therapies underway. However almost all of them are being conducted by doctors. At least as many should be done by non-medically qualified practitioners who have a different appreciation of the subtle aspects and synergy of the therapies - but that is up to us!.

We need your help.
You have already helped by buying a copy of this book, as all the profits go straight to the All Hallows House Foundation for the research trials mentioned below. So thank you.

Unfortunately we cannot invite you to be part of any trials or you would be described as "self selected" and this would bias the outcome. Where you can help is to encourage your practitioner and your GP in investigating different approaches, to take part in one of the trials below, or in the UK candidiasis audit. And/or, you could make a donation to the All Hallows House Foundation. This can be in the form of cash (see below), your time and expertise in statistical inputting or analysis ,or in donating any computer hardware you have access to. Many practitioners will need to buy computers to participate in the audits or trails or to upgrade their existing systems. (Practitioners, please see appendix 3 for how you can be involved - and how we can help you.)

Proposed research projects - to take place in 1995-8
Most of these will be arranged in co-operation with orthodox researchers, existing specialist associations concerned with these symptoms, so they will all be subject to their approval and to that of the Research Council of Complementary Medicine.
- Recurrent thrush
- Irritable Bowel Syndrome
- Fibromyalgia Syndrome
- Candidiasis and ME
- The incidence, diagnosis and treatment of candidiasis in general practice
- Alternatives to oral antibiotics
- Large scale audits of holistic treatment of candidiasis/gut dysbiosis

Donations:
If you are wondering about making a donation and would like to know more, or would like to support a particular project, please write to me (a s.a.e. would be much appreciated) at the address below.

Donations can be made in three ways:

1 Single donations. Please send cheques made payable to All Hallows House Foundation and send to the address below.

2. Donation by Deed of Covenant. These must be made for the same amount over a period of a minimum of 4 years. The big advantage of doing it this way is that because the Foundation is a registered charity, we can reclaim all the tax you will have paid on this amount. Whether you pay tax at 25% or 40%, this is worth having. Please ask for a Deed of Covenant Form.

3. Standing Order. You can also choose to pay monthly or quarterly, by standing order if you prefer.

For example, if you wanted to donate £10 per month for 4 years, we would actually receive £600 if you pay tax at 25% and £672 if you pay tax at 40%.

All donors will receive the candida newsletter automatically and will receive an annual report from the Foundation - and MUCH appreciation and gratitude!

The address to send enquires and donations to is:

The All Hallows House Foundation, Idol Lane, London EC3R 5DD.

Please mark any enquiries for my attention (Jane McWhirter).

CHAPTER 11.

A BRIEF BACKGROUND TO THE THE COMPLEMENTARY THERAPIES.
How do they work, how are the practitioners trained and how do I contact one?

Trying to find your way to the "right therapy" and a good therapist through the maze of complementary therapies can seem like a jungle even to its own inhabitants - so it is no wonder that would-be clients and doctors exploring it for the first time can find it a little bewildering. But it is actually a very fascinating and loving place - especially if you have an experienced 'guide' or a word of mouth recommendation to help you make your first contact. If not, hopefully this chapter plus the Directory in the next section will be the next best thing.

Where to start.
Chapter 3 introduced you to the different philosophy and approach to medicine, and explained why there is no such thing as "The Right Therapy" for any particular symptom(s) because all the therapists treat *you* as a whole rather than your symptoms. The introduction to the Directory gives you some step by step suggestions and answers some queries you may have such as 'what can I get on the NHS?'

As I've said, anyone wishing to clear their candidiasis will probably do best by seeing a practitioner trained in one of the three "baseline" therapies (nutrition, naturopathy or medical herbalism) as they will be able to help you sort out your diet. I have covered these first. (see below). However about 15% of sufferers are so disabled by another symptom, such as back pain or depression for instance, that it is sensible to start tackling that symptom directly first. If this applies to you, check under your symptom(s), listed alphabetically in Chapter 4, bearing in mind that my suggestions there are by no means comprehensive. If you have heard of a really good therapist locally, more likely than not, they will help whatever the symptom and whatever their therapy. Ring them up and discuss it. However, do remember that while most of your other symptoms will improve significantly or go away all together within 6 weeks or less of starting the anti-candida programme (assuming you have candidiasis rather than something else), this does not work the other wayy around. In our experience, until you tackle the underlying yeast and gut problem directly, any treatment for other symptoms is likely to help, but only in the short term.

If you know you want a particular therapy and there is not a practitioner listed in your area in this Directory, contact their national head office for a complete register (most professional associations will charge £1.50 - £2.50 for this service).

Most holistic practitioners are eclectic and have added further training, formally or informally to their main discipline. Each therapy has several different schools all over the country, each with their different emphasis. Therefore, the experience you might have in going to one nutritionist, for example, may be quite different from that with another. Also, the same practitioner will use different approaches for different individuals. *So the notes below are to help you know what to expect in theory rather than in practice.*

For more detailed information on the following therapies see Ann Woodham's excellent HEA Guide to Complementary Medicine and Therapies.

THE THREE BASE LINE THERAPIES FOR TREATING CANDIDIASIS

Nutritional Therapy

We will have less than optimum health if either our diet is deficient in vitamins, minerals and enzymes; if we cannot absorb them (either at a cellular level or because of a damaged gut), or if the amount of toxins we have ingested through our food or our environment are too much for our system to eliminate on a daily basis, so that a toxic overload builds up in our tissues. People suffering from candidiasis are likely to have problems in all three of these areas. Nutritionists will use a combination of dietary advice and specific supplements *in therapeutic doses* to correct these imbalances, deficiencies and disfunctions. Identifying and finding alternative foods for anything to which you are intolerant or allergic is also crucial. Some nutritionists use laboratory testing, and others are skilled in one of the diagnostic techniques mentioned below - many use both.

Generally speaking, nutritionists ask you to fill out a detailed questionnaire, which you return before seeing them for your initial consultation. Then they will go through your medical history with you and the practicalities of the dietary changes they recommend and the dosages of any supplementation in detail. This usually lasts. about 1 ½ hours. Second appointments are shorter and between 3 weeks and 3 months later, with telephone contact in between if necessary.

Note that hospital dieticians have a completely different approach and may not even recognise candidiasis at all. Medically qualified practitioners are trained and listed at the BSAEM or the BNA - see under *Clinical Ecology.*

There are several registers of trained nutrition consultants:

The Council for Nutrition Education and Therapy, is based at the Institute for Optimum Nutrition. (CNEAT/ ION,)
Blades Court,
Deodar Road,
London SW5 2NU
Please send £2 payable to the ION Trust.

The Register of Nutritional Therapists (RNT)
Penny Woollie
01926 484 449

Society for the Promotion of Nutritional Therapy, (SPNT)
Linda Lazarides,
First Floor, The Enterprise Centre,
Station Parade,
Eastbourne BN21 1BE
Tel: 01323 430 203
Please send £2 for their list of members.

Medical Herbalism

Herbs have been used medicinally from our earliest beginnings. In fact many pharmaceutical drugs started life as herbs, but their active ingredient has been isolated and synthesised so that it can be mass produced in a standardised way. The difference is that pharmaceuticals are compounds not known to the body, designed to suppress any symptoms, thus allowing the habits that caused the problem to continue. When you take the whole root or plant however, the body can use the natural and complete chemicals to heal and rebalance itself, while the buffering of all the various compounds present reduces immediate side effects and the body is able to benefit from the support that the plants can give the other systems overall. However, it is important to be aware that just because something is natural or herbal does not necessarily mean that it is safe. This is why it is usually essential to consult a trained herbalist rather than try to self-medicate. They will also be skilled in combining remedies to enhance their synergy. Members of the NIMH will have completed a four year intensive course, so they will probably be able to help with most of your secondary symptoms as well as the candidiasis itself. Herbs are given in the form of teas, creams or tinctures, though since tinctures are based in alcohol, they may not prescribe these for you. Another advantage is that herbal remedies from a practitioner often work out considerably cheaper than over the counter remedies and nutritional supplements. Most herbal practitioners will recommend probiotics as well.

The National Institute for Medical Herbalists
Hon. General Sec,
56 Longbrook Street
Exeter
EX4 6AH
Tel: 01392 426022

NB the NIMH has nearly 200 members in the UK of which only a fraction are listed in this edition of the directory because we were not able to circulate to their full list.

Naturopathy

Naturopathy is also known as 'nature cure' or natural medicine. It is based on the observation that the body has the ability to heal itself with the help of the healing powers of Nature. Trained naturopaths integrate the use of clean, simple food, rest, exercise and hydrotherapy. They are usually well versed in a broad spectrum of natural therapies including herbalism, homoeopathy and of course nutrition. Many are also trained in osteopathy. Naturopathy is a general term that anyone can use, so to make sure that they have passed the complete four year full time course. Look for the letters ND and MRN.

The General Council and Register of Naturopaths
The British Naturopathic and Osteopathic Association
Frazer House
6 Netherhall Gardens
London   NW3 5RR

DIAGNOSTIC THERAPIES

All the following techniques, whether ancient or more recent, work on the principle that our body-minds have an 'innate intelligence', and that we, or a skilled practitioner, can access this for information. This can often be more accurate, complete and subtle than diagnoses offered by the high technology of modern medicine. It is also a great deal cheaper. Unfortunately the power invested in anything high-tech by our culture tends to overwhelm and belittle anything low-tech. That said, modern technology is very valuable as well, and these diagnostic tests are discussed in chapter 2.

Iridology
Trained iridologists can tell the state of your physical and mental health in amazing detail just by studying the iris and pupils of your eyes. They often diagnose problems long before they could be spotted by orthodox medicine. In candidiasis this is particularly useful as they will be able to tell whether your main problem stems from a toxic bowel, an overloaded liver, a weakened pancreas or adrenal glands and so on. The iris is said to represent a body map, different areas representing different parts and systems of the body. But it also shows your constitutional type and strengths and vulnerabilities in general. Practitioners who have completed a 12-18 month course are registered with:

National Council and Register of Iridologists
998 Winbourne Road
Bournemouth BH9 2DE
Tel: 01202 518 078

Kinesiology

Also known as 'muscle testing' and 'touch for health', or applied kinesiology. It is both a diagnostic tool and a means of treatment and is particularly useful for identifying specific food intolerances and allergies. The practitioner will test the strength of a muscle, such as in the arm as a baseline. You will be given particular substances to hold or tiny amounts to put under your tongue, and you will find - to your amazement - that an arm which was previously strong and could resist his gentle pressure goes limp however hard you try to resist. Kinesiologists correct imbalances, blockages and weaknesses by 'reprogramming circuits' which correspond almost exactly to the 12 energy meridians of traditional Chinese medicine (see acupuncture and TCM).

There are several kinesiology schools in the UK, but to be sure the practitioner has completed at least 150 hours training and 200 hours clinical experience within two years, contact either of the following:

The Kinesiology Federation/Touch for Health
30 Sudley Road
Bognor Regis
West Sussex
PO21 1ER
Tel: 01243 841 689

The Assoc. for Systematic Kinesiology
39 Browns Road
Surbiton
Surrey
KT5 8ST
Tel: 0181 399 3215

Dowsing

Dowsing is the ability of the human body to pick up vibrations from unseen energy sources. We all know about water diviners being able to tell whether or not there is water under them by using a hazel twig (companies as 'established' as the water boards emply lots of them). A dowser will use a pendulum or L shaped rods to do the same, testing for a whole host of 'good' or 'bad' energy fields. They can also test for specific food intolerances and get a yes or no answer, as well as the level of severity of your intolerance (which of course will change over time as you get better). Note that pendulums or L Rods are simply tools to aid the practitioner's intuition. So, although they might use a very fancy looking pendulum, a ball of putty on a string might work just as well!

Radionics uses the same principle, but practitioners can diagnose and heal at a distance. This is explained by the fact that we are universally connected to all living things in a subtle way. People are often convinced because it works extremely well with animals. Of course, since it works at a distance this is particularly helpful if you happen to live miles away from any practitioners. After an initial telephone contact, you will be asked to fill out a questionnaire and send in a 'witness', i.e. a lock of your hair or a drop of your blood or even a signature. They may also ask for a sketch of where you work and sleep to check for negative energy fields (see chapter 9). They go into a very detailed analysis which may take 2 hours initially and then broadcast the healing energy waves to you rather like radio waves, to correct any imbalances in your energy fields. Practitioners train over 4 years and use the letters MRadA

Confederation of Radionics and Radiaesthetic Organisations
The Maperton Trust
Wincanton
Sommerset BA9 8EH
Tel: 019 6332 651

Vega Test Machine

This machine achieves very similar things to the above two diagnostic techniques but uses electronic equipment to measure the changes in electric frequencies when different substances are introduced into the circuit and react with your energy fields. Experienced practitioners can work extremely fast, covering a vast array of substances and come up with very specific readings. These include a phial called 'candida albicans' and your sensitivity to it can be measured on the dial from low (which everybody has) up to high. Treatment often involves homoeopathy. NOMA have trained 300 practitioners and there are other schools in Poole and Yorkshire. To find your nearest practitioner trained by NOMA, contact:

Sylvia Austen,
NOMA, Unit 3, 1-16 Hollybrook Road
Upper Shirley
Southamptom SO16 6RB
Tel: 01703 770513

The twelve pulses and tongue reading

Acupuncturists, shiatsu practitioners and traditional Chinese medicine practitioners are all trained in the taking of the 12 pulses. They palpate (feel) both wrists for the 6 deep and 6 superficial pulses. From these they can glean an amazing amount of information about your whole constitution, both in general and on that particular day, and about particular groups of organs and whether they are *'yin' or 'yang' or 'full' or 'empty'*. See the individual therapies below.

Clinical Ecology is from the modern western stable and uses many sophisticated laboratory tests and techniques (some of which are mentioned in chapter 2.)to identify allergens and toxic build up, whether from foods or the environment. All full members of the BSAEM and the BNM are medically qualified, though they are regarded as pretty alternative by some of their MD colleagues. You will need a referal from your GP.

British Society for Allergy and Environmental Medicine & the British Society for Nutritional Medicine,
Acorns,
Romsey Road,
Cadnam,
Southampton,
Hants, SO4 2NN

THE OTHER THERAPIES

The following list of therapies that will help other related symptoms in candidiasis sufferers is not comprehensive but chosen for those who, in our experience, have provided the most help to candida sufferers for their related symptoms. For more details see the HEA Guide as above.

Acupuncture

This Chinese system of medicine is over four thousand years old and has a philosophy and way of looking at the human body in health and disease that is complete in its own right. As well as the 12 pulses and tongue reading, diagnosis can be made from acupressure points. If they are tender then it confirms that there is a blockage or imbalance in the associated meridian. Treatment consists in inserting needles in specific points along one of the 12 meridians or energy channels of *qi* (pronounced chee). The needles are so fine that you generally do not even feel when they have been put in. They are always sterile and used only once so there is no chance of any infection. If, however, you are really terrified of needles try *Shiatsu* which uses similar principles but with finger pressure instead.

Once the needles are in you may well feel an ache or a tingling as the energy begins to flow between them. They will be left in for anything between a few minutes to half an hour.

Acupuncture is becoming more widely accepted by GPs, particularly as a means of pain control and you may even be be able to get it on the NHS. However, do find out how long a session will be and how they are trained because it is often used inappropriately by doctors, in the sense that sessions lasting only 5 or 10 minutes are not suitable for a condition such as candidiasis, which really needs a full hour's holistic approach. The Directory of British Acupuncturists which combines the registers of five member associations in the UK is available from:

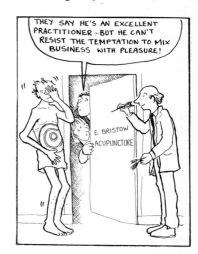

Council for Acupuncture
179 Gloucester Place
London NW1 6EX
Tel: 0171 724 5756

For a list of medical doctors who are trained in acupuncture contact:
The British Medical Acupuncture Society
Newton House, Newton Lane
Lower Whitley, Warrington
Cheshire, WA4 4JA
Tel: 019 2573 0727

Anthroposophical Medicine

This is a whole system of medicine, based on the philosophy and teaching of the Austrian scientist Rudolf Steiner. He taught that as well as our physical bodies we have subtle bodies (such as the etheric and astral) and that all these should be in balance with our spiritual consciousness for perfect health. As well as many of the naturopathic remedies, anthroposophical doctors often recommend art therapy, music and speech therapy and creative eurythmy in which movement is linked to speech and music. If a physical approach to your candida treatment has only got you so far after many months, you might well have a breakthrough with this approach.

The Anthroposophical Association
Rudolf Steiner House
35 Park Road
London NW1 6XT
Tel: 0171 723 4400

Specialised treatments (in and out patients)
The Park Attwood Clinic
Trimpley
Bewdley
Worcestershire DY12 1RE
Tel: 01299 86144

Aromatherapy

Now one of the most popular complementary therapies (in terms of numbers of practitioners trained), this combines a wide range of specific massage techniques with the whole spectrum of essential aromatic oils, many of which share common roots with herbal and homoeopathic remedies. This therapy is not only sheer bliss to receive at the time, but received regularly over several weeks will have deep and lasting effects. It is particularly good as a support to the dietary changes you will be making as it relieves stress, enhances well being and helps in the rejuvenation and regeneration of your body. Your aromatherapist will also advise you on many self-help techniques you can use if you suffering from thrush or cystitis, chest or nasal infections, depression, anxiety or skin problems and many more.

The Aromatherapy Organisations Council (AOC) has set a minimum training standard of 180 hours in class. For a list of member associations contact:

Aromatherapy Organisations Council
3 Latymer Close
Bay Brooke
Market Harbour
Leicester LE16 8LN
Tel: 01858 434 242

Autogenic Training

AT is one of the most practical of *stress management and relaxation techniques* available. It is a medically validated series of mental exercises designed to switch off the stress 'flight or fight' response and to bring about and maintain a balance in the body-mind. The effect is similar to yoga or meditation, though once you have practised and learnt the technique you can get real benefit in 10-15 minutes or even less - though a minimum of 20 minutes per day is ideal. The exercises are easy to do virtually anywhere and anytime. Used regularly over six months and more, people report really remarkable benefits. AT will benefit candida sufferers whether they have any other symptoms or not, since enhancing your abilities to cope with stress will speed up your healing process. However, if you do suffer from depression, anxiety, eating or sleep disorders, or addiction for example, it will be particularly beneficial. If appropriate the trainer will help you to add any special formulae to the basic exercises for your own personal needs. People often notice that it enhances the benefits of other treatments and once you have learnt the technique, it is as if you have it 'in your pocket' for the rest of your life.

After an initial one to one consultation with your trainer, you generally learn the technique in a small group with an hour to an hour and a half long sessions weekly for nine weeks. Most practitioners are doctors, nurses and psycotherapists and they have completed a two year part-time training course. For a list of practitioners, contact:

The Hon.Sec. British Association for Autogenic Training and Therapy (BAFATT)
Heath Cottage
Pitch Hill
Ewhurst
Nr Cranleigh
Surrey GU6 7NP

Ayurvedic Medicine

Ayurveda is Sanskrit for 'the science of life' and is the ancient Indian equivalent of traditional Chinese medicine. It is nearly 3000 years old and considered just as sophisticated and comprehensive. As with TCM, the underlying philosophy is that of a balance between the energies of five elements or *(Doshas)*, Earth, Water, Fire, Air and Ether. Deepak Chopra has written many best-selling books in which he clearly describes the three body types *Vata, Pitta and Kapha*. Understanding . your type is very helpful in understanding how your body works and how to bring it back into balance. Ayurvedic practitioners may well integrate your astrological charts and the seasons, time of day and the climate into your treatment as well as the usual patterns of your constitution and habits.

Training is a five and a half year degree course (Bachelor of Ayurvedic Surgery and Medicine) which includes a basic study of western medicine.

International Association of Ayurveda
PO Box 3043
Barnet
Herts EN4 0QZ

Bach Flower Remedies

Dr Edward Bach, a bateriologist, physician and homoeopath practising in London earlier this century, found that energies from 38 flowers, when taken homoeopathically in sunlight, could restore the balance of specific states of mind and emotions necessary for good health. Bach Flower Remedies are a wonderful adjunct to other therapies and in the hands of experienced practitioners can have really remarkable results. The other advantages are they are so gentle and cheap. Rescue Remedy which combines five of the flower essences is recommended for shocks and stresses, whether physical, mental or emotional, and particularly for times when you are feeling very vulnerable.

The Bach Centre
Mount Vernon
Sotwell
Wellford
Oxon OX10 0PZ
Tel: 01491 834 678

Colonic irrigation

In experienced hands this can be of considerable help to candidiasis sufferers, as it will flush out years of waste material built up in the bowel that might be causing 'auto intoxication' or self poisoning. A toxic and sluggish bowel is a haven for candida albicans and can sabotage your chances of recovery.

Most people do not like the sound of having a tube inserted into their rectum and warm water flowing up into their colon, but actually it should not be in the least bit embarrassing or degrading and it is certainly not an unpleasant feeling, though it can be similar to feeling uncomfortably full after too big a meal. People often report feeling wonderfully light and cleaner afterwards - even 'high'. A course of 4-8 colonics are recommended. It is very important that the healthy bowel flora are replaced, but all good practitioners will include this in the herbal mixture in the water. To be sure of getting a well trained therapist, contact:

Colonic International Association
50a Morrish Road
London SW2 4EG
Tel/Fax: 0171 483 1595

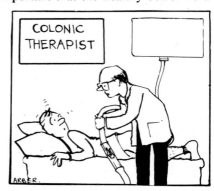

YOU REMEMBER THOSE CAR-KEYS
YOU SAID YOU LOST SIX MONTHS AGO?

Healing

Anyone who has rubbed a child's sore knee better will have a sense of everyone's ability to heal. Healers have simply developed and trained this ability further. The Confederation of Healing Organisations thinks of healing as 'a transference of harmonizing paraphysical (ie beyond the physical) energies'. Whether you call this healing energy, or *qi*, or *Prana* (as the Indians call it), Love energy or God (whether he is Christian, Moslem, Islam, Buddhist or Jewish,) it is all the same thing.

Healers are sometimes confused with "faith healers", implying that if you do not believe in a cure then you will not get one. It is true that if you have a good rapport with your practitioner you will often do better, but healing is certainly much more than a placebo response.

Dr Daniel Benor, an American psychiatrist, who started the Doctor-Healer Network in the UK, has collected a arge of examples of controlled scientific studies demonstrating the positive effects of healing. Many healers do not charge a fee as they regard healing as a gift.

For general information contact:

Confederation of Healing Organisations,
Suite J, 2nd Floor, The Red and White House,
113 High Street,
Berkhamstead,
Herts HP4 2DJ.
Tel: (01442) 870 660

To find a CHO healer, contact the following
member organisations:

For spiritual healing:
The British Alliance of Healing Associations,
26 Highfield Avenue,
Herne Bay,
Kent CT6 6LM.
Tel: (01227) 373 804
Non-denominational:
The College of Healing,
3 Runnings Park,
Croft Bank,
West Malvern, Worcs.
Tel: (01684) 565 253.

Maitreya School of Healing,
2 Jeymer Avenue,
London NW2 4PL.
Tel: (0181) 452 2882.

Sufi Healing Order of Great Britain
29 Grosvenor Place,
London Road,
Bath, Avon BA6 6BA.
Tel: (01225) 312 694

Non-denominational distant healing:
The Radionics Association,
Baerlein House, Goose Green, Deddington,
Banbury, Oxon OX15 0SZ
Tel: (01869) 38852

Non-denominational Christian:
The White Eagle Lodge,
Brewells Lane,
Rake, Liss,
Hants GU33 7HY
Tel: (01730) 893 300.

Mahi Kari *('True Light')*

A spiritual practice from Japan that has helped many people with chronic illness. Light cleanses the spirit and because of the principle 'spirit first, mind follows, body belongs' a person who receives Light may experience a profound benefit mentally and physically. Light can also help people realise that paying attention to spiritual aspects is important for the sake of their health and well-being.

There are 300 trained members, 150 of whom are in and around London. They give Light voluntarily though you may make a donation to their centre if you wish.

For a practitioner, write to

Dr Sidney Chang
12 Kemplay Road
London SW3 1SY
Please send an s.a.e. and include your phone number.

Homoeopathy

According to the principle that "like cures like", homoeopaths prescribe a substance designed to produce the same symptom pattern in a healthy person as that which they want to cure in a sick one. What you are actually given is not the substance itself, but a dilution of it that is so weak that none of the original physical substance remains. Only its unique energetic pattern is imprinted in the water. This imprint stimulates the 'vital force' of the body-mind to respond in an equally specific way, i.e. to produce the symptoms associated with the healing process of the particular disease or imbalance they are trying to cure. Your personality type, constitutional and genetic factors are all as important to a homoeopath as the problem in question. Since there is no physical substance present, there cannot be any toxic side effects. However, the reactions can occasionally be suprisingly dramatic (a good sign), so be warned.

Homoeopathy is best for chronic conditions, allergies and psychological disorders and digestive and reproductive imbalances. However, since it aims to trigger the immune system into action, it often is not so successful in cases such as prolonged candidiasis or ME where the immune and detoxification systems are badly damaged.   Having said this, in combination with a candida programme, homoeopathy can be very powerful for rebalancing the psychological patterns underlying the physical candidiasis. It is also helpful in a supportive role for other troubling symptoms. It is particularly good for children. I know many who have never had an antibiotic or vaccination in their lives thanks to their homoeopath.

Initial consultations go into fascinating detail, and will probably last one and a half hours plus. If the homoeopath is prescribing constitutionally, there will be no quick fix - rather, if you want, an ongoing life process that unfolds and changes as you do.

The above describes classsical homoeopathy where one or two remedies are chosen. Complex homoeopathy uses remedies in combinations. The Reckweg remedies are good.

EPD (enzyme potentiated desensitisation) is a technique commonly used by medical homoeopaths which aims to desensitise you to environmental allergens. A combination of 80 standard allergens, including yeasts in very low dilutions, plus enzymes is given as an injection into a muscle and the idea is that it helps your immune system to build up its defences against allergens that had been upsetting it, rather like a vaccination. It is said to be particularly useful when you are being exposed to allergens that you cannot escape, such as an airborne ones, as it suppresses the reaction while you get well. EPD holds a necessary and important place in the armoury of techniques available. However it is surrounded by quite some controversy, particularly with ME and chronic fatigue patients because it is found in *some* people, not to work, or, as far as one can tell, to give them new sensitivites. Many practitioners do not feel it is appropriate to introduce allergens into anybody's system - let alone a very sensitive one. And the 'blanket'approach does mean that the patient can and does become sensitised to other, new substances. Contact Action for ME (address in Appendix 2) or see Dr Brostoff's book for more details.

More than 600 medical doctors have trained in homoeopathy and are mostly in private practice, but there are five Royal hospitals in London, Glasgow, Bristol, Tunbridge Wells and Liverpool to which you may be refered by your GP on the NHS.

British Homoeopathic Association,
27a Devonshire Street,
London W1N 1RJ
Tel: (0171) 935 2163

For non medically qualified homoeopaths who have completed 4 years of training plus a year's clinical supervised practice, contact:

Society of Homoeopaths,
2 Artizan Road,
Northampton NN1 4HU.
Tel: (01604) 21400

Further information is also available from
The Hahnemann Society,
2 Powis Place,
Great Ormond Street,
London WC1N 3HT
Tel: (0171) 837 3297

Light Therapy

If you have lethargy, depression, PMS, or a tendency to binge that is noticeably worse during the winter, this could be very helpful. Also if you work night shifts or have sleep reversal (common in ME). Increased levels of melatonin which induces drowsiness have been identified in sufferers of seasonal affective disorder (SAD). This is secreted by the pineal gland which governs all our daily (circadian) rhythms and is stimulated by daylight (via the eyes). You sit beside a box for about 2 hours every morning which emits 2500lux. (Daylight is 5000lux while indoor lighting is usually only 500lux).
SAD Association, Box 989, London SW7 2PZ

The Manipulative Therapies: Chiropractic/Osteopathy/Physiotherapy

More people by far use the manipulative therapies than any other type of non-conventional therapy. I have grouped these three manipulative therapies together because, when asked, 'What is the difference?' I always feel bound to reply, 'There is as much difference between individual practitioners trained together as there is between different schools and the entire therapies.' While the three disciplines certainly have their distinct philosophies, in practice what I say is true. If you have candidiasis which is manifesting as chronic back or neck pain or fibromyalgia (fibrocytis) i.e. tenderness in the muscles or muscle fatigue, it is very important that you find a practitioner who uses very gentle manipulative techniques. First, because bodies that are already imbalanced on several levels and overloaded with toxins simply cannot take the short, sharp adjustments that other people do so well on. Second, because generally, the gentler the approach, the deeper and subtler are the levels at which clients are helped. In my eight years of experience in this field, I have found that in these types of cases, you will benefit most from a whole body approach which is only normally practised by about 25% of practitioners. This is because whether by realigning the spine and the skeleton you improve the function of the nervous system (as chiropractors believe) or improving the blood and lymph systems as well (as osteopaths believe), having and maintaining a good total structural alignment will improve your body's ability to heal and stay healthy. In other words, if you have pain only in your neck, this will ensure that your sacral and lumbar vertebrae are well aligned and you will actually improve your digestive and reproductive systems into the bargain - which is just what all candida sufferers need. Manipulative therapists should also be able to give you a sound analysis and advice on your posture, which is particularly valuable if you have a sedentary job.

The only way you can be sure that an individual practitioner uses gentle techniques, has a sensitive touch and has a whole body approach is through a word of mouth recommendation. While the schools not mentioned here do marvellous things for most people, generally speaking the following should be a safer bet for candidiasis sufferers and those with ME, fibromyalgia, arthritis and other such tender conditions.

McTimoney and McTimoney Corley chiropractors

Osteopaths who have also trained in naturopathy

Anyone who is also trained in cranial osteopathy

NB   Many manipulators are also trained in applied kinesiology, massage or shiatsu.

Osteopathy and chiropractic are both on the way to being regulated by law. Each should have their national registers, covering all their schools, set up by 1997 at the latest.

Physiotherapy is widely available on the NHS, but be warned that the therapists are usually restricted by time and by doctors' instructions, so are you are unlikely to find one with a holistic approach unless they are in private practice.

McTimoney Chiropractic Association
21 High Street
Enysham
Oxon
OX8 1HE
Tel: 01865 880 970

The British Association of Applied Chiropractic
(McTimoney Corley)
The Old Post Office
Stratton Audley
Bicister, Oxon OX6 9BA
Tel: 01869 277111

For Cranial Osteopaths contact
The Osteopathic Information Service
PO Box 2074
Reading, Berks RG1 4YR
Tel: 01432 356 655

The Osteopathic Centre For Children
Tel: 0171 414 1231

The Bowen Technique

is a very gentle, precise soft tissue technique that is quite newly arrived from Australia. I have not experienced it yet, but hear very good reports from patients with joint and muscle pains and tenderness.
Ring Julian Baker on 01373 461873 for your nearest practitioner.

Massage

This is one of the most ancient forms of healing of all, and it is now being rediscovered by Western medicine. Unfortunately, many people still think of massage 'parlours', or associate massage with self-indulgence . They don't know what they are missing. Although it does not claim to be a cure for any particular complaint, gentle massage can be very helpful for candida sufferers by reducing stress and anxiety and strengthening the nervous, lymphatic and immune systems.
Manual Lymphatic Drainage is a specialised and very gentle technique for detoxifying and reducing fluid retention. Joint and muscle pain and tenderness is very common among candida sufferers, so you could benefit enormously from this approach. More generally it may be referred to as *holistic massage*. However the deep tissue, more vigorous style of *remedial massage* is better left for other people with specific sports injuries.
While you are usually asked to undress for a whole body massage, this is not in the least embarrassing as you are kept covered up all the time, except for the bit of you being worked on. Immediately afterwards, you may feel exhilarated and high, light-headed or emotional, or pleasantly relaxed to knocked out, but quite achy next day. If you are very ill, a whole body treatment at one session is not advisable until you are used to it. There is nothing better than having a partner or member of the family who can give you a good massage. At All Hallows House we have run short 'Free Massage for Life' courses, for partners and couples to

learn basic massage techniques with essential oils, which have been tremedously popular. Suggest that your therapist does the same.

There are too many weekend courses around, so pick your therapist with care. ITEC (International Therapy Examinations Council) is a recognised, basic qualification in anatomy, physiology and massage. The ICM holds a register . The newly formed umbrella group that aims to regulate minimum training standards is:

Massage Therapy Council,
3 Woodhouse Cliff,
Headingley, Leeds L56 2HF
Tel: (01532) 785 601

Clare Maxwell-Hudson School of Massage,
PO Box 457,
London NW2 4BR
Tel: 0171 731 7520

Meditation

Far from being "flakey", cranky or woolly, regular meditators seem to have far greater powers of concentration and a sense of control, clarity and efficiency in their busy lives. You certainly do not have to be religious to meditate, although people often find that they develop a new awareness of their spiritual side. Now that it is shaking off its cranky image, more and more people are using it as a powerful tool (and a means of survival) in the business world.

Meditation changes the brainwave frequency to the long alpha waves that are a sign of deep relaxation coupled with a state of mental alertness and receptivity. It has been shown to lower blood pressure, pulse and breathing rate, and to decrease the metabolic rate to levels otherwise only seen in deep sleep and hibernation. Therapeutically it is invaluable, as this is the level at which our bodies do their best healing and repair work.

Meditation is best learned from a trained teacher, although there are some good books on it. As with anything, you only get out as much as you put in and it needs practice and patience to start with - but then you will be richly rewarded.

See relaxation techniques and Autogenic Training.

Osteopathy - see manipulative therapies

Polarity Therapy

is a fascinating and powerful therapy which marries Western and Eastern medicine. Its roots lie in chiropractic and osteopathy, naturopathy and yoga and Chinese medicine. Using just the hands, underlying energy blocks are released and the positive and negative polarities of energy (known as air, fire, water, earth and ether corresponding to the Eastern chakras) are rebalanced. As the treatment progresses, the practitioner will also be analysing the subtle energy anatomy.

Stretching and vocalisation, diet and cleansing techniques are all used, with counselling to explore any negative attitudes if appropriate.

A course of at least 6 treatments is generally recommended. Training is 2-3 years part-time in one of three schools. The full register is held at:
British Polarity Council,

Monomark House,
27 Old Gloucester Street,
London WC1N 3XX

Psychotherapy

In the "olden days" if ever we were overwhelmed by a crisis, grief, anxieties, stress, phobias or depression, we could turn to the village priest, the family GP, or a wise old relative or neighbour - all of whom would have known us and our general ups and downs, all our lives. But in modern society, the general pace seems to get faster by the week and we do not have time for anything - let alone for listening to people's troubles. We also move around so much that there is precious little continuity anywhere.

While many people still regard psychotherapists as only for their neurotic American cousins, thousands of us are turning to cousellors and psychotherapists in the UK. The number of GP practices providing their services is growing annually as they recognise the value of getting the root of an emotional or personal problem rather than suppressing it with drugs (which may then be needed indefinitely). Companies too are employing counsellors and running confidential "Employment Assistance Programmes" as they appreciate the direct relationship between employees' performance at work and their general happiness and emotional well-being. Companies calculate that the cost of hidden losses saved is between two and *sixteen* times the cost of the counsellors.

UKCP,
Regent's College,
Inner Circle, Regent's Park,
London NW1 4NS
Tel: (0171) 487 7554

Association of Psychotherapists,
37 Mapesbury Road,
London NW2 4HJ
Tel: (0181) 452 9823

British Association for Counselling,
1 Regent Place,
Rugby , Warwickshire CV21 2PJ
Tel: (01788)_ 578 328

Free or much cheaper treatment is available through:
Westminster Pastoral Foundation,
23 Kensington Square,
London W8 5HN
Tel: (0171) 937 6956

Qi Gung (pronounced Chee Goong)

literally means 'storing of energy' and is an ancient Chinese system of flowing exercises in breathing, posture and focusing the mind that aims to strengthen and control the circulation of the life force Qi. Unfortunately not very widely availble yet. See also T'ai chi ch'uan which is a form of Qi Gong.

Healing Tao Foundation (England),
PO Box 195,

85 Marylebone High Street,
London W1M 3DE.
Tel: (0171) 224 1817

The Community Health Foundation,
188-196 Old Street,
London EC1V 9FR
Tel: (0171) 251 4076.

Reflexology (or Zone Therapy)

Our Western minds may find it difficult to see how massaging the roots of our toes can possibly make a sinus headache go away, or how pressing around the ankle can reduce symptoms of PMS by 30%, but once people have experienced how reflexologists can both identify problems elsewhere in the body with uncanny accuracy and then treat them, they are usually hooked.

Reflexologists see the feet as a map of the body, which are connected to it via ten vertical lines of energy rather like the Chinese meridians or energy channels. Foot massagers appear in Ancient Egyptian tomb paintings, though the modern system was only developed in the USA this century. It was brought to the UK by Doreen Bayly in the 1960s and has been popular ever since.

During a treatment which lasts 45 to 60 minutes, the practitioner will cover all of both feet systematically, producing an toning, relaxing and balancing effect all over. He or she will concentrate on the areas in which the crystaline deposits beneath the skin indicate imbalance in the corresponding organ or part of the body. These are often exquisitely tender, but this sharpness melts away quite quickly as the deposits are dispelled. Reflexology can be particularly useful when someone is in too much pain to be treated on the spot itself, or where the deep organs need help. The after-effects can sometimes be quite acute, but well worth it. It is particularly helpful for candidiasis sufferers with symptoms such as constipation or IBS, menstrual problems, joint and muscle pains, allergies, toxic overload, migraine and any other stress related problems. A course of 4-8 treatments is generally recommended.

Though teaching is often only 60 hours, subsequent experience is emphasised and many trainees are already qualified in another therapy. (Many nurses are now training).

Association of Reflexologists,
25 Friars Walk,
Lewes, BN7 2LF
Tel: (01273) 479 020

Shiatsu

is another therapy developed into its present form this century that is said to combine some of the best of Western and Eastern medicine. It is also ideal for people who would benefit from acupuncture but can't stand needles. The word is Japanese for 'finger pressure' and it combines Chinese diagnosis, pressure on the TCM acupoints with elements of the manipulative tecniques.

184

For treatment you wear loose, longsleeved , cotton clothes such as a track suit and lie on a mat or futon on the floor. While there can be a few sore spots, (indicating that they need working on) it is a deeply relaxing therapy with long lasting benefits after a course of several treatments.

The Shiatsu Society,
5 Foxcote,
Wokingham, Berks, RG11 3PG.
Tel: (01734) 730 836

T'ai Chi Ch'uan

This is a stunningly beautiful set of exercises to watch and to perform. Its flow and serenity is a perfect antidote to the crazy hussle of modern living and has a powerful healing effect at all levels. It is often called 'meditation in motion' and is said to have developed out of a blend of the Taoist philosophy and the martial arts in eleventh century China.(t'ai chi means 'wholeness' or 'ultimate' and ch'uan means 'fist'). It should be performed outside, where the earth forces of universal Qi can be drawn up and expressed throught the hands. It is best learned in a class with an experienced teacher. The 'short form' of 37 movements can be done in under ten minutes while the 'long form' of 108 movements takes 20-40 minutes.

The School of T'ai Chi Ch'uan,
5 Tavistock Place,
London WC1H 9SN
Tel: (0181) 444 6445

Traditional Chinese Medicine

Chinese medicine is an independent system of practice evolved over 4000 years into a very detailed and complex system. A doctor aims to find 'the pattern of disharmony' and regards illness as a result of an imbalance in the flow of qi through the body and the constant movement of energy between yin and yang. (See acupuncture and Chinese diagnosis). While it comes from a completely different tradition and way of looking at the body from our Western perspective, it certainly has remarkable results.

The Register of Chinese Herbal Medicine,
21 Warbeck Road,
London W12 8NS

Yoga

There are now over half a million people practising yoga regularly in the UK. However, not all teachers give much time to the philosophy and spiritual aspects that should be integral to the physical business of keeping fit and supple. The word is Sanskrit for 'union' and the system has been developed over 6000 years -

so no wonder it is so powerful. I have to confess, being a philistine ex-sprinter, I thought yoga was for people wanting to pretend they were keeping fit - until I tried it last September. I realised within 20 minutes how very wrong I had been and have been completely hooked ever since. Like all the other systems with their roots in the East, they are a powerful antidote to the crazy pace, emotional hassles and left-brain thinking of the West. You actually seem to get more energy out than you put in. And the thing about yoga is that all ages, levels of fitness and physiques can benefit and you take it at whatever level is right for you. If you are fit and in robust health and you really go for it, an hour's yoga will leave you with the same tired but exhilarated glow one gets after a six mile run. Anyone with stress-related problems such as migraine, tense neck and shoulders, high blood pressure, or IBS will benefit tremendously with better energy levels all round Even people who never dreamed that they could take any form of exercise whose health is very shaky and energy reserves depleted will find that yoga done gently and in small doses can be of tremendous therapeutic value and give their quality of life a real boost. It is as if it taps into your hidden reserves, leaving you with a much deeper, more integrated sense of well-being on all levels - spiritual, emotional, mental and subtle as well. Classes for people with physical handicaps and ME and MS are flourishing (see Yoga for Health Foundation below) and many of the world's top sports and businessmen and women are finding it enhances their performance significantly.

Yoga can really only be learned properly in a class to start with. Do go to some trouble to find a teacher who suits you. All you will need is some loose comfortable clothes and a rubber or 'sticky' mat.

British Wheel of Yoga,
1 Hamilton Place, Boston Road,
Sleaford, Lincs, NG34 7ES.
Tel: (01529) 306 851

Iyengar Yoga Institute,
223a Randolph Avenue,
London W9 1NL
Tel: (0171) 624 3080.

Yoga for Health Foundation,
Ickwell,
Bury, Biggleswade,
Beds SG18 9EF.
Tel: (01767) 627 271

An excellent video by Maxine Tobias and John Patrick Sullivan is available for £10.99

RECOMMENDED READING

*NB Many of these books are available by mail order through **The Green Library** who are distributing this Directory and Guide. Phone 0171 385 0012 Both **The Nutrition Line Bookshop** and the **Institute for Optimum Nutrition** have very good lists and mail order services.*

GENERAL BOOKS ON CANDIDA

CANDIDA ALBICANS - A USER'S GUIDE TO TREATMENT AND RECOVERY, by Gill Jacobs. Optima, 1994 ISBN 0-356-21088-X

CANDIDA ALBICANS - COULD YEAST BE YOUR PROBLEM, by Leon Chaitow Thorsons 1985, revised 1991. ISBN 0-7225-2452-8 (New Edition in early 1996)

CANDIDA - A PRACTICAL GUIDE FOR SUFFERERS, Angela Kilmartin, Bloomsbury 1995

CANDIDA - THE SYMPTOMS, THE CAUSES, THE CURE Revised version, by Luc De Schepper, M.D. PhD, C.A. 1990. ISBN 0-942501-08-X

THE MISSING DIAGNOSIS, by C Orian Truss, M.D. The Missing Diagnosis Inc, PO Box 26508, Birmingham, Alabama 35226 USA 1983. ISBN 0-9615758-0-8

CHRONIC FATIGUE AND THE YEAST SYNDROME, W G Crook, Professional Books, 1992

LAMBERTS HEALTHCARE LTD BULLETIN, by Erica White Dip I.O.N (from Lamberts or Erica)

WTDDTY GUIDE TO CANDIDA AND ME - POSSIBLE CAUSES AND LIKELY TREATMENTS, The Wallace Press, Editor and Co-Publishers: Lynne McTaggart., 1994.

THE YEAST SYNDROME, J P Trowbridge and M Walker, Bantam, New York, 1987

THE WAY BACK, The A-Z of coping with ME candida and allergies, Jo Hampton, 1993 available from Jo - she is in the Directory

SELECTED 'MUST HAVE' BOOKS (GENERAL)

FOOD ALLERGY AND INTOLERANCE, Dr Jonathan Brostoff and Linda Gamlin, Bloomsbury 1989 ISBN 0-7475-05666-7

ALL DAY ENERGY - THE STRESS FREE WAY TO REVITALISE YOUR HEALTH-, by Kathryn Marsden, Bantam Books; Transworld Publishers Ltd 1995. ISBN 0-553-40849-6.

BETTER HEALTH THROUGH NATURAL HEALING - HOW TO GET WELL WITHOUT DRUGS OR SURGERY, by Ross Trattler ND, DO, Thorsons. ISBN 0-7225-1382-8

THE HEA GUIDE TO
COMPLEMENTARY MEDICINE AND
THERAPIES, Anne Woodham, Heath
Education Authority 1994 ISBN 1-
85448-903-8

RAW ENERGY, Leslie and Susannah
Kenton, Arrow Books 1988 ISBN 0-09-
946810-7

FURTHER READING - Listed under each chapter

Chapter 1
THE LACTIC ACID BACTERIA -
THEIR ROLE IN HUMAN HEALTH,
by Dr Nigel Plummer BSc PhD,
BioMed Publications Ltd 1992. ISBN
0-9520440-0-5

SUPERBUG - NATURE'S REVENGE,
Geoffrey Cannon, Virgin Publishing
1995
ISBN 1-85227-364-X

THE COMPLETE GUIDE TO FOOD
ALLERGIES AND ENVIRONMENTAL
ILLNESS, by
Dr Keith Mumby, Thorsons, an imprint
of Harper Collins 1993. ISBN 0-7225-
2504-4

A CANCER THERAPY, Results of fifty
cases, Dr Max Gerson, 1958 (Out of
print)

Chapter 2
THE BEAT FATIGUE WORKBOOK,
How to identify the cause and discover
new vitality, Leon Chaitow, Thosons
1988

TIRED ALL THE TIME, by Dr Alan
Stewart, Optima Books 1993. ISBN 0
356 20763 3

HYPOTHYROIDISM: THE
UNSUSPECTED ILLNESS, by Broda
Barnes and Lawrence Galton, Harper &
Row
The Broda Barnes Research
Foundation, PO Box 98, Trumbull,
Connecticut 06611, USA, is a research
organisation involved in thyroid
research. If you write to them for
information, please send international
reply coupons with your self-addressed
envelope.

Chapter 3
MEDICINE FOR THE 21ST CENTURY,
The key to healing with vibrational
medicine, Keith Mason, Element Books
1992

VIBRATIONAL MEDICINE, Richard
Gerber, Bear and Company, 1988

AGELESS BODY, TIMELESS MIND,
Depak Chopra. Rider 1993

Chapter 4
AROMATHERAPY - A GUIDE FOR
HOME USE, by Christine Westwood,
Amberwood Publishing

NUTRITIONAL MEDICINE The drug
free guide to better family health, Dr
Stephen Davies & Dr Alan Stewart, Pan
1987

HOMOEOPATHY FOR THE FAMILY,
The Homoeopathic Development
Foundation, Wigmore Publications
£1.50

THE GOOD HEALTH HANDBOOK,
Help yourself get better, Dr Peter
Mansfield, Grafton Books, 1988 ISBN
0-246-13169-1

OVERCOMING FOOD ALLERGIES, YOU DON'T HAVE TO 'LIVE WITH IT'. Gwynne Davies ND MTOS, Ashgrove 1993

YOU DON'T HAVE TO FEEL UNWELL, NUTRITION, LIFESTYLE, HERBS AND HOMOEOPATHY, A HOME GUIDE. Robin Needes ND SRN, Gateway Books 1994.

WOMEN'S BODIES WOMEN'S WISDOM, The Complete Guide to Women's Health and Wellbeing, Dr Christiane Northrup, Piatkus Books, 1995 ISBN 0-7499-1484-X

THE BOOK OF PAIN RELIEF, Leon Chaitow, Thorsons 1993 (very good chapter on hydrotherapy)

THE COMPLETE BOOK OF WATER THERAPY. Dian Dincin Buchman, Keats Publishing 1994.

THE A-Z GUIDE OF MODERN HERBALISM, by Simon Y Mills, Thorsons

FOLK REMEDIES FOR COMMON AILMENTS, by Anne McIntyre, Gaia Books Limited 1994.
 ISBN 1-85675-086-8

BEATING STRESS AT WORK, Anne Woodham, HEA

BACK IN ACTION, by Sarah Key, Random Century 1991, ISBN 0 71 26 4990 5
(see chapter 6 for exercises)

THE BACK AND BEYOND, The hidden effects of back problems on your health, Dr Paul Sherwood, Arrow 1992

ARE YOU SITTING COMFORTABLY?, by Andrew Wilson, Optima

BALANCE HORMONES NATURALLY, by Kate Neil, ION

NATURAL PROGESTERONE: The multiple roles of a remarkable hormone, JOHN r Lee MD, BLL Publishing, California 1993

SEXUAL CHEMISTRY - UNDERSTANDING OUR HORMONES, THE PILL AND HRT, by Dr Ellen Grant, Cedar Mandarin.

ME: HOW TO LIVE WITH IT, A Macintyre, Thorsons, 1992

MENTAL ILLNESS NOT ALL IN THE MIND - A MENTAL HEALTH PROJECT PUBLICATION, Edited by Patrick Holford, Published by ION Press £1.00, 1995. ISBN 1-870976-11-8
(Very good on low blood sugar and depression)

THE BITTER PILL, Dr Ellen Grant, Corgi, London, 1985

PERFECT WEIGHT -The complete mind-body programme for maintaining your ideal weight, by Deepak Chopra, Quantum 1991. ISBN 0-7126-7405-5.

DIETING MAKES YOU FAT, Geoffrey Cannon,

A HANDBOOK OF HOMOEOPATHIC ALTERNATIVE TO IMMUNISATION, Susan Curtis, Winter Press 1994

CHEMICAL CHILDREN, how to protect your family from harmful pollutants, Dr Peter Mansfield & Dr Jean Munro, Century 1987

HOW TO STOP SMOKING AND STAY STOPPED FOR GOOD, by Gillian Riley, Vermilion an imprint by the Random Century Group. ISBN 0-09-175178-0

COMING OFF TRANQUILISERS, Shirley Trickett, Thorsons

Chapter 5
THE FOOD COMBINING DIET, by Kathryn Marsden, Thorsons ISBN 0 7225 2790 X
FOOD COMBING IN 30 DAYS, by Katherine Marsden, Thorsons 1994 ISBN 0-7225-2960-0
FOOD COMBINING FOR HEALTH, by Doris Grant and Jean Joice Thorsons, ISBN 0 7225 2506 0

10 DAY CLEAN-UP PLAN, by Lesley Kenton, Ebury Press, ISBN 0 09 178617 7
10 DAY DE-STRESS PLAN, by Lesley Kenton, Ebury Press, £5.99
THE BIOGENIC DIET, L Kenton, Arrow, London, 1986

A HARMONY OF SCIENCE AND NATURE, Ways of staying healthy in a modern world, John & Lucy Davidson, 1986, The Wholistic Research Company ISBN 0-948071-01-0

TISSUE CLEANING THROUGH BOWEL MANAGEMENT, Bernard Jensen (1981) , available from: Box 52, Route 1, Escondido, CA 92025 USA.

E FOR ADDITIVES. THE COMPLETE E NUMBER GUIDE. everything you should know about additives in your food, by Maurice Hanssen with Jill Marsden, Thorsons 1984. ISBN 0-7225-1150-7.

COMPLETE STRETCHING, by Maxine Tobias and John Patrick Sullivan, Dorling Kindersley, ISBN 0 8631 8832 X

STRETCH AND RELAX, by Maxine Tobias & Mary Stewart, Dorling Kindersley, ISBN 0863181155

VIDEO: BASIC YOGA FOR TODAY, Pickwick , £10.99 from John Lewis, Virgin Megastore etc.

HEALING WITH LOVE, Leonard Laskow MD, 1992 Harper San Fransisco

CREATIVE VISUALISATION, by Shakti Gawain, Bantam Books

THE MEDITATOR'S HANDBOOK, Dr David Fontana,1992, Element

HOW TO MEDITATE, by Lawrence LeShan, Crucible/Turnstone Press

MEDITATION, THE MOST NATURAL THERAPY, Judy Jacka, Lothian, Australia 1990 ISBN 0-85091-393-4

Chapter 6 - Recipe Books
<u>Cooking for candida</u>

COPING WITH CANDIDA, RECIPES TO HELP YOU RECOVER, Sue Elliot. Copies are available from 92 Roman Road, Shrewsbury, SY3 9AL. £7.00 + £1.50 p&p

BEAT CANDIDA COOKBOOK, Erica White, 22 Leigh Hall Road, Leigh-on-Sea, Essex SS9 1RN

RECIPES FOR CANDIDA ALBICANS, Shirley Trickett, Thorsons, 1995

Corrine Sergeant is producing a lovely looking book that should be ready before the end of 1995, contact All Hallows House

Jo Hampton and Luc de Shepper's books also include recipes.

Ordinary Cookery Books that are particularly good on healthy ideas.

RAW ENERGY, by Leslie & Susannah Kenton, Arrow Books Limited 1986. ISBN 0-09-946810-7

FOOD COMBINERS' MEAL PLANNER, by Kathryn Marsden, Thorsons

COOKING WITHOUT, Barbara Cousins, Moorside Natural Healing Centre, 177 Moorside Road, Swinton, Manchester, M27 34D

SUGAR-FREE DESSERTS, DRINKS AND ICES, Elbie Lebrecht, Faber & Faber, 1993
SUGAR-FREE CAKES AND BISCUITS, Elbie Lebrecht, Faber & Faber, 1993

WHEATLESS COOKING (INCLUDING GLUTEN-FREE RECIPES), by Lynette Coffey. Greenhouse Publications Pty Ltd, Melbourne, Australia, 1984. ISBN 0-89815-156-2.
THE COMPLETE WHEAT-FREE COOKBOOK - COULD WHEAT INTOLERANCE BE YOUR PROBLEM?

by Dr Sheila Gibson, Louise Templeton and Dr Robin Gibson. Thorsons 1986. ISBN 0-7225-2317-3

MACRO-BIOTIC COOKING, Misho Kushi

SUPERFAST FOODS, by Michael Van Stratten and Barbara Griggs, Dorling Kindersley 1994. ISBN 0-7513-0088-8.

HOW TO DINE LIKE THE DEVIL AND FEEL LIKE A SAINT, by Luc De Schepper Full of Life Publishing, Sante Fe, USA;

Books for Cooks have a mail order service: 4 Blenheim Crescent,London W11 2EE 0171 221 1992

Chapter 8
(see also under Journals and Appendix 2, useful contacts and addresses)

THE JOKE'S ON ME, by Martin and Yvonne Arber. Cartoons from Interaction, used in this book. Available from Action for ME

HOLISTIC LONDON - Comprehensive and easy to use listings of psychotherapy, alternative health and spiritual centres in the capital, by Kate Brady &
Mike Considine, Brainwave 1995. ISBN 0 9513347 7 8.

HOW TO BE GREEN, John Button, 1989 Random Century

Chapter 9
ARE YOU SLEEPING IN A SAFE
PLACE? by Rolf Gordon (write to him
c/o 130 Gypsy Hill, London SE19 1PL;
£5.95.

RADIATION PROTECTION MANUAL,
by Dr Lita Lee (available from
Grassroots Network, 2061 Hampton
Avenue, Redwood City CA 94061 USA;
$6.95 plus postage.
THE NATURAL HOUSE, by David
Pearson, Gaia
ELECTROHEALING - THE MEDICINE
OF THE FUTURE, Roger Coghill,
Thorsons

THE CREATION OF HEALTH, by
Norman Shealy & Caroline Myss,
Stillpoint 1993, ISBN 0 913299 94 4

MEANING AND MEDICINE, by Larry
Dossey MD Bantam 1991, ISBN 0 553
07869 0
HEALING WORDS: THE POWER OF
PRAYER AND THE PRACTICE OF
MEDICINE, by Larry Dossey MD,
Harper Collins

HEALING AND THE MIND, by Bill
Moyers (Ed), Bantam Doubleday 1993,
ISBN 0 385 46870 9

YOU CAN HEAL YOUR LIFE, Louise
Hay, Eden Grove Editions, London,
1988

LOVE YOURSELF, HEAL YOUR LIFE
WORKBOOK, Louise Hay, Eden grove
Editions

THE ROAD LESS TRAVELLED, M
Scott Peck, Rider 1983

AN AUTOBIOGRAPHY OF A YOGI, P
Yogananda, Rider

LIVING THE MINDFUL LIFE, a
handbook for living in the present
moment, Charles Tart, Shambala 1994

LOVE IS LETTING GO OF FEAR, by
Gerald G Jampolsky MD, Celestial
Arts, California

FRONTIERS OF HEALTH FROM
HEALING TO WHOLENESS, by
Christine R Page, The C W Daniel
Company Limited, 1992. ISBN 0-
85207-256-2

LOVE, MEDICINE AND MIRACLES, B
Siegel, Arrow, London, 1988

MEDITATIONS FOR WOMEN WHO
DO TOO MUCH, by Anne Wilson
Schaef, Harper San Francisco

FAMILIES AND HOW TO SURVIVE
THEM, Robin Skynner & John Cleese,
Cedar 1983

YOU JUST DON'T UNDERSTAND,
Women and men in conversation,
Deborah Tannen, 1990, Ballantine

PROPHET FOR OUR TIMES, The life
and teachings of Peter Deunov, Ed.
David Lorimer, 1991, Element ISBN 1-
85230-211-9 (This includes a lot of
simple, everyday advice on living
healthily)
GEMS OF LOVE, Prayers and
Formulas, by Beinsa Douno, translated
by David Lorimer, available from the
Grain of Wheat, 258 Kew Road,
Richmond, Surrey TA9 3EG

SPIRIT RELEASEMENT THERAPY, a technical manual. William J Baldwin 1992 Centre for Human Relations

Self development, psychology and spiritual books mail order services: Wrekin Trading Company, Keepers Cottage, 114 Upton Road, Clevelode, Malvern Worcs WR13 6PB Tel: 01905 830132

Compendium Bookshop, 234 Camden High Street London NW1 8QS Tel: 0171 485 8944
Watkins Books, 22 Cecil Court, London WC2N 4EZ Tel: 0171 836 2182

Chapter 12
HEALING WITH RADIONICS - THE SCIENCE OF HEALING ENERGY, by A L G Dower, Thorsons 1988. ISBN 0-7225-1541-3

THORSONS INTRODUCTORY GUIDE TO KINESIOLOGY, Maggie la Tourelle with Anthea Courtenay, Thorsons, 1992

JOURNALS AND MAGAZINES

WHAT DOCTORS DON'T TELL YOU (WDDTY), 4 Wallace Road, London, N1 2PG

BERRYDALES SPECIAL DIET NEWS, edited by Michelle Berrydale-Johnson

(available on subscription from Berrydale Publishers, Berrydale House, 5 Lawn Road, London NW3 2XS.

NUTRITIONAL THERPAY TODAY The official newspaper of the SPNT

BIOMED NEWS, Available through BioCare Ltd

POSITIVE HEALTH, Ed Sandra Goodman, Health Research Ltd, Tel: 0117 963 5109

JOURNAL OF ALTERNATIVE AND COMPLEMENTARY MEDICINE, Green Library, 0171 385 0012 This is for practitioners, though it is full of material you'll find interesting as well.

HOLISTIC HEALTH, The Newsletter for members of the BHMA

BEYOND NUTRITION MAGAZINE, from Higher Nature.

CADEUCEUS, Healing into Wholeness, Quarterly, Tel: 01926 451897

LIVING EARTH, The Magazine of the Soil Association

INTERACTION, The Journal of Action for ME

NMS NEWS, Natural Medicines Society

APPENDIX 2

USEFUL CONTACTS AND ADDRESSES

NB When sending for information please remeber to include an s.a.e

Several booksinclude particularly useful resource lists.

*Food Allergy & Intolerance, Brostoff
Nutritional Medicine, Davies & Stewart
All Day Energy, Katherine Marsden
How to be Green by John Button,*

4. TRAVELLING

See Ainsworths under Homoeopathy, who sell travel kits including anti-radiation drops for long haul flights.
Alternatives to vaccinations - see Sue Curtis' book

Biocare do Jetzyme enzymes to mitigate the free radical activity during long haul flights.

4. BABIES& CHILDREN

The Active Birth Centre
55 Dartmouth Road
London NW5 1SL
Tel: 0171 267 4239

National Childbirth Trust
Alexandra House
Olham Terrace
London, W3 6NH
Tel: 0181 992 8637

La Leche League (Breastfeeding advice)
BM 3424
London, WC1N 3XX

INFORMATION ON VACCINATIONS

The Informed Parent
29 Greyhound Road,
Sutton, Surrey, SM1 4BY

The Assoc for Parents of Vaccine Damaged Children
2 Church Street
Warwickshire CV36 4AP

SEASONAL AFFECTIVE DISORDER

See Wholistic Research Co

Full Spectrum Lighting Ltd
Unit 1 Riverside Business Centre
Victoria Street
High Wycombe
Bucks HP11 2LT

F.S.I. Scotland
Unit 11 42 Dalsetter Avenue
Glasgow G15 8SL

5. HEALTH FOOD MAILORDER

Wild Oats
220 Westborne Grove
London W11 2RH
Tel: 0171 229 1063
fAX: 0171 243 0988
*Three times winner of Health Food shop of the
Year - a feast of goodies with very helpful and
knowledgeable staff. Open on Sundays.
ALL PRODUCTS INGREDIENTS ARE
MARKED*

Anglo-Dutch Rye Company
11a Park Crescent
Worthing
W Sussex BN11 4AH
Tel: 01903 237 664
*A small company making delicious wheat and
yeast-free rye bread. New cake recipes are
being developed. Please send an s.a.e. for
their leaflet and order form.*

5. ORGANIC FOOD

The Real Meat Company
Warminster BA12 7BZ
Tel: 01985 840436
Friends of the Real Meat Company,
membership free to customers and includes
copies of Real Meat News.

Compassion in World Farming
20 Lavant Street
Petersfield
Hampshire, GU32 3EW

Free-Range Egg Association
37 Tanza Road
London, NW3 2UA

Henry Doubleday Research Association
National Centre for Organic Gardening
Ryton-on-Dunsmore
Coventry, CV8 3LG

The Soil Association Ltd
86-88 Colston Street
Bristol, BS1 5BB
Membership to this wonderful organisation is
currently £16 (concessions). Excellent
publications include
- *Living Earth, (members' magazine)*
- *Directory of Farm Shops and Box*
  Schemes £2.50
- *Go Organic! Regional Guide to buying*
  Organic produce £2.50
- *Local Food Links, New ways of getting*
  Organic food from farm to table. £3.00
- *Extensive book list available.*

5. EQUIPMENT SUPPLIERS

The Wholistic Research Company
Bright Haven, Robin's Lane,
Lolworth, Cambridge CB3 8HH
Tel: 01954 781074
Run by John and Lucie Davidson, who
produce a whole range of essential and
fascinating products and information
including
- *juicers,*
- *water distillers,*
- *rebounders,*
- *ionizers*

- *electromagnetic pulsors,*
- *tip-u-ups (for bad backs),*
- *enema kits,*
- *full spectrum lighting,*
- *anti-allergy products,*
- *Aloe vera mother plants.*

JUICERS

Kenwood, Braun and Moulinex are all
available from department stores. £38-£45

See the Wholistic Research Co. for powerful
ones

or for cancer patients, juicers from the States
used for the Gerson therapy. Contact
The Gerson Trust, Lesley Pearce
013720 375912

WATER FILTER UNITS

Brita's systems are widely available,
Information line: 01932 770599
Also **Crystal Waymaster**

See Wholistic Research Co

5. RELAXATION TAPES

Aurora
16A Neal's Yard
Covent Garden
London WC2

New World Cassettes
Paradise Farm
Westhall, Halesworth
Suffolk, IP19 8RH

5. EXCERCISE

Rebounders - see Amway
The Wholistic Research Co

Cycling - see Friends of the Earth Cycling
Campaign

Sustrans, Paths for People,
0117 926 8893

Cyclists' Touring Club, 69 Meadrow,
Godalming, Surrey GU7 3HS

5. PRODUCTS TO MINIMISE ALLERGENS

VACUUM CLEANERS -
recommended for asthmatics and allergy
sufferers, especially for dustmites.
Medivac is widely available

Worwerk UK Ltd *imports a brilliant*
machine from Germany that is expensive but
pays for itself in saved cleaning bills
(household and clothes).
Vorwerk House,
Toutley Road
Wokingham
Berks RG11 5QN
Tel: 01734 794878

The National Bed Federation Ltd
251 Brompton Road
London SW3 2EZ
0171 589 4888
Produce a very useful self-help guide to
minimising allergens including house-dust
mites.

Ecover
Mouse Lane, Steyning
West Sussex' BN4 3DF
(manufacturers of eco-friendly household
cleaning products - available in Health food
stores and supermarkets.)

Faith Products Ltd (Clear Spring)
Unit 5, Kay Street
Bury , Lancs BL9 6BU

The National Society for Clean Air
136 North Street
Brighton, East Sussex, BN1 1RG
Membership and information leaflets.

Amway
Snowdon Drive
Winterhill
Milton Keynes, Bucks,. MK6 1AR
Tel: 01908 679888
Suppliers of environmentally-friendly house
hold cleaning products. Local distributors.

The Little Green Shop
16 Gardner Street
Brighton
East Sussex BN1 1UP
01273 571221Mail order catalogue
Offer a range of household products for
allergy sufferers.

5. HOLIDAYS, RETREATS, CLINICS

Places to Be 95/96 £6.50 inc p&p
A guide to retreats, vegetarian and distinctive
B&Bs from
Edge of Time Ltd. FREEPOST MK 1659
PO Box 1808, Winslow, Bucks MK18 3BR

See AfME's travel club for winter holidays

Working Weekends on Organic Farms
19 Bradford Raod
Lewes Sussex BN7 1RB

If you need in patient care:

Tyringham Clinic (Naturopathic)
Newport Pagnell
Bucks MK16 9ER
Tel: 01908 610450

The Raphael Medical Centre
Hollanden Park,
Coldharbour Lane,
Hildenborough
Tonbridge, Kent TN11 9LE
Tel: 01732 833924

See **Park Attwood Clinic** page 174.

Forest Mere Health Hydro,
Liphook, Hants GU30 7JQ
Tel: 01428 722051

5. BACK CARE PRODUCTS

David and Moira McDonald
The Total Back Care Company
505 Hagley Road
Bearwood
BIRMINGHAM B66 4AX
Very good brochure. David is an excellent
speaker for compaines and groups. He comes
to London weekly.

Pelvic Support Chairs
New Mill Lane
Eversley
Hants
RG27 0RA
Chairs and working stools (like the godsend one this book was written on) designed by an engineer turned Mctimoney chiropractor

Alternative Sitting
PO Box 19
Chipping Norton
Oxford
OX7 6NY

Anatomia Ltd
21 Hampstead Road
London NW1 3JA
Tel: 0171 387 5700

The Back Shop
24 New Cavendish Street
London W1M 7LH
0171 935 9120

7. SUPPLEMENT SUPPLIERS

BioCare Ltd
Lakeside
180 Lifford Lane
Kings Norton
Birmingham B30 3NT
Tel: 0121 433 3727
Fax: 0121 433 3879
BioCare cannot give adivce or send supplements direct to patients.

Blackmores UK
They are moving shortly, but thier fax number stay
Tel: 01753 683815
Fax: 01753 684663

Higher Nature Ltd
The Nutrition Centre
Burwash Common
East Sussex TN19 7LX
Tel: 01435 882880
Fax orders: 01435 883720

Lamberts Healthcare Ltd
1 Lamberts Road
Tunbridge Wells
Kent TN2 3EQ

Tel: 01892.513116
Direct orders: 01892.546488
Fax: 01892.515863

Nature's Way
Hebron Rd
Kilkenny
IRELAND
Mail order Tel: 00353.5651498
Head office: 00353.14513619

The NutriCentre (ace mail order service)
7 Park Crescent
London W1N 3HE
Tel: 0171 436 5122
Fax: 0171 436 5171

HOMOEOPATHY

Weleda and Nelsons are widely available
Ainsworths Homoeopathic Pharmacy
38 New Cavendish Street
London W1M 9FG
0171 935 5330 **Mail order**
Can offer a certain amount of help over the phone. ask about their first aid and travel kits.

8. SUPPORT GROUPS

Action for ME and Chronic Fatigue
PO Box 1302
Wells
Somerset BA5 2WE
A charitable trust that provides support services to people with ME and their families, friends and carers. It also funds research and campaigns to change attitudes towares the disease. Membership is £15.00 per year. There are over 7,000 members and 140 local groups and contacts all over the UK..
Members also have access to a Therapy and Information Helpline, advocacy and a Counselling Helpline.
The 24 hour helpline is on 0891 122976 (calls are charged at 39p per minute cheap rate or 49p at all other times). 30% of the profit will go to AfME to contribute to research and support service funding.
Interaction their excellent journal comes out 3 times a year. It regularly reviews books on Candida, and features articles on the latest treatments.

The trading arm of AfME has launched a mail order nutritional supplement service (mainly BioCare) at very competitive prices, with a number of Special Offers, including a Candida starter pack for £45.
AfME's Travel Club is able to offer special prices for winter holidays in ME friendly climates. Ring 01749 670799 for details.

Action for ME in Scotland
PO Box 45
Edinburgh EH7 4EJ

Action Against Allergy
24-26 High Street
Hampton Hill
Middlesex TW12 1TD
Some local groups, newsletter

Springhill Centre
Cuddington Road
Dinton
Aylesbury
Buckinghamshire HP18 0AD
A centre for relief care for chronically sick children with disabling and life limiting desease. Set up by Dr Nadya and Hugh Coates. Conductive education and seminares on diet and candidiasis.

Hyperactive Children's Support Group
Sally Bunday
71 Whyke Lane
Chichester
West Sussex PO21 2DE
Lots of local groups and a journal. Wide experience of treating children with candidiasis. Also supplies supplements (mostly BioCare).

National Society for Research into Allergy
PO Box 45
Hinckley
Leicestershire   LE10 1JY
Local groups

The National Back Pain Association
16, Elmtree Road,
Teddington, Middlesex TW11 8ST
Tel: 0181 977 5474

Women's Health & Information Centre
52 Featherstone Street
London EC1
Advice and library

Alcoholics Anonymous (GB) Ltd
PO Box 1, Stonebow House
Stonebow
York YO1 2NJ
Tel: 01904 644026

Overeaters Anonymous
for local groups, phone:
Tel: 01426 984674

Action on Smoking and Health
5-11 Mortimer Street
London W1N 7RH

The Vegetarian Society
Parkdale
Dunham Road
Altrincham
Cheshire WA14 4QG

The Vegan Society
33-35 George Street
Oxford OX1 2AY

The Breakthrough Centre
7, Poplar Mews, London W12 7JS
Tel: 0181 749 8525
If you live in London, and want to meet others who are interested in personal development and conscious business, this 'home of holistic enterprise and new ideas' is a must. Run by Andrew Fergusson.

8. GENERAL ORGANISATIONS

Friends of the Earth
26-28 Underwood Street
London N1 7JQ
(a wealth of information and advice on all "green" issues, suppliers etc)

Energy Inform
9-10 Charlotte Square
Newcastle upon Tyne, NE1 4XF

Consumers' Association (publishers of Which?)
2 Marylebone Road
London NW1 4DX

The Solar Trade Association
Brackenhurst
Greenham Common South
Newbury, Berks RG15 8HH

Noise Abatement Society
PO Box 8
Bromley
Kent, BR2 0UM

8. GENERAL SOCIETIES

British Holistic Medical Association
Trust House
Royal Shrewsbury Hospital South
Shrewsbury, SY3 8XF
01743 261155

The McCarrison Society
24 Paddington St
London W1M 4DR
Tel: 0171 935 3924
*This pioneering society studies the
relationship between nutrition and health.
Regualar Journal*

Natural Medicines Society (NMS),
Edith Lewis House,
Ilkeston,
Derbyshire, DE7 8EJ.

**Research Council for Complementary
Medicine (RCCM),**
60 Great Ormond Street,
London WC1N 3JF
Tel: (0171) 833 8897

**Institute for Complementary Medicine
(ICM),**
PO Box 194,
London SE16 1QZ.
Tel: (0171) 237 5165.
*The ICM holds a General Register of
practitioners send an s.a.e. for a copy*

9. ELCTROMAGNETIC FIELDS

*See also under recommended reading in
Appendix 1*

The Radon Survey
National Radiological Protection Board
Chilton
Didcot
Oxfordshire OX11 0RQ

9. MERCURY FREE DENTISTRY

**International Academy of Oral Medicine
and Toxicology,**
Tony Newbury, President
72 Harley Street,
London W1N 1AE
Tel: 0171 580 3168
or via Alan Hibberd in the Directory

**Society The British Society for Mercury
Free Dentistry (incorporating the British
Dental for Clinical Nutrition)**
see Jack Levenson's entry in the Directory
*They will be able to recommend dentists who
are experienced in replacing mercury fillings.*

Robert Hempleman (dentist),
221 Old Brompton Road,
London SW7.
Tel: 0171 370 0055

Rating 0/10 - 10/10

	Date:	Date:	Date:	Date:	Date:	Date:	Date:	Date:	Date:	Date:	Date:
Abdominal ache:											
Abnormal thirst:											
Aching joints:											
Anal itching: –											
Anxiety/Panic attacks:											
Asthma:											
Athletes Foot:											
Belching during / after meals:											
Bloating:											
Constipation:											
Cystitis:											
Depression:											
Depression:											
Diarrhoea:											
Dry skin:											
Ear ache / Ear infections:											
Energy swings:											
Fatigue:											
Feeling of incomplete bowel movement:											
Feeling Spaced out / Haziness:											
Fluid retention:											
Flushing / perspiring after meals:											
Food cravings:											
Foul taste in mouth:											
Frequent Urination:											
Halitosis:											
Headaches:											
Heartburn:											
Heavy/aching muscles:											
Inability to concentrate:											
Indigestion:											
Inflamed digestive tract/stomach:											
Insomnia / Disturbed sleep:											

Symptoms of Candida Overgrowth continued:

	Week 1	Week 2	Week 3	Week 4	Week 6	Week 8	Month 3	Month 4	Month 6
Irritability:									
Lethargy:									
Menstrual cramps:									
Mood swings:									
Mouth ulcers:									
Nausea:									
PMT:									
Sinus Problems:									
Spots / pimples:									
Thrush:									
Weight problems:									
Wind:									
Other:									
Other:									
Other:									
Food intolerance 1)									
Food Intolerance 2)									
Food Intolerance 3)									
Food intolerance 4)									
Food intolerance 5)									

Continued:	Date:	Date:	Date:	Date:	Date:	Date:	Date:	Date:	Date:	Date:
Abdominal ache:										
Abnormal thirst:										
Aching joints:										
Anal itching:										
Anxiety/Panic attacks:										
Asthma:										
Athletes Foot:										
Belching during / after meals:										
Bloating:										
Constipation:										
Cystitis:										
Depression:										
Depression:										
Diarrhoea:										
Dry skin:										
Ear ache / Ear infections:										
Energy swings:										
Fatigue:										
Feeling of incomplete bowel movement:										
Feeling Spaced out / Haziness:										
Fluid retention:										
Flushing / perspiring after meals:										
Food cravings:										
Foul taste in mouth:										
Frequent Urination:										
Halitosis:										
Headaches:										
Heartburn:										
Heavy/aching muscles:										
Inability to concentrate:										
Indigestion:										
Inflamed digestive tract/stomach:										
Insomnia / Disturbed sleep:										

Symptoms of Candida overgrowth continued:

	Month 7	Month 8	Month 9	Month 10	Month 11	Month 12	Month 14	Month 16	Month 18
Irritability:									
Lethargy:									
Menstrual cramps:									
Mood swings:									
Mouth ulcers:									
Nausea:									
PMT:									
Sinus Problems:									
Spots / pimples:									
Thrush:									
Weight problems:									
Wind:									
Other:									
Other:									
Other:									
Food intolerance 1)									
Food Intolerance 2)									
Food Intolerance 3)									
Food intolerance 4)									
Food intolerance 5)									

THE UK DIRECTORY OF PRACTITIONERS WHO TREAT CANDIDA ALBICANS HOLISTICALLY

CONTENTS

APPENDIX III

YOUR SYMPTOMS DIARY

With kind permission of Anya Harris.

● Remember to fill in your symptoms in the Diary in Appendix III which precedes this page. Score them out of ten for frequency and severity if you like. You will be very glad to be able to look back at how much you have improved over the months. It is amazing how quickly and completely we forget. You may find that you notice new symptoms as your old ones get better.

INTRODUCTION TO THE UK DIRECTORY

The following pages list *over 200 practitioners at nearly 300 different clinic addresses* who are qualified and experienced in treating people suffering from candidiasis. There is a pretty even spread around the UK, although you are spoilt for choice if you live in London. In this first edition, at least, it is often Hobson's choice if you are in Scotland, Ireland, Wales, or parts of the North of England. However we hope to list many more practitioners in future editions.
Updates to the directory will be published regularly in between editions. Please send an s.a.e. plus 2 x first class stamps to "Directory Update, All Hallows House, Idol Lane, London EC3R 5DD".

The practitioners are listed alphabetically under the counties then towns in which they practise. In London, they are under Central, North, East, South, West, by postcode. If you know a practitioner you want by name, see the index at the back.

To make sure that everyone listed here is properly qualified, we only approached practitioners through their professional associations or through the leading supplement suppliers. The professional bodies who mailed all their members individually were: *The Institute for Optimum Nutrition and The British Register of Naturopaths.* The members of the *National Institute for Medical Herbalists* were reached via their local practitioner groups rather than an individual mailing. Other practitioners to whom we wrote individually, have been personally recommended or are well known experts in the field.

Each practitioner was asked to fill in a detailed pro forma giving their qualifications, experience and how they treat candida. While we reserved the right to vet entries *PLEASE NOTE THAT THIS IS NOT AN OFFICIAL VALIDATED REGISTER THAT GUARANTEES THE QUALITY OF PRACTITIONERS' TRAINING AND TREATMENT.*

We have included several practitioners on the strength of their long experience or because they were candida sufferers themselves, even though their formal training may not have been ideal. Where a practitioner has no official qualification in a therapy, but has studied it and recommends it as an important part of their overall approach, the therapy has been shown in brackets. eg. (Nutrition). You may check the qualifications of the practitioners you are considering by cross referring to the *glossary of qualifications* at the back which gives what their letters mean. More details of the training at the main schools are included under the description of the therapies in chapter 11.

- Talk to other candida sufferers and, if possible, get a word of mouth recommendation.

- Scan the practitioners listed in your area (and any in the Late Additions page).

- *Start with a baseline therapy: ie nutrition, herbal medicine or naturopathy - see the "Which Therapy?" in chapter 11..* Any of these will be thoroughly trained in giving the dietary advice you need for beating candidiasis.

- If, however, you have *related symptoms* (such as back pain or depression) which are so severe that you really cannot entertain the idea of making any changes to your diet or lifestyle at this stage, then start with a therapist who may not have training in the dietary side of things, but who will nonetheless be able to help you regain enough quality of life to start on the candida programme as a whole a bit later on. It is important that you choose someone who appreciates what having candidiasis can mean, since some psychotherapists or chiropractors, for example, may not. We have included several practitioners who are especially helpful for related symptoms and appreciate the need to temper their treatment for people with candida. See chapter 4 on" Other Symptoms or Conditions often Associated with Candidiasis", for suggestions as to which therapy may be most appropriate.

- It is very helpful to get a specific diagnosis, particularly about any individual food intolerances. The *diagnostic therapies* are grouped together in the second section of chapter 11. If you can find a baseline practitioner who also uses one of these diagnostic techniques, so much the better. . But if not and you can afford it, it may be worth seeing somebody else separately. See chapter 2 for details on the common diagnostic tests.

- If you want to see more than one practitioner, whether you see them simultaneously or in sequence is entirely up to you and may well depend on your time and finances. Remember this is all going to take some time, so doing everything at once is not necessarily better or faster. Always tell practitioners about any other treatment you are having (whether complementary or from your GP).

- You can gauge the experience and popularity of practitioners by how many hours they work (remember most work in more than one clinic) and the length of their waiting lists if mentioned. Understandably lists will generally be longer if they are covered by private medical insurance or the NHS.

- In general, the longer the consultation, particularly the initial one, the more holistic the approach is likely to be, although some practitioners' diagnostic and intuitive skills and/or technology mean they can sum up clients much faster than others.

- Generally speaking, the practitioners mentioned as also treating CFS(ME) will be more experienced. Some practitioners call it something else, or regard it in rather a different way according to their tradition, so don't be put off. They will treat your individual needs anyway.

- *How much will it all cost? As you can see, fees vary enormously. Remember any laboratory tests, supplements or remedies will be in addition* (nutritional supplements will start at about £30-40 per month, herbal, homoeopathic remedies will probably be less - though many practitioners will recommend you use both). If you have a tight budget, tell the practitioner at the beginning and ask him or her to aim to stick to it. Taking less than the optimum number of supplements means you will probably have to work harder with your diet. Many practitioners will agree to concessionary rates for genuine cases and/or to trying to get your supplements at a reduced rate.

- *If there is not a listing for the therapy of your choice in your area, contact their head office* (details are under the therapies in chapter 11.). Just because a particular therapist is not listed in this directory does not necessarily mean anything. They may have not heard about it, or have simply not got round to sending their application back. The professional associations will give you your nearest practitioner over the phone or send you their whole register. *NB There is usually a charge of £1.50-£2.00 for this.*

- If you are in any doubt, ask to speak to the practitioner on the phone before booking an appointment, or ask that your first consultation be an exploratory one. It is important that you feel you have a good rapport with your practitioner.

- Do not expect practitioners to follow the guidelines in this guide to the letter. Their background, training and experience will differ and they will be tailoring their recommendations to you as an individual. If you find a treatment or remedy that we have not mentioned that works well, please write and tell us about it.

With your help, we aim to improve and expand this Directory regularly. If you have any feed back about any practitioner - whether they are listed here or not - please let us have it. We estimate that the next edition will be published in Spring/Summer 1996, but updates will be available in the meantime.

The use of Nystatin, Dyflucan and other anti-fungal drugs.
Although we have said that this is a directory of practitioners who treat naturally, which may imply that they do not use drugs, we have listed several doctors who do recommend drugs on occasions since there is always a time and a place for them. We have made this clear in the directory and it is up to you to read the pros and cons on the use of drugs in the treatment of candidiasis and how long you should continue to take them in chapter 3. Discuss this with your practitioner and decide for yourself.

Can I get this treatment on the NHS?
A few of the supplements are listed on the NHS's drugs tariff, so you should be able to get them on prescription. Ask your pharmacist, but check with your practitioner before accepting alternatives as there may be a big difference in strength or quality.

As for the treatments, there are two main ways that you could get them on the NHS:
a) if your GP is a fundholder, he might already have contracts with alternative practitioners. If not, you or your practitioner may be able to convince him that it will be cheaper for his practice to offer alternative approaches for you and similar cases. We aim to have cost effectiveness statistics from a study in a GP fund holding practice available by mid-1996.

b) if your GP is not a fundholder, you may be able to get approval through the Family Health Services Authority. But both these options will take time and persistence if they are not already in place.

Student clinics
This is a very good wheeze to get cheaper treatment. Provided these are well supervised, you will do well, and they often are only too glad for the extra clients. Phone the professional body's head office listed here for the locaton of their schools and student clinics.

Can I claim this treatment on my private medical insurance?
Candida will not be an accepted diagnosis, and be aware that any chronic condition you had before you started your policy will not be covered. We have

also heard of many instances of long term treatment for chronic conditions being discontinued. If you also have symptoms that are recognised by mainstream medicine, such as IBS, back or neck pain, severe thrush, depression, severe headaches etc, you should be able to get the appropriate referral from your GP to a recognised specialist or to one of the practitioners listed in this directory. Any of the medical doctors listed here should be accepted by all the insurance companies. Otherwise it depends on the company and your particular policy. PPP have their own lists and criteria as to which complementary practitioners they will cover, although they will not release this to the public. BUPA apears more flexible but you have to go through a consultant, who will probably need some persuasion to refer you to a complementary practitioner. OHRA, HSA, Crusader, WPP and many other independent or local companies are now covering an increasingly wide range of complementary therapies. NB Most companies do not cover the cost of supplements.

If you have a private policy and want to claim on it, read the small print and GO TO YOUR GP FIRST! Check his recommendation with the company itself (most have good helplines). But in the end, do what you feel will get to the root of your problem, whether you have to pay for it or not. Life is too short and your health is too precious to compromise.

Finally, if you have had expensive tests, treatments or operations and can show that your insurance company would have saved money by covering you to see an alternative practitioner at the outset, write and tell them, or they will be none the wiser.

AVON

Jackie Melling, DiplON

Bath Natural Health Clinic, James Street West, Bath, Avon BA1 2BP ☎01225-313 153
Nutrition, Kinesiology, Supplements.
Jackie also treats ME and is an ex-sufferer herself. Fri 9am-1.30pm, plus as required.
Initial Consultation: £25-00 / 1½ hrs
Subsequent visits: £20-00 / 1 hr

Cilla Moncrieff, DThD DNMed MCSR

MRxS MIAT
30 West Way, Clevedon, Bristol BS21 7XN
☎01275-897 810
Nutrition, Reflexology, Allergy Testing.
Treats some ME patients. Mon-Fri 9am-5.30pm.
Initial Consultation: £40-00 / 1½ hrs
Subsequent visits: £25-00 / 45 mins

Rainer Trebuth, HP (Germany) CHT

(USA) MRN
Natural Health Clinic, 39 Cotham Hill, Bristol BS6 6JY ☎0117-974 1199
Natural Medicines, Hypnotherapy, Healing, Bach Flower Remedies, Celloid Minerals. Available Fridays.
Initial Consultation: £40-00 / 1½
hrsSubsequent visits: £30-00 / 45mins-1 hr

Sarah Bunting, DThD DO DIrid

18 St Helena Road, Westbury Park, Bristol BS6 7NR ☎0117-973 9538
Nutrition, Iridology, Osteopathy, Reflexology. 9am-6pm.
Initial Consultation: £40-00 / 1½ hrs
Subsequent visits: £20-00 / 45 mins

Sarah Bunting, DThD DO DIrid

The Natural Therapy Centre, 126 Whiteladies Road, Bristol BS8 2RP ☎0117-946 6035
Nutrition, Iridology, Osteopathy, Reflexology. 9am-6pm.
Initial Consultation: £40-00 / 1½ hrs
Subsequent visits: £20-00 / 45 mins

Cilla Moncrieff, DThD DNMed MCSR

MRxS MIAT
(Neals Yard) Natural Therapy Centre, 126 Whiteladies Road, Bristol BS8 2RP
☎0117-946 6035
Nutrition, Reflexology, Allergy Testing.
Treats some ME patients. Mon 9am-1pm.
Initial Consultation: £40-00 / 1½ hrs
Subsequent visits: £25-00 / 45 mins

Pauline Noakes, BA (Hons) DipAPI

LicASK RCT MCIA
10 Eastfield Road, Westbury-on-Trym, Bristol BS9 4AD ☎0117-962 8302
Colonic Hydrotherapy, Kinesiology, Supplements, Allergy Testing.
Pauline also treats ME. **Support Group Initial Contact.** Mon-Sat 10am-6pm.
Initial Consultation: £45-00 / 1½ hrs
Subsequent visits: £38-50 / 1 hr

BERKSHIRE

Jennifer A Harper, DipDTh DipNatMed

MBRCP MRNT
Royal Berkshire Racquet and Health Club, Nine Mile Ride, Bracknell, Berks. RG12 7PB
☎01344-869 066
Nutrition, Kinesiology, Bach Flower Remedies.
Jennifer Harper is qualified in nutrition and natural therapies. She has developed her own system, combining holistic therapies and healing in a unique way to help re-balance the body and achieve high levels of health and wellbeing. Ms Harper has lectured and written articles for a number of well-known magazines and has a BBC radio phone-in programme. Tuesdays.
Initial Consultation: £40-00 / 1 hr
Subsequent visits: £25-00 / ½ hr

Alberto Nafig, ITEC MRA

Castle Hill Clinic, 1c Tilhurst Road, Reading, Berks. RG1 7TW ☎01734-586 766
Nutrition, Reflexology, Kinesiology, Iridology, Remedial Massage.
Alberto uses iridology and urinalasys diag-

nostically. He also uses aromatherapy.
Mon-Fri 9am-4.30pm; Sat 9am-12pm.
Initial Consultation: £25-00 / 1½ hrs
Subsequent visits: £20-00 / 1 hr

Peter Bartlett, DO DipRM MNTOS MCO
MCrOA
Harwood, Shurlock Road. Waltham St. Lawrence,
Reading, Berks. RG10 0HN ☎01734-344 203
Osteopathy, Nutrition, Biological
Medicine, Complex Homoeopathy.
Peter qualified from the McTimoney Chiropractic
School and is also trained in remedial massage.
He treats ME and lectures on the subject in UK
and Ireland.
Mon 9am-11am; Wed 9am-5pm; Fri 9am-1pm.
Initial Consultation: £45-00 / 1 hr
Subsequent visits: £25-00 / ½ hr

Gillian Lidbetter, Dip ION
54 South View Avenue, Caversham, Reading,
Berks. RG4 5AJ ☎01734-475 358
Nutrition, Supplements.
Support Group Initial Contact. Days and
evenings.
Initial Consultation: £30-00 / Up to 1½ hrs
Subsequent visits: £20-00 / 45 mins

Alberto Nafig, ITEC MRA
6 Palmerstone Road, Earley, Reading, Berks.
RG6 1HL ☎01734-265 158
Nutrition, Reflexology, Kinesiology,
Iridology, Remedial Massage.
Alberto uses iridology and urinalasys diagnos-
tically. He also uses aromatherapy.
Mon-Fri 9am-6.30pm; Sat 9am-1pm.
Initial Consultation: £25-00 / 1½ hrs
Subsequent visits: £20-00 / 1 hr

Ms Deenah Sing, CNH MHPA RIPHH
91 Marescroft Road, Slough, Berks. SL2 2LN
☎01753-739 917
Nutrition, Complex Homoeopathy, Bio-
Resonance Therapy. Available any Time.
Initial Consultation: £35-00 / 1 hr
Subsequent visits: £25-00 / 1 hr

Mrs Clare De Freitas, BA MSc CHM
NIMH
Morrell Room Cottage, Church Lane, Streatley,
Berks. RG8 9HT ☎01491-875 347
Herbal Medicine, Nutrition, Massage.
Tue/Thur 9am-5pm.
Initial Consultation: £25-00 / 1 hr
Subsequent visits: £15-00 / ½ hr

Sandy Treweeke, SRN DHD ANM IFA
MICRA
20 Foxglove Close, Wokingham, Berks.
RG41 3NF ☎01734-792 173
Nutrition, Iridology, Aromatherapy,
Reflexology.
Sandy is a nurse who became interested in na-
tural therapies through her own health problems
when orthodox medicine failed to help her. Since
then she has trained in a number of therapies and
keeps up to date with the latest world-wide
research through seminars.
Tue-Fri 9am-5pm. Evenings by arrangement.
Phone Mon-Fri 9am-9pm.
Initial Consultation: £20-00 / 1hr
Subsequent visits: £10-00 / ½ hr

Grace Hall, MBRI DISc IACT
89 Windmill Avenue, Wokingham, Berks.
RG41 3XG ☎01734-786 727
Iridology/Nutrition, Homoeopathy,
Counselling.
Grace also offers computerised EAV tests for
nutritional deficiencies and allergies. She treats
M.E and is currently also doing research into this
as well as candida, allergies and ME. (3-4 weeks
waiting list.) Mon-Sat 8am-8pm.
Initial Consultation: £35-00 / 1 hr
Subsequent visits: £15-00 / ½ hr

BUCKINGHAMSHIRE

Jane McWhirter, MA (Hons) MC
Lesser Halings, Tilehouse Lane, Denham, Bucks.
UB9 5DG ☎01895-832 495
McTimoney Chiropractic, Celloid
Minerals, Advice on complementary
therapies.
Clients frequently come with long term back or

2

neck pain that is due to underlying candida and respond to Jane's eclectic approach. (Jane is expecting a baby in October and will not be available from Oct to Dec '95).
Mon/Tue/Fri 2.30-7pm.
Initial Consultation: £30-00 / 1 hr
Subsequent visits: £25-00 / 45 mins

Helen Johnson, DO MRO ND MRN
Holmer Farm, Holmer Lane, Booker, High Wycombe, Bucks. HP12 4QA
☎01494-473 414
Naturopathy, Diet, Homoeopathic Nosodes, Osteopathy.
Helen also treats ME. Weekdays 9am-5pm.
Initial Consultation: £40-00 / 1 hr
Subsequent visits: £20-00 / ½ hr

Ruth Patience, DipION
49 Partridge Way, Downley, High Wycombe, Bucks. HP13 5JX ☎01494-446 896
Nutrition, Supplements.
Ruth encourages her clients to take active responsibility for their health. Her previous experience in the food industry as a food technologist and nutritionist enables her to offer effective advice and support. Each client will receive a detailed report and a letter on her findings and recommendations. Ruth also treats ME. By appointment only.
Initial Consultation: £35-00 / 1 hr
Subsequent visits: £35-00 / per hour, pro rata.

Karin Czapnik, DipION
The Old Barn, Town Farm, Beacon Hill, Penn, Bucks. HP10 8NJ ☎01494-817 317
Dietary Therapy, Supplements.
Patients with long term eating disorders will sometimes be referred to colleagues for hypnotherapy or psychotherapy, to heal the 'child' within. Mon-Fri 9am-7pm.
Initial Consultation: £35-00 / Min 1½ hrs
Subsequent visits: £25-00 / 1 hr

CAMBRIDGESHIRE

Lyn Barnes, DipION
St Martin's Cottage, 36 Apthorpe Street, Fulbourn, Cambridge CB1 5EY

☎01233-880 474
Nutrition, Supplements.
Free 20 minute appointment offered (with no obligation) so that you can find out what nutritional therapy involves and whether you feel it is the right therapy for you. First two treatments will take 1½ hrs each. Lyn also treats ME.
Mon/Tue/Thu/Fri 9am-4pm.
Initial Consultation: £20-00 / 1½ hrs
Subsequent visits: £18-00 / 1 hr

Alison Davies, BSc (Hons) MNIMH
19 Swaynes Lane, Comberton, Cambridge CB3 7EF ☎01223-246 159
Herbal Medicine, Nutrition, Aromatherapy.
Herbs combined with natural nutritional remedies, which aid the holistic dimensions of improving the vital force and balancing the emotional aspects of the condition. Alison also treats ME.
Tue/Thu 9am-6pm.
Initial Consultation: £25-00 / 1 hr
Subsequent visits: £12-50 / ½ hr

CHESHIRE

Ms Jules Miller, MNIMH
15 Newry Park, Chester CH2 2AR
☎01244-371 114
Herbal Medicine, Nutrition, Counselling.
Ms Miller also treats ME. Mon/Thu 9am-6pm; Wed 9am-5pm; Fri 9am-2pm.
Initial Consultation: £25-00 / 1 hr
Subsequent visits: £12-00 / ½ hr

Margaret Pardoe, RIr MH SRN
Balance Complementary Therapy Centre, Cumberland Offices, 19 King Edward Street, Macclesfield, Cheshire SK10 1AQ
☎01625-619 836
Iridology, Herbal Medicine, Supplements.
Margaret is also a nurse and a midwife. Fri 9.30am-5.30pm.
Initial Consultation: £40-00 / 1½ hrs
Subsequent visits: £20-00 / 45 mins

CLEVELAND

Rosalind Ridley, DipION DipNIM MRNT
21 Chingford Grove, Elm Tree Farm, Stockton-on-Tees, Cleveland TS19 0OD
☎01642-603 100
Vega Tests, Nutrition, Reiki, Reflexology.
Initial consultation includes two hours of Vega testing. Rosalind also treats ME. After 7pm usually.
Initial Consultation: £50-00 / 3 hrs
Subsequent visits: £20-00 / 1 hr

CUMBRIA

Selina Import, DipION
The Old Rectory, Dufton, Appleby-in-Westmorland, Cumbria CA16 6DA
☎01768-351 635
Nutrition, Bowen Technique, Kinesiology. Weekends & evenings.
Initial Consultation: £30-00 / 1½ hrs
Subsequent visits: £15-00 / 45 mins

DERBYSHIRE

Margaret Pardoe, RIr MH SRN
Natural Choice Therapy Centre, 24 St John Street, Ashbourne, Derbys. DE6 1GH
☎01335-346 096
Iridology, Herbal Medicine, Supplements.
Margaret is also a nurse and a midwife Thu 9.30am-2.30pm. Sometimes 9.30am-6.30pm.
Initial Consultation: £40-00 / 1½ hrs
Subsequent visits: £20-00 / 45 mins

Heather Lyons, DipION MNCA
St Wilfrid's Rectory, West Hallam, Ilkeston, Derbys. DE7 6GR ☎0115-944 3493
Nutrition, Supplements.
Diagnosis includes evaluation of Dr Crook's Candida Questionnaire. Heather's advice includes measures for intestinal cleansing, detoxification, anti-fungal therapy, food intolerance testing, reflorestation with probiotics and healing of the gut wall. This is done through a careful food programme, pulse challenge test, stress management and a supportive on-going dialogue. Mon-Thu 9am-5pm.
Initial Consultation: £28-00 / 1hr
Subsequent visits: £23-00 / 1 hr

DEVON

Sue Griffin, KFRP FICGT MIACT MBAPS
Natural Health Practice, 2 Spicer Road, Exeter, Devon EX1 1SX ☎01392-832 005
Kinesiology, Colour Therapy.
Sue uses S.E.T (a Kinesiology technique) to teach the body to regulate the levels of candida istelf. She is also a trained yoga teacher and treats ME. Mon-Wed 10am-5pm.
Initial Consultation: £25-00 / 1½ hrs
Subsequent visits: £20-00 / 1 hr

Derek Wolfe, DBM DiplSc ND BNA MCIA
"Newton Mill", Newton-St Petrock, Holsworthy, Devon EX22 7LP ☎01409-281 454 (& Fax) 0378-673 983 (Mobile)
Naturopathy, Oxygen Therapy, Colonic Hydrotherapy, Herbal Medicine.
Derek is a qualified Heilpraktiker (Holistic Therapist) in Germany (1982). He also treats ME and sometimes uses Nystatin. All week & weekends.
Initial Consultation: Free / 1½-2 hrs
Subsequent visits: £30-00 / 1 hr

Dr Dorothy West, MRCS ENG LRCP MFHom FH BSENM
Rutt House, Ivybridge, Devon PL21 0DQ
☎01752-892 792 Fax 896 547
Homoeopathy, Nutrition, Kinesiology.
Dr West has been in practice for nearly 40 years. She also treats ME. Mon-Fri 9am-5.30pm; Sat 9am-12.30pm.
Initial Consultation: £50-00 / 1 hr
Subsequent visits: £25-00 / ½ hr

Michael Ash, DO DipION MCO
The Eldon Health Clinic, 20 South Road, Newton Abbot, Devon TQ12 1HO ☎01626-332 574
Osteopathy, Nutrition, Naturopathy, Clinical Testings.

Michael also treats ME. Mon-Fri 9am-6pm.
Initial Consultation: £25-00 / ½ hr
Subsequent visits: £20-00 / 20-30 mins

DORSET

Martin L Budd, ND DO LicAc MRO
29 Ferncroft Road, Bournemouth BH10 6BY
☎01202-578 640
Osteopathy, Naturopathy, Acupuncture.
Martin has a special interest in functional hypo-glycaemia and also treats ME. Mon/Fri 9.30am-5.30pm; Wed 2-9pm.
Initial Consultation: £25-35 / ½-1 hr
Subsequent visits: £20-00 / 20 mins.

Dr D K Owen, MBBS MRCS LRCP
MFHom
Bowood House, 3 Wellington Road, Bournemouth
BH8 8JQ ☎01202-558 986
Homoeopathic Physician, Dietary Therapy, Supplements.
Dr Owen is a homoeopathic physician who also treats ME. By appointment.
Initial Consultation: £65-00 / 1hr
Subsequent visits: £35-00 / 20 mins

Dr Robert C Kelvinson, PhD RGN
RCT BSc (Hons) DHM ND (USA) DSc (India)
IFR
Dorset Natural Health Clinic, 32A Wessex Road
Parkstone, Poole, Dorset BH14 8BQ
☎01202-717 727
Naturopathy, Diet, Herbal Medicine, Homoeopathy.
First Tue of every month.
Initial Consultation: £25-00 / 1 hr
Subsequent visits: £18-50 / ½ hr

Janet Andrew, DiplON MLSR
4 Greenwood Avenue, Lilliput, Poole, Dorset
BH14 8QD ☎01202-707 074
Reflexology, Nutrition, Supplements.
Flexible appointments.
Initial Consultation: £20-00 / 1 hr
Subsequent visits: £10-00 / ½ hr

Bill Rhys, DiplSM MBSR PKP
6 Church Street, Poole, Dorset BH15 1JP
☎01202-678 947
PKP Kinesiology, Stress Management, Reflexology, Dowsing.
Anytime by phone. Clinic Tuesdays.
Initial Consultation: £15-00 / 1 hr
Subsequent visits: £15-00 / 1 hr

EAST SUSSEX

Penny Davenport, RNT
Woodlands, London Road, Battle, E Sussex
TN33 0LP ☎01424-774 103
Nutrition, Supplements, Herbal Medicine.
Penny also offers extensive laboratory testing for food sensitivity, candida and helico-bacter, as well as various kinds of literature.
Mon-Wed.
Initial Consultation: £30-00 / 1½ hrs.
Subsequent visits: £15-00 / 1 hr

Anya Harris
Shamballa Healing Centre, 4 Little East Street,
Brighton BN1 1HT ☎01273-724 172
(Nutrition), Healing, (Colour Therapy).
Anya is and experienced healer and has in-depth knowledge of treating candida, having suffered herself. She was a founder member of the Candida Support Group at All Hallows House.
Support Group Co-ordinator. Wed/Thu.
Initial Consultation: £25-00 / 1-1½ hrs
Subsequent visits: £15-00 / ½ hr

Sharon Kaye, DiplON
'Healing Hands', 10 Bond Street, Brighton
BN1 1RD ☎01273-601 140/735 323
Nutrition, Supplements, Herbal Remedies.
Ms Kaye also offers extensive laboratory testing for food sensitivity, candida and helicobacter, as well as various kinds of literature. Concessions

available. By appointment.
Initial Consultation: £25-00 / 1hr-1hr 15 mins
Subsequent visits: £18-00 / 45 mins

Matthew Bennett, DC
The Sundial House Chiropractic Clinic, 118
Queens Road, Brighton BN1 3XF
☎01273-774 114
Chiropractic, Kinesiology, Nutrition.
Mon/Tue/Thu/Fri 10am-7pm; Wed/Sat 9am-2pm.
Initial Consultation: £28-00 / 40 mins
Subsequent visits: £22-00 / 20 mins

Penny Davenport, RNT
The Nutrition Line, Burwash Common, E Sussex
TN19 7LX ☎Enq: 01435-882 964
Premium: 0891-615 522
*Nutrition, Supplements, Herbal
Medicine.*
Penny both sees people for individual
consultations at the Higher Nature clinic and
consults over the phone. She also offers
extensive laboratory testing for food sensitivity,
candida and helicobacter, as well as various kinds
of literature.
Initial Consultation: £35-00 / 1 hr
Subsequent visits: £20-00 / 1 hr

Penny Fox, DiplON
7 East Drive, Brighton BN2 2BQ
☎01273-684 141
Nutrition, Supplements.
Penny specialises in ME. Mon-Fri 10am-7pm.
Initial Consultation: £25-00 / 1½ hrs
Subsequent visits: £15-00 / 30-45 mins

Sharon Kaye, DiplON
The Nutrition Line, Burwash Common, E Sussex
TN19 7LX ☎Enq: 01435-882 964
Premium: 0891-615 522
*Nutrition, Supplements, Herbal
Remedies.*
Sharon both sees people for individual
consultations at the Higher Nature clinic and
consults over the phone. She also offers
extensive laboratory. She also ofters extensive
laboratory testing for food sensitivity, candida and
helicobacter, as well as various kinds of literature.

Concessions available. Mon-Wed 10am-7pm,
occasional Sat.
Initial Consultation: £35-00 / 1-1½ hrs
Subsequent visits: £20-00 / 1 hr pro rata.

Dyan Wilson, DNMed DIrid DR BANMA
"Munnings", Shepherds Hill, Buxted, E Sussex
TN22 4PX ☎01825-890 582
*Naturopathic Diet, Herbal Medicine,
Homoeopathy.*
Mon-Sat 9am-12 noon.
Initial Consultation: £30-00 / 2 hrs
Subsequent visits: £20-00 / 30-45 mins

Judy Richardson, DThD DNMed
'Stepping Stones', Saxonbury Close,
Crowborough, E Sussex TN6 1EA
☎01892-662 374
*Dietary Therapy, Supplements, (Naturo-
pathy).*
Judy is an ex-sufferer of chronic fatigue, migraine, candida and gut dysbiosis and therefore
has first-hand knowledge of and can advise
patients on the healing power of good nutrition and
supplements, colonic hydrotherapy; chiropractic,
homoeopathy and counseling. She treats each
client individually, giving on-going support during
their healing journey.
Mon-Fri 8.30am-9pm; Saturdays if required.
Initial Consultation: £20-00 / 2½ hrs
Subsequent visits: £10-00 / 1 hr

Miss E Williams, BSc DiplON
Flat 27, Arlington House, Upperton Road,
Eastbourne BN21 1LR ☎01323-733 133
*Nutrition/Diet, Supplements,
Counselling.*
Miss Williams has worked with Dr Belinda Dawes,
who specialises in ME and is now working with
GPs in Polegate, Hastings and Alfriston. She also
treats privately chronic fatigue, irritable bowel
syndrome and candidiasis. Fee for the third visit
onwards is £12-50.
Mon-Sat 10am-5pm.
Initial Consultation: £25-00 / 1 hr
Subsequent visits: £20-00 / 45 mins

Ben Edwards, MNIMH FDZ Ass.BAFATT
Herbal Health Clinic, Place Farm Cottages
Fairlight Place, Hastings, E Sussex TN35 5DT
☎**01424-812 761**
Herbal Medicine, Massage, Reflexology,
Healing. Ben also treats ME. Wed-Sun 7.30am-
9pm.
Initial Consultation: £23-00 / 1 hr
(Concessions).
Subsequent visits: £12-00 / ½ hr (Concessions)

Anya Harris
Complementary Health Centres, 73 Western
Road, Hove, E Sussex ☎**01273-724 172**
(Nutrition), Healing, (Colour Therapy).
Anya is an experienced healer and has in-depth
knowledge of treating candida, having suffered
herself. She was a founder member of the Can-
dida Support Group at All Hallows House.
Support Group Co-ordinator.
Available Mondays.
Initial Consultation: £25-00 / 1-1½ hrs
Subsequent visits: £15-00 / ½ hr

Roberta Morgan, DiplON
Flint House, 41 High Street, Lewes, E Sussex
BN7 2LU ☎**01273-473 388**
Nutrition, Iridology, Dowsing.
Roberta also treats ME. Thu 9.30am-3.30pm.
Initial Consultation: £25-00 / 1 hr
Subsequent visits: £18-00 / ½ hr

Ben Edwards, MNIMH FDZ Ass.BAFATT
Rye Osteopathic Practice, 16 Ferry Road, Rye,
E Sussex TN31 7DN ☎**01797-225 099**
Herbal Medicine, Massage, Reflexology,
Healing.
Ben also treats ME. Mon 9am-7pm.
Initial Consultation: £23-00 / 1 hr (Concessions)
Subsequent visits: £12-00 / ½ hr (Concessions)

William Balcombe, LCH
Kings Road Natural Health Clinic, St Leonards-
on-Sea, E Sussex TN37 6EA
☎**01424-714 800**
Homoeopathy, Nutrition, Supplements.
Many local GPs who have no effective treatment
for the various gut/digestive/candida problems etc.

recommend their patients to Mr Balcombe, who is
himself a sometime sufferer from candida and
IBS. He also treats ME. Tue-Fri all day.
Initial Consultation: £35-00 / 1½ hrs
Subsequent visits: £20-00 / 45 mins

Roberta Morgan, DiplON
15 London Road, Uckfield, E Sussex TN22 1JB
☎**01825-767 168**
Nutrition, Iridology, Dowsing.
Roberta also treats ME. Mon/Tue/Wed/Fri
9.30am-5pm and 7pm.
Initial Consultation: £25-00 / 1 hr
Subsequent visits: £18-00 / ½ hr

ESSEX

Lesley Croft, ITEC AIPTI
Gloucester Park Swimming Pool, Broadmayne,
Basildon, Essex SS14 2EV ☎**01268-767 727**
Nutrition/Diet, Aromatherapy,
Reflexology.
Tue-Thu 1.30-8.30pm; Sat 10.30am-1.30pm.
Initial Consultation: £15-£25 / 45-75 mins
Subsequent visits: £15-£25 / 45-75 mins

M F Chen, MA Oxon DCHM LicAc
Westbury, 2Cliff Way, Frinton-on-Sea, Essex
CO13 9NL ☎**01255-675 526**
Acupressure, Acupuncture, Chinese
Herbal Medicine, Supplements.
Ms Chen also treats ME. **Support Group Initial**
Contact. 15th of every month to end of month, by
appointment only.
Initial Consultation: £15-00 / 1 hr
Subsequent visits: £15-00 / 1 hr

Julia Johnson, ASK
43 Woodside, Leigh-on-Sea, Essex SS7 4QX
☎**01702-525 391**
Kinesiology. Tue-Fri.
Initial Consultation: £30-00 / 2 hrs
Subsequent visits: £20-00 / 1½ hrs

Erica White, DiplON
22 Leigh Hall Road, Leigh-on-Sea, Essex
SS9 1RN ☎**01702-720 85**

Nutrition, Supplements.

Erica has a very busy practice; she uses a detailed questionnaire for postal and personal consultations with careful analysis of answers. Fees include professional report plus audiotape and three months' support, followed by re-assessment and advice. An ex-sufferer herself, Erica is author of "Beat Candida Cookbook", lecturer and tutor at the Institute for Optimum Nutrition and a committed Christian. She also has many ME. patients.
Mon-Fri 9am-12; 2pm-5pm.
Initial Consultation: £45-00 / 1 hr
Subsequent visits: £45-00 / 1 hr

Dr Kai Kermani, MB BS LRCP MRCS DRCOG MRCGP

10 Connaught Hill, Loughton, Essex IG10 4DU
☎0181-508 9712
Spiritual Healing, Holistic General Practice, Autogenic Training.
Dr Kermani offers concessionary fees. He is the author of 'Autogenic Training; the effective way to conquer stress', published by Thorson's. He also treats ME. Every day;
Mon/Tue/Thu until 10 pm.
Initial Consultation: £20-00 / 1½ hrs
Subsequent visits: £20-00 / 1½ hrs

Susan Allshorn, NIMH

'Hillside', Clay Tye Road, Ockendon, Essex RN14 3PL ☎01708-226 061
Herbal Medicine, Supplements, (Counselling).
Susan also treats ME. By arrangement.
Initial Consultation: £30-00 / 1½ hrs
Subsequent visits: £15-00 / 45 mins

GLOUCESTERSHIRE

Carol Townend, DipION MIIR MIAT

Natural Therapy Centre, 24 Castle Street, Cirencester, Glos. GL7 5PR ☎01285-656 393
Reflexology, Nutrition, Allergy Testing.
Carol also treats ME. Mon 9am-1.30pm; Wed 9am-6pm; Thu 2pm-6pm.
Initial Consultation: £30-00 / 1hr
Subsequent visits: £20-00 / 45 mins

HAMPSHIRE

Dr Anthony Dunstan Fox, BSc

MBBS DCH DRCOG RCGP
54 Barton Court Avenue, Barton-on-Sea, Hants.
BH25 7HG ☎01425-618 801
Homoeopathy, Diet, Herbs, Vega Test, Bach Flower Remedies.
Dr Fox treats a large number of patients with ME.
Mon/Wed; some Sats.
Initial Consultation: £46-00 / 40 mins
Subsequent visits: £30-00 / 20 mins

Richard W. Block, DipION LCSP

AccHyp NCP
'Integration', 42 Kingsway, Chandler's Ford, Hants. SO53 1EN ☎01703-266 263
Massage, Hypnotherapy, Nutrition.
Richard integrates nutrition, massage and hypnotherapy to encourage the body to attain homeostasis, the state in which the complex mechanisms of the body permit it to adapt continually to the various stresses and pressures which assaults it from all sides, inwardly and outwardly.
Mon-Fri 9.30am-630pm; Sat/Sun emergencies only.
Initial Consultation: £30-00 / 1 hr
Subsequent visits: £20-00 / ½ hr

Dr Anthony Dunstan Fox, BSc

MBBS DCH DRCOG RCGP
The Wessex Nuffield Hospital, Winchester Road, Chandler's Ford, Eastleigh, Hants. SO5 2DW
☎01703-266 377
Homoeopathy, Diet, Herbs, Vega Test, Bach Flower Remedies.
Dr Fox treats a large number of patients with ME.
Tuesdays.
Initial Consultation: £46-00 / 40 mins
Subsequent visits: £30-00 / 20 mins

Dedj Leibbrandt, MNIMH

75 Newtown Road, Eastleigh, Hants. SO50 9BX
☎1703-619 776
Herbal Medicine, Naturopathy,Nutrition.
Dedj has trained as a nurse and also treats ME.
Mon-Thu 9am-5pm.
Initial Consultation: £30-00 / 1½ hrs
Subsequent visits: £15-00 / ½ hr

Keith Mason, PhD BRCP
The Mill House, Breamore, Fordingbridge, Hants.
SP6 2AF ☎01725-513 018
Radionics, Metaphysical Assessment,
Element Therapy, Celloid Minerals, Diet,
Homoeopathy.
Keith investigates the underlying biochemical and
metaphysical (ie energetic or pre-physical) influ-
ences on your character. These may include
electromagnetic fields. Suggestions for treatment
will often be at an energetic level. Keith has written
and researched widely on omplementary
medicine. He also treats ME. Mon-Fri 11am-5pm.
Initial Consultation: £45-00 / 1 hr
Subsequent visits: £17-50 / ½ hr

Martin L Budd, ND DO LicAc MRO
Keston North, Greenlands, Lymington, Hants.
SO41 8BB ☎01590-676 117
Osteopathy, Naturopathy, Acupuncture.
Martin has a special interest in functional hypo-
glycaemia and also treats ME. Tue 9.30am-
5.30pm; Thu 9.30am-12.30pm.
Initial Consultation: £25-35 / ½-1hr
Subsequent visits: £20-00 / 20 mins

Anne Donelan, DHH CertEd DipCN MIAT
18 Whitefield Road, New Milton, Hants.
BH25 6DF ☎01425-638 474
Kinesiology, Nutrition, Allergy Testing.
Anne is very aware of the need to detoxify gently,
especially where depression is involved. She also
treats for co-habiting parasites. **Support Group**
Initial Contact. Available two days a week -
flexible.
Initial Consultation: £22-£24 / 2 hrs
Subsequent visits: £20-00 / 1½-2 hrs

Ann Rowland, DipION MNCA
Old Bell Cottage, Rogate, Petersfield, Hants.
GU31 5EF ☎01730-821 725 (& Fax)
Nutrition, Bach Flower Remedies.
Anne also treats ME. **Support Group Co-**
ordinator. By Appointment.
Initial Consultation: £30-00 / 1 hr
Subsequent visits: £18-00 / ½ hr

Anne Smithells, DO MGO MIFA EHP
NLP
BioTech Health and Nutrition Centre, 12 High
Street, Petersfield, Hants. GU32 3JG
☎01730-233 414
Iridology, Electro-Dermal Screening,
Osteopathy, (Manual Lymphatic
Drainage).
Anne uses massage for lymphatic drainage. She
also uses the LISTEN system, a sophisticated
computer screening device that checks the body
for food sensitivities and vitamin/mineral defi-
ciencies. This may allow the patient a more lenient
'candida diet'. Full body screenings are also
available to detect metal, virus, bacteria, parasites
and fungus toxicity. Mon-Fri 9.30am-6pm
Saturday by appointment only.
Initial Consultation: £55-00 / 1 hr
Subsequent visits: £30-00 / 45 mins

Richard W. Block, DipION LCSP
AccHyp NCP, 'Integration', The Mill, Shawford,
Hants. SO21 2BP ☎01703-266 263
Massage, Hypnotherapy, Nutrition.
Richard integrates nutrition, massage and hypno-
therapy to encourage the body to attain homeo-
stasis, the state in which the complex
mechanisms of the body permit it to adapt
continually to the various stresses and pressures
which assaults it from all sides, inwardly and
outwardly.
Wed 9.30am-6.30pm.
Initial Consultation: £30-00 / 1hr
Subsequent visits: £20-00 / ½ hr

Dr Julian K Kenyon, MB ChB MD
FRCS BMAS BSAEM
The Centre for Study of Complementary Medicine,
51 Bedford Place, Southampton SO15 2DT
☎01703-334 752
Homoeopathy, Acupuncture,
Manipulative Therapy, Herbal Medicine.
Dr Kenyon practises complex and classical
homoeopathy as well as environmental medicine.
Patients wishing to see him on the NHS must
have a GP referral under special funding
arrangements. He sees hundreds of ME. patients
and has researched widely. (He has a 4 week
waiting list in London, 2-3 in Southampton.)
Mon/Wed/Thu/Fri 9am-4.30pm.
Initial Consultation: £42-00 / 15 mins
Subsequent visits: £42-00 / 15 mins

George T Lewith, BA MB BChir MRCP
MRCGP DM
The Centre for the Study of Complementary
Medicine, 51 Bedford Place, Southampton
SO15 2DT ☎01703-334 752
*Environmental Medicine, Homoeopathy,
Herbal Medicine.*
Dr Lewith recommends drugs for about about
20% of his candida patients. Patients wishing to
see him on the NHS must have a GP referral
under special funding arrangements. He has
written and lectured extensively on com-
plementary medicine. Five days a week.
Initial Consultation: £42-00 / 15 mins
Subsequent visits: £42-00 / 15 mins

Dr Erik B Holm, DC ND
Simcoe Clinic, 29 Archers Road, Southampton
SO16 2NB ☎01703-227 200
*Chiropractic, Nutrition, Naturopathic
Diet, Herbal Remedies, Homoeopathic
Remedies.*
Mon/Wed/Thu 8.45am-8pm; Tue/Fri 9am-6pm.
Initial Consultation: £20-00 / Varies.
Subsequent visits: £17-00 / Varies.

Dr Deborah Thomson, MB BChir
LicAc MAc
7 St James Terrace, Winchester, Hants.
SO22 4PP ☎01962-865 560
Acupuncture.
Dr Thomson is a medical doctor practising pri-
vately as an acupuncturist. All week.
Initial Consultation: £60-00 / 1-1½ hrs
Subsequent visits: £30-00 / ½ hr approx.

Dr D K Owen, MBBS MRCS LRCP
MFHom
Bradford House, 106 Stockbridge Road,
Winchester, Hants. SO22 6RL
☎01962-856 310
*Homoeopathic Physician, Dietary
Therapy, Supplements.*
Dr Owen is a homoeopathic physician who also
treats ME. By appointment.
Initial Consultation: £65-00 / 1 hr
Subsequent visits: £35-00 / 20 mins

Jane Colebourn, DipAdEd
Winchester Natural Therapy Centre, 6 Hatherley
Road, Winchester, Hants. SO22 6RT
☎01962-866 302 Fax: 01962-884 466
Reflexology, Reiki, Polarity Therapy.
Treatment has an ayuervedic influence and is
tailored to individual needs often involving other
practitioners, eg homoeopaths and chiropractors.
Jane is trained in reflexology by Janice Ellacott
and also treats ME. **Support Group Initial
Contact.**
Initial Consultation: £30-00 / 2 hrs
Subsequent visits: £20-00 / 1 hr

HEREFORDSHIRE

Liz Thearle, DipION
2 Wye Gnat Cottage, Lane Head, Eaton Bishop,
Herefordshire HR2 9QE ☎01981-251 780
*Nutrition, Allergy Testing,
Aromatherapy.*
Liz also treats ME. Mon/Thu/Fri (Variable).
Initial Consultation: £30-00 / 1 hr
Subsequent visits: £20-00 / ½ hr

Liz Thearle, DipION
The Hereford Centre for Natural Health,
Eastholme Avenue, Belmont, Hereford
HR2 7XT ☎01432-279 653
*Nutrition, Allergy Testing,
Aromatherapy.*
Liz also treats ME. Tue/Wed 9am-7pm.
Initial Consultation: £30-00 / 1 hr
Subsequent visits: £20-00 / ½ hr

HERTFORDSHIRE

Jacqueline Young, BAAR
"In Essence", Hadley Works, Old Fold Lane,
Hadley Highstone, Herts. EN5 4QN
☎0181-449 7771
*Oriental Medicine, Nutrition, Self-care
techniques.*
'Healthcheck' offers total health consultations
utilising the Japanese AMI diagnostic device to
assess immune function; nervous system imbalance; energy levels; internal organ function,
acupuncture meridians and spinal alignment. The
test is simple, non-invasive and very accurate.

Treatment and self-care recommendations are given based on the test results. Jacqueline also treats ME. Wed and occasional Sat.
Initial Consultation: £35-00 / 1 hr
Subsequent visits: £25-00 / ½ hr

Elizabeth Halford, BSc (Hons) DO MCO
Osteopathic Practice, 145 Bengeo Street,
Hertford SG14 3EY ☎01992-586 294
Osteopathy, Naturopathy, Nutrition.
Elizabeth also treats ME. Mon-Fri 9am-6pm.
Initial Consultation: £25-00 / 45 mins
Subsequent visits: £20-00 / ½ hr

Roger Newman Turner, BAc ND DO
MRO MRN
111 Norton Way South, Letchworth, Herts.
SG6 1NY ☎01462-684 232
Osteopathy, Naturopathy, Acupuncture, Clinical Tests.
Roger recommends drugs to about 10% of his patients. He is the author of many best selling books and the chairman of the Research Council for Complementary Medicine.
Tue/Thu/Fr.
Initial Consultation: £36-00 / 45 mins
Subsequent visits: £22-00 / ½ hr

Alison Davies, BSc (Hons) MNIMH
Healthwise Clinic, Old Police Station, 8 Priory Lane, Royston, Herts. SG8 9DU
☎01763-247 944
Herbal Medicine, Nutrition, Aroma-therapy.
Herbs combined with natural nutritional remedies, which aids the holistic dimensions of improving the vital force and balancing the emotional aspects of the condition. Alison also treats ME. Wednes-days.
Initial Consultation: £25-00 / 1 hr
Subsequent visits: £12-50 / ½ hr

Katie Bolland, DThD GNI
22 Heathfield Road, Bushey, Watford, Herts.
WD2 2LJ ☎01923-222 327
Nutrition, Iridology, Colonic Hydrotherapy.
A consultation with Katie consists of iris diagnosis and a photo of the eye serving as a record. A

detailed case history is taken and the client may be referred for tests to his/her doctor or an independent laboratory. Advice on diet, supplements and probiotics is individual. Colonic therapy is optional but usually highly recommended. Tue/Thu.
Initial Consultation: £40 approx / 1½ hrs
Subsequent visits: £30 approx / 1 hr

HUMBERSIDE

Rex E Newnham, PhD ND DO DHom
6 The Cloisters, Grimsby, Humberside
DN37 9QX ☎01472-882 074
Mineral Nutrition, Homoeopathy, Herbal Medicine. By arrangement.
Initial Consultation: £25-00 / 1 hr
Subsequent visits: £5-£30 / Varies

Trudy Norris, BA ITEC NIMH
93 Morwell Road, Scunthorpe, Humberside
DN17 2SX ☎01724-867 385
Herbal Extracts, Supplements, Essential Oils, Topical Preparations.
Mon-Fri 9am-5pm
Initial Consultation: £25-00
Subsequent visits: £10-00

KENT

Kirsten Blaikie, DiplON
24 Mount Pleasant, Aylesford, Kent ME20 7BE
☎01622-719 409
Dietary Therapy, Supplements.
Mon-Fri 9am-9pm.
Initial Consultation: £25-00 / 1 hr
Subsequent visits: £10-00 / ½ hr

Mary Cannon, DiplON CertEd
CertHealthEd
8 South Canterbury Road, Canterbury, Kent
CT1 3LJ ☎01227-470 111
Nutrition, Vega Tests, Supplements.
Most days. Mon-Fri 9am-8pm; Sat morning.
Initial Consultation: £20-£30 / 1 hr
Subsequent visits: £10-£15 / ½ hr

Jon Leigh, ND DO MRN
Canterbury Clinic of Herbal Medicine,
15 Ethelbert Road, Canterbury, Kent CT1 3ND
☎01227-766 797
Naturopathy, Osteopathy.
Jon also treats ME. Tue pm, Fri am.
Initial Consultation: £22-00 / ½ hr min.
Subsequent visits: £22-00 / ½ hr min.

James Jewell, BSc ITEC MRS
Complementary Health Practice,
11 Earls Avenue, Folkestone, Kent CT20 2HW
☎01303-850 234
Reflexology, Celloid Mineral Therapy, Nutrition, Herbal Medicine.
James had ME for three years and is now totally healed, thus having invaluable experience in the field of ME and candida. He offers empathy, inspiration and understanding towards fellow sufferers. In his experience an energetic approach (Reflexology) plus nutritional support provide the best results. He is also a Samaritan. Tue 9am-12 noon Thu 2pm-5pm; Fri/Sat 9am-5pm.
Initial Consultation: £28-00 / 1½ hrs
Subsequent visits: £20-00 / 1 hr

Jon Leigh, ND DO MRN
Gillingham Clinic of Complementary Medicine,
50 Watling Street, Gillingham, Kent ME7 2YN
☎01634-576 292
Naturopathy, Osteopathy.
Jon also treats ME. Mon/Tue/Sat am; Wed am & pm; Thu pm.
Initial Consultation: £22-00 / ½ hr min.
Subsequent visits: £22-00 / ½ hr min

Amanda Reuter, DiplON MRNT MNCA
Riseden Cottage, Goudhurst, Kent TN17 1HJ
☎01580-212 207
Nutrition, Supplements.
Amanda uses laboratory testing to detect systemic candidiasis as well as urine checks for bowel toxicity. **Support Group Initial Contact.** Wed 9am-1pm; Fri 9am-5pm; eves 6-9pm; some Sats.
Initial Consultation: £25-00 / 1 hr
Subsequent visits: £15-00 / ½ hr

Kirsten Blaikie, DiplON
Lifeforce, Roderick O'Driscoll & Partners
23 Union Street, Maidstone, Kent ME14 1EB
☎01622-690 444
Dietary Therapy, Supplements.
Thu, by appointment only.
Initial Consultation: £25-00 / 1 hr
Subsequent visits: £10-00 / ½ hr

Mary Cannon, DiplON CertEd CertHealthEd
Hawley Health Centre, 7-9 Hawley Square, Margate, Kent CT9 1PF ☎01843-292 056
Nutrition, Vega Tests, Supplements.
Mon/Wed afternoon.
Initial Consultation: £25-£30 / 1 hr
Subsequent visits: £12-50 / ½ hr

Sherridan L. Stock, BSc (Hons) CBiol IOB ASK BCMA MIBiol
Medway Clinic of Nutritional and Bioenergic Medicine, 28 The Precinct, Rainham, Kent ME8 7HW ☎01634-362 267
Vitamin/Mineral Therapy, Herbal Medicine, Kinesiology.
A Chartered Biologist, Mr Stock has developed relevant products for Nutriscene. He is also scientific adviser for the Society for the Promotion of Nutritional Therapy and professional Member of the Association of Systematic Kinesiology.
Support Group Initial Contact. Tue/Thu/Fri.
Initial Consultation: £47-00 / 1 hr, pro rata incl. VAT.
Subsequent visits: £47-00 / 1 hr, pro rata incl. VAT.

Gaynor Greber, DipNut DiplON MNCA
'Clemency', 5 The Shambles, Sevenoaks, Kent TN13 1AL ☎01732-450 049
Candida Questionnaire, Nutrition, Supplements.
Thu 9am-2pm or home visits any day.
Initial Consultation: £30-00 / 1 hr
Subsequent visits: £22-00 / ½ hr

Christine Todd, DNMed DIrid IFADip
BAMA IFA
Kemsing, Sevenoaks, Kent TN15 6PA
☎01732-762 999
Naturopathic Diet, Supplements,
Aromatherapy.
Supplements include nutritional, herbal and
homoeopathic remedies. Aromatherapy may also
be used. Mon-Fri 9am-6pm.
Initial Consultation: £35-00 / 2 hrs
Subsequent visits: £20-00 / 30-45 mins

Amanda Reuter, DiplON MRNT MNCA
'Metabolics', 14 Mount Pleasant Road, Tunbridge
Wells, Kent TN1 1QU
☎01892-542 609
Nutrition, Supplements.
Amanda uses laboratory testing to detect sys-
temic candidiasis as well as urine checks for
bowel toxicity. Mon/Tue/Thu 9am-5pm.
Initial Consultation: £45-00 / 1 hr
Subsequent visits: £45-00 / per hour, pro rata.

Lynda Vaughan, RAWNutDip ITEC
St Marks Clinic of Natural Medicine, 65 Frant
Road, Tunbridge Wells, Kent TN2 5LH
☎0892-541 161/01483-761 312
Nutrition, Iridology, Kinesiology.
Thu 1pm-6pm.
Initial Consultation: £40-00 / 1½ hrs
Subsequent visits: £20-00 / ½ hr

Dr E Schellander, MD (Vienna) LMSSA
(London)
Liongate Clinic, 8 Chilston Road, Tunbridge
Wells, Kent TN4 9LT ☎01892-543 535
Fax: 01892-545 160
Chelation Therapy, Medical Ozone,
Orthomolecular Medicine.
Dr Scellander recommends drugs and also treats
ME. Mon-Fri 9am-5pm.
Initial Consultation: £60-00 / 1 hr
Subsequent visits: £60-00 / 1 hr, pro rata.

LANCASHIRE

Helen Duxbury, MNIMH RGN RHV
74 New Bank Road, Blackburn, Lancs. BB2 6JW
☎01254-261 026
Medical Herbalism, Diet, Supplements.
Support Group Initial Contact. Most days.
Initial Consultation: £25-00 / 1 hr
Subsequent visits: £15-00 / ½ hr

Marian Whitsey, RIr RCTh SI MHA
21 York Street, Clitheroe, Lancs. BB7 2DH
☎01200-442 102
Iridology, Celloid Mineral Therapy,
Homoeopathy.
You may be able to see Marian on the NHS. Mon-
Fri 9am-5.30pm; Sat 9am-12.30pm.
Initial Consultation: £35-00 / 1 hr
Subsequent visits: £19-95 / ½ hr

Janet Fazackerley, DHD
The Marian Whitsey Practice, 21 York Street,
Clitheroe, Lancs. BB7 2DH ☎01200-442 102
Dietary Therapy, Nutrition, Reiki.
Ms Fazackerley has found that dietary treatment
alone is not enough to treat candida. Her pro-
gramme combining nutritional and herbal supple-
mentation with a specialised diet aims to ease
symptoms and improve the patient's health in the
shortest possible time. She also treats ME. Mon-
Thu 9am-5.30pm.
Initial Consultation: £39-95 incl. VAT / 1 hr
Subsequent visits: £19-95 incl. VAT / ½ hr

Dr Vincent G Mainey, MB BS MRCGP
DRCOG PSI
Withnell Health Centre, Withnell, Nr Chorley,
Lancs. PR6 8UA ☎01254-831 877
Allopathy, Homoeopathy, Acupuncture.
Dr Mainey also offers Bach flower remedies,
organo-therapy, shiatsu and auricular therapy. He
sees patients on the NHS. His private patients
tend not to receive allopathic care, but benefit
from the more effective naturopathic treatments,
though he does also recommend drugs for most
cases of candida. (He has a 2 week waiting list).
Mon/Wed/Thu/Fri 11-1pm; Mon/Wed 3-4pm.
Initial Consultation: £40-00 / 40 mins
Subsequent visits: £30-00 / 30 mins

Dr Vincent G Mainey, MB BS MRCGP
DRCOG PSI
Landau Chapel Lane, Hoghton, Preston, Lancs.
PR5 0RY ☎01254-853 605
Allopathy, Homoeopathy, Acupuncture.
Dr Mainey also offers Bach flower remedies, organo-therapy, shiatsu and auricular therapy. He sees patients on the NHS. His private patients tend not to receive allopathic care, but benefit from the more effective naturopathic treatments, though he does also recommend drugs for most cases of candida. (He has a 2 week waiting list).
Tue 10am-12pm; & 1.30-4pm.
Initial Consultation: £40-00 / 40 mins
Subsequent visits: £30-00 / 30 mins

LEICESTERSHIRE

Ann Chester, MNIMH
12 Watson Avenue, Market Harborough,
LE16 9NA ☎01858-431 929
Herbal Medicine, Nutrition, Bach Flower Remedies.
The aim of the treatment is to treat the whole person, as the suppression of symptoms will not rid the body of disease. The use of different remedies to restore the balance of the body enables it to harness its own healing powers. Ann also treats ME. **Support Group Co-ordinator.**
8.30am-5pm, plus evenings if required.
Initial Consultation: £30-00 / 1½ hrs
Subsequent visits: £15-00 / 45 mins

LINCOLNSHIRE

Anne Betz, MNIMH
Eastview, Donington Road, Kirton End, Boston, Lincs. PE20 1PB ☎01205-724 054
Medical Herbalism, Dietary Advice.
Anne also treats ME. Mon-Thu 9am-7pm; Fri 9am-4pm; Sun 10am-6pm.
Initial Consultation: £30-00 / 1 hr
Subsequent visits: £15-00 / ½ hr

Vivienne Bradshaw, MRNT
3 Maltings Cottages, Gonerby Hill Foot, Grantham, Lincs. NG31 8JF ☎01476-67 420
Kinesiology, Vega Tests, Nutrition, Manual Lymphatic Drainage, (Homoe-
opathy).
Ms Bradshaw is a health consultant who also practises Emotional Stress Release and Lymphatic Drainage. By appointment only. Some eves and weekends.
Initial Consultation: £20-00 / 1 hr
Subsequent visits: Pro rata / Variable.

Mrs Jo Hampton, MRNT
46 Wainfleet Road, Skegness, Lincs. PE25 3QT
☎01754-768 336
Nutrition/Diet, Vega Test, Aromatherapy, Counselling.
Jo Hampton specialises in candida, ME and allergies and has published articles and books on her own work. She began treating herself 20 years ago and is now known for her success in treating inflammatory bowel diseases by natural means, eg Crohn's and colitis. IBS also responds to her treatment. She has her own nutritional formula. Weekdays 1-5.30pm. Answerphone 24 hrs.
Initial Consultation: £35-00 / 40 mins
Subsequent visits: £25-00 / 40 mins

Mrs Sue Fuller, DHom FIGN (Med)
Church Farm, Great Hale, Sleaford, Lincs.
NG34 9LL ☎01529-460 536
Vibronics Homoeopathy, Vitamin/Mineral Therapy, Bach Flower Remedies.
The treatment involves the use of specially formulated homoeopathic preparations, known as Vibronics, at £2 a bottle.
Initial Consultation: £25-00 / 1 hr at least.
Subsequent visits: £10-00 / ½-1 hr

Annette Rawlings, MIr ISPA
The Coxon Clinic, 7 London Road, Spalding, Lincs. PE11 2TA ☎01775-710 734
Nutrition, Iridology, Aromatherapy.
Ms Rawlings is trained in nutrition and iridology and also practises aromatherapy. She is especially interested in detecting health imbalance due to vitamin/mineral deficiencies and problems relating to the gut, eg malabsorbtion and candidiasis. By appointment.
Initial Consultation: £35-00 / 1½ hrs
Subsequent visits: £20-00 / 1 hr

CENTRAL LONDON

Dr Siggy Trefzer, MSc MD MFHom
All Hallows House Centre for Natural Health and Counselling, Idol Lane, London EC3R 5DD
☎0171-283 8908
Naturopathy, Osteopathy, Nutrition.
Siggy is a medical doctor with an eclectic and integrated knowledge of natural medicine. He also sees many patients with ME. Thursdays.
Initial Consultation: £40-00 / 1 hr
Subsequent visits: £35-00 / 45 mins

Gillian Hamer, BSc DipCNS MAR
All Hallows House Centre for Natural Health and Counselling, Idol Lane, London EC3R 5DD
☎0171-283 8908 *Nutrition, Reflexology.*
Gillian and her grateful clients were the inspiration behind All Hallows support group and this book. Thur 8am-7pm.
Initial Consultation: £45-00 / 1½ hrs
Subsequent visits: £31-00 / 45 mins

Jane McWhirter, MA (Hons) MC
All Hallows House Centre for Natural Health and Counselling, Idol Lane, London EC3R 5DD
☎0171-283 8908
McTimoney Chiropractic, Celloid Minerals, Advice on complementary therapies.
While not qualified in nutrition herself, Jane is part of a formidable team of holistic therapists at AHH, which she set up in 1990. Clients frequently come with long term back or neck pain that is due to underlying candida and respond to Jane's eclectic approach. (Jane is expecting a baby in October and will not be available from Oct to Dec '95.) Wed/Thu.
Initial Consultation: £38-00 / 1 hr
Subsequent visits: £31-00 / 45 mins
General advice: £25-00 / ½ hr

Maxine Tobias
All Hallows House Centre for Natural Health and Counselling, Idol Lane, London EC3R 5DD
☎0171-283 8908
Iyengar Yoga, Macrobiotics.
Maxine is one of the leading Yoga teachers in the UK. She has written two books and made a video. Classes every Thursday 1-2 pm.
Fee: £7-00 / 1 hr

Gaye Annand, MFPhys MISPA MAR
All Hallows House Centre for Natural Health and Counselling, Idol Lane, London EC3R 5DD
☎0171-283 8908
Dowsing, Reflexology, Aromatherapy.
Gaye has success countering the effects of vaccinations, anaesthetics. Wed 10am-1pm.
Initial Consultation: £38-00 / 1 hr
Subsequent visits: £38-00 / 1 hr

Susan Allshorn, MNIMH
All Hallows House Centre for Natural Health and Counselling, Idol Lane, London EC3R 5DD
☎0171-283 8908
Herbal Medicine, Supplements, (Counselling).
Susan also treats ME. Tue 10am onwards.
Initial Consultation: £45-00 / 1½ hrs
Subsequent visits: £20-00 / 45 mins

Jill Tompson, BA LFRSH LCH
All Hallows House Centre for Natural Health and Counselling, Idol Lane, London EC3R 5DD
☎0171-283 8908
Homoeopathy, (Nutrition).
Jill had ME herself for two years and has studied it in depth. Her classical approach to taking case histories in detail includes plenty of personal support where appropriate. Wed 1-6pm.
Initial Consultation: £50-00 / 1½ hrs
Subsequent visits: £38-00 / 1 hr

Dr John Briffa, BSc (Hons) MBBS BMA BSNM BSAEM
Cannons Health Enhancement Centre, Cousin Lane, London EC4 3TE ☎0171-283 0105
Cytotoxic Blood Testing, Electro-Dermal Screening, Biochemical Blood Testing.
Dr Briffa is a qualified doctor specialising in the nutritional management of a wide range of conditions including candida, PMS, bloating and fatigue. He is generally opposed to the widespread use of drugs in orthodox medicine and prefers to identify and correct the underlying

cause for each individual's symptoms. He also treats ME and chronic fatigue syndrome.
Tue/Wed 8.30am-5.30pm.
Initial Consultation: £50-00 / 1 hr
Subsequent visits: £50-00 / 1 hr

Margie Finchell, RCT MCIA MAVR
5 Jacobs Well Mews, George Street, London W1H 5PD ☎0171-935 5401
Colonic Therapy, Vacuflex Reflexology.
Margie Finchell, Registered Colonic Therapist, recommends whenever possible a special cleanse consisting of vegetable juices and broth, water and herbal teas, psyllium husks and bentonite and a daily colonic (or two enemas) for seven days. This is then followed by a proper diet and the BioCare programme in four phases. Mon-Sat.
Initial Consultation: £50-00 / 1½ hrs
Subsequent visits: £45-00 / 1 hr approx.

Grace Hall, MBRI DISc IACT
10 Duke Street, London W1M 5AA
☎01734-786 727
Iridology/Nutrition, Homoeopathy, Counselling.
Grace also offers computerised EAV tests for nutritional deficiencies and allergies. She treats ME and is currently also doing research into this as well as candida, allergies and ME. (3-4 weeks waiting list.) Three Mondays a month.
Initial Consultation: £50-00 / 1 hr
Subsequent visits: £40-00 / 30-45 mins

Jack Levenson, LDS RCS
1 Welbeck House, 62 Welbeck Street, London W1M 7HB ☎0171-486 3127
Mercury-Free Dentistry, Vega Test, Nutritional Supplements.
Jack G Levenson is president of the British Society for Mercury Free Dentistry and has lectured extensively on published research implicating mercury from dental fillings in numerous health conditions. He is recognised internationally as a pioneer and expert in this field. Mon-Fri 9am-5pm.
Initial Consultation: £90-00
Subsequent visits: £50-00

Dr Alice Greene, MB BCh BAO
DipCouns DipObs DCH MRCGP MFHom mBAFATT
86 Harley Street, London W1N 1AE
☎0171-580 4188
Psychotherapy, Homoeopathy, Autogenic Relaxation.
Dr Greene prescribes Nystatin for about 80% of candida patients. Mon-Fri 9am-6pm.
Initial Consultation: £80-00 / 1 hr
Subsequent visits: £50-00 / ½ hr min

Deborah Beswick, BSc (Hons) DThD
BDA MNS
12 Harley Street, London W1N 1CD
☎0171-323 4664
Nutrition, Naturopathy, Probiotics.
Deborah is particularly interested in diet, nutritional supplements, herbs and probiotics for candida, exhaustion, digestive complaints, skin conditions and food allergies. She helps people with restricted diets such as vegan, gluten free, low saturated fat or low sugar and combines this with advice on gut dysbiosis as necessary. Tues afternoons & evenings.
Initial Consultation: £40-00 / 1 hr
Subsequent visits: £35-00 / 1 hr

Roger Newman Turner, BAc ND DO
MRO MRN
1 Harley Street, London W1N 1DA
☎0171-436 1446
Osteopathy, Naturopathy, Acupuncture, Clinical Tests.
Roger recommends drugs to about 10% of his patients. He is the author of many best selling books and the chairman of the Research Council for Complementary Medicine. Mon/Wed.
Initial Consultation: £48-00 / 45 mins - 1hr
Subsequent visits: £30-00 / ½ hr

Rosemary Burr
28 Weymouth Street, London W1N 3FA
☎0171-636 2400
Kinesiology, Bach Flower Remedies, Aura Soma Therapy.
Mon-Fri 10am-6pm; Sat 10am-1pm.
Initial Consultation: £40-00 / 1 hr
Subsequent visits: £40-00 / 1 hr

Peter Bartlett, DO DipRM MNTOS MCO MCrOA

The Hale Clinic, 7 Park Crescent, London
W1N 3HE ☎0171-631 0156
Osteopathy, Nutrition, Biological Medicine, Complex Homoeopathy.
Peter qualified from the McTimoney Chiropractic School and is also trained in remedial massage. He treats ME and lectures on the subject in UK and Ireland. Mon 1pm-8pm; Thu 9am-5pm.
Initial Consultation: £50-00 / 1 hr
Subsequent visits: £30-00 / ½ hr

Dr Mosaraf Ali, MD (Med) DAc PGAc

The Hale Clinic, 7 Park Crescent, London
W1N 3HE ☎0171-631 0156/637 3377
Fax 0171-323 1693
Naturopathic Diet, Herbal Medicine, Physical Therapy, Yoga, Ayurveda.
Dr Ali is the Head of the Department of Integrated Medicine at the Hale Clinic. By appointment.
Initial Consultation: £42-00 / ½ hr
Subsequent visits: £36-00 / ½ hr

Harald Gaier, ND DO DHomM DipAc

Allergy & Nutrition Clinic, 7 Park Crescent,
London W1N 3HE ☎0171-631 0604
Naturopathy, Homoeopathy, Herbal Medicine.
Harald is author of the "Encyclopaedic Dictionary of Homoeopathy" (London: Harper Collins, 1991) and monthly 'alternatives' columnist in "What Doctors Don't Tell You". He has researched and written widely on gut dysbiosis and ME.
Mon-Thu 9.15am-5.15pm.
Initial Consultation: £58-00 / 40 mins
Subsequent visits: £34-00 / 20 mins

Colin Nicholls, BA DipPhyt MNIMH

The Hale Clinic, 7 Park Crescent, London
W1N 3HE ☎0171-631 0156
Herbal Medicine, Essential Oils, Supplements/Probiotics.
Colin treats ME and is also editor of the British Journal of Phytotherapy (Herbalism). Monday afternoons.
Initial Consultation: £47-00 / 1hr
Subsequent visits: £25-00 / ½ hr

Leon Chaitow, ND DO MRO

The Hale Clinic, 7 Park Crescent, London
W1N 3HE ☎0171-631 01 56
Nutrition/Herbal, Stress Management, Osteopathy.
Leon Chaitow treats people with candidiasis and chronic fatigue holistically, working to enhance the individual's overall health status, immune function and stress coping abilities. He uses nutrition, herbal medicine, detoxification strategies, osteopathy, soft tissue manipulation, hydrotherapy and stress reduction techniques. Tue/Thu.
Initial Consultation: £75-00 / 1hr
Subsequent visits: £65-00 / 45 mins

Ursula Gateley, MCIA MHPA NFSH

The Hale Clinic, 7 Park Crescent, London
W1N 3HE ☎0171-631 0156
Colonic Hydrotherapy, Nutrition, Healing, Lymphatic Drainage.
Ursula sees many patients with ME and also for gut parasites. Mon-Fri 9am-5pm.
Initial Consultation: £58-00 / 1 hr 15 mins
Subsequent visits: £58-00 / 1 hr

Andrew J Bates, DO BSc MCO CCAM

Centre for Health and Healing, 197 Piccadilly,
London W1V 0LL ☎0171-437 7118
Cranial Osteopathy, Naturopathy, Counselling.
The gentle technique of cranial osteopathy brings about structural balance and enables the body, mind and spirit to heal in a natural way. Body awareness and counselling are also integrated into the treatment. 30-minute consultations available at £20-00. Mr Bates operates a sliding scale.
Tue-Thu.
Initial Consultation: £35-00 / 1 hr
Subsequent visits: £30-00 / 50 mins

Genevieve De Wynter, ND DO

Cameo House, 11 Bear Street, Leicester Square,
London WC2H 7AS ☎0171-930 6996
Osteopathy, Naturopathy, Supplements.
Support Group Co-ordinator.
Tue-Fri 9am-6pm.
Initial Consultation: £40-00 / 1 hr
Subsequent visits: £25-00 / ½ hr

LONDON NORTH

Helios Centre (& HIV Service)
61 Collier Street, London N1 9BE
☎0171-713 7120
A range of therapies available.
The centre has 48 practitioners and spiritual healers qualified in a variety of therapies. Most charge £25-00 per hour. The HIV service is funded by the Health Authority. Eighty per cent of the centre's work is with people who are HIV+, most of whom also have candida. They also treat many people with hepatitis, ME and cancer. The choice of therapist(s) is discussed individually. By appointment only.

Joanna Knight, DipION RN RM HV
Clissold Park Natural Health Centre, 154 Stoke Newington Church Street, London N16 0JU
☎0171-249 2990
Nutrition, Supplements, Celloid Minerals.
Joanna's programme consists of a yest and sugar-free diet and a tailor-made supplement program-me, followed by probiotics and anti-fungal remedies, usually Mycopryl. For milder cases a regular cleansing programme would be sufficient, sometimes with the use of celloids.
Support Group Initial Contact.
Tue eve; Fri morning by appointment.
Initial Consultation: £27-00 / 1 hr
Subsequent visits: £16-00 / ½ hr

Julio da Costa, DNMed DThD
5 Somerfield Road, London N4 2JN
☎0171-226 7634
Nutrition, Counselling, Iridology.
Mon-Fri 9am-6pm.
Initial Consultation: £38-00 / 1½ hrs
Subsequent visits: £25-00 / 50 mins

Dr David Dowsen, MB ChB
14 Harley House, Upper Harley Street, London NW1 4PR ☎0171-935 7848
Dietary Therapy, Desensitisation, Complex Homoeopathy, Acupuncture.
Dr Dowsen treats many hundreds of ME patients every year and is currently doing research on gut dysbiosis. Patients can be seen on the NHS under special funding arrangemements. Thursdays.
Initial Consultation: £58-00 / 20 mins
Subsequent visits: £58-00 / 20 mins

George T Lewith, BA MB BChir MRCP MRCGP DM
The Centre for the Study of Complementary Medicine, 14 Harley House, Upper Harley Street, London NW1 4PR ☎0171-935 7848
Environmental Medicine, Homoeopathy, Herbal Medicine.
Dr Lewith recommends drugs for about about 20% of his candida patients. Patients wishing to see him on the NHS must have a GP referral under special funding arrangements. He has written and lectured extensively on comple-mentary medicine. Five days a week.
Initial Consultation: £58-00 / 20 mins
Subsequent visits: £58-00 / 20 mins

Dr Julian K Kenyon, MB ChB MD FRCS BMAS BSAEM
The Centre for Study of Complementary Medicine, 14 Harley House, Upper Harley Street, London NW1 4PR ☎0171-935 7848
Homoeopathy, Acupuncture, Manipulative Therapy, Herbal Medicine.
Dr Kenyon practises complex and classical homoeopathy as well as environmental medicine. Patients wishing to see him on the NHS must have a GP referral under special funding arrangements. He sees hundreds of ME patients and has researched widely. (He has a 4 week waiting list in London, 2-3 in Southampton.)
Tue 9am-5pm.
Initial Consultation: £58-00 / 15 mins
Subsequent visits: £58-00 / 15 mins

Veronica Wolseley, DipION
60a St. Augustine's Road, Camden Town, London NW1 9RP ☎0171-485 5823
Nutrition, Kinesiology, Biochemical Testing. Weekdays.
Initial Consultation: £30-00 / 1½ hrs
Subsequent visits: £20-00 / 1 hr

Sharon Black, DipION
36A Nant Road, Child's Hill, London NW2 2AT
☎0181-209 1142
Nutrition, Supplements.
Support Group Initial Contact.
Generally Mon & Wed.
Initial Consultation: £30-00 / 1 hr
Subsequent visits: £20-00 / ½ hr

Rainer Trebuth, HP (Germany) CHT
(USA) MRN
Heath Health Care, 5 Elm Terrace, Constantine
Road, Hampstead, London NW3 2LL
☎0171-974 1199
*Natural Medicines, Hypnotherapy,
Healing, Bach Flower Remedies, Celloid
Minerals.* Wednesdays.
Initial Consultation: £50-00 / 1½ hrs
Subsequent visits: £40-£50 / 45 mins - 1 hr

Andrew J Bates, DO BSc MCO CCAM
12 Lawn Road, Hampstead, London NW3 2XS
☎0171-722 8178
*Cranial Osteopathy, Naturopathy,
Counselling.*
The gentle technique of cranial osteopathy brings
about structural balance and enables the body,
mind and spirit to heal in a natural way. Body
awareness and counselling are also integrated
into the treatment. 30-minute consultations
available at £20-00. Mr Bates operates a sliding
scale. Fridays.
Initial Consultation: £35-00 / 1 hr
Subsequent visits: £30-00 / 50 mins

M Limnios, DipION
12 Spaniards End, Hampstead, London
NW3 7JG ☎0181-458 3032
*Nutrition, Biological Testing,
Supplements.* Thu afternoon.
Initial Consultation: £38-00 / 1 hr
Subsequent visits: £28-00 / ½ hr

Joseph Goodman, ND DO DrAc
11 Alderton Crescent, Hendon, London
NW4 3XU ☎0181-202 6242
Naturopathy, Osteopathy, Acupuncture.

Joseph also treats people with ME. Mon/Wed/Fri.
Initial Consultation: £56-40 / 1 hr
Subsequent visits: £48-18 / ½ hr

Dr John Briffa, BSc (Hons) MBBS BMA
BSNM BSAEM
20 Croftdown Road, Parliament Hill Fields,
Dartmouth Park, London NW5 1EH
☎0171-284 3569
*Cytotoxic Blood Testing, Electro-
Dermal Screening, Biochemical Blood
Testing.*
Dr Briffa is a qualified doctor specialising in the
nutritional management of a wide range of conditions including candida, PMS, bloating and
fatigue. He is generally opposed to the widespread use of drugs in orthodox medicine and
prefers to identify and correct the underlying
cause for each individual's symptoms. He also
treats ME and chronic fatigue syndrome.
Mon/Thu/Fri 8.30am 7pm.
Initial Consultation: £70-00 / 1½ hrs
Subsequent visits: £45-00 / 1 hr

Maria Davies, DipION
Flat C, 28 Lady Somerset Road, Kentish Town,
London NW5 1UP ☎0171-267 1354
*Dietary Therapy, Nutrition, Supple-
ments.* Evenings and Saturdays.
Initial Consultation: £35-00 / 1 hr
Subsequent visits: £20-00 / ½ hr

Veronica Wolseley, DipION
Muswell Healing Arts, 169 Avenue Mews,
Muswell Hill, London NW10 3NN
☎0181-365 3545
*Nutrition, Kinesiology, Biochemical
Testing.* Mon pm.
Initial Consultation: £30-00 / 1½ hrs
Subsequent visits: £20-00 / 1 hr

Joanna Knight, DipION RN RM HV
17 Woodside Park, North Finchley, London
N12 8RT ☎0181-445 0678
*Nutrition, Supplements, Celloid
Minerals.*
Joanna's programme consists of a yeast and
sugarfree diet and a tailor-made supplement
programme, followed by probiotics and anti-fungal

remedies, usually Mycopryl. For milder cases a regular cleansing programme would be sufficient, sometimes with the use of celloids. By appointment only.
Initial Consultation: £27-00 / 1 hr
Subsequent visits: £16-00 / ½ hr

Sharon Black, DipION
'Natural Health', Ballards Lane, North Finchley, London N12 8LT ☎0181-445 4397
Nutrition, Supplements. Mondays.
Initial Consultation: £25-00 / 1 hr
Subsequent visits: £20-00 / ½ hr

Fiona Robertson, DO MRO ND RGN
Sunstone Health and Leisure Club, 16 Northwold Road, Stoke Newington, London N16 7HR
☎0171-923 1991
Osteopathy, Naturopathy.
Tue 3-9pm; Thu 9am-2pm.
Initial Consultation: £25-00 / 1 hr
Subsequent visits: £20-00 / ½ hr

Elizabeth Halford, BSc (Hons) DO MCO
Bickerton House, 25-27 Bickerton Road, Upper Holloway, London N19 5JT ☎01992-586 294
Osteopathy, Naturopathy, Nutrition.
Elizabeth also treats ME.
Tues 12-7pm; Sat 9am-12.
Initial Consultation: £25-00 / 45 mins
Subsequent visits: £25-00 / 45 mins

Mervyn D Cole, SRN MSoc BioMed DTCM
Wood Street Clinic, 133 Wood Street, Barnet, Herts. EN5 4BX ☎0181-441 0231/ 449 7656/449 5656
Vega Machine Tests, TCM, Supplements.
Initial consultation involves vitamin, mineral, candida and allergy tests. Mr Cole uses complex homoeopathic preparations (Rekewig) and other supplements. Mervyn Cole is also secretray of The Foundation of Biological Medicine.
Mon 2pm-8pm; Tue/Fri 9am-6pm; Thu 9am-8pm Sat 9am-2pm.
Initial Consultation: £70-00 / 1½ hrs
Subsequent visits: £25-00 / ½ hr

LONDON EAST

Veronica Wolseley, DipION
Bodywise, 19 Roman Road, London E2 0QN
☎0181-981 6938
Nutrition, Kinesiology, Biochemical Testing. Wed pm.
Initial Consultation: £30-00 / 1½ hrs
Subsequent visits: £20-00 / 1 hr

Lisa Harris, GCRO MRN
The Feel Good Factor, ASDA, 151 East Ferry Road, Isle of Dogs, London E14 3BT
☎0171-537 1114
Osteopathy, Naturopathy, Supplements.
Ms Harris also offers acupuncture in conjunction with nutritional supplements and Chinese herbs. Mon-Fri 9am-8pm.
Initial Consultation: £20-00 / 1 hr
Subsequent visits: £20-00 / ½ hr

LONDON SOUTH

Deborah Beswick, BSc (Hons) DThD BDA MNS
New Cross Natural Therapy Centre, 394 New Cross Road, New Cross, London SE14 6TY
☎0181-469 0858
Nutrition, Naturopathy, Probiotics.
Deborah is particularly interested in diet, nutritional supplements, herbs and probiotics for candida, exhaustion, digestive complaints, skin conditions and food allergies. She helps people with restricted diets such as vegan, gluten free, low saturated fat or low sugar and combines this with advice on gut dysbiosis as necessary. Thurs am and by arrangement.
Initial Consultation: £30-00 / 1 hr
Subsequent visits: £25-00 / 1 hr

Jean Clarke, LCSP RCT MCIA DHD
50a Morrish Road, Brixton Hill, London SW2 4EG ☎0181-671 7136
Colonic Hydrotherapy, Dietary Therapy, Massage, Supplements. Mon-Fri 10am-8pm.
Initial Consultation: £55-00 / 1½ hrs
Subsequent visits: £45-00 / 1 hr

Marcia M Harewood, DO ND MCO

255A Lavender Hill, Battersea, London
SW11 1JD ☎0171-498 9966/978 5538
*Cranial/Osteopathy, Naturopathic Diet,
Healing.*
Marcia also treats people with ME. Avail: Every
weekday, one Sat morning per month.
Initial Consultation: £28-00 / 1 hr
Subsequent visits: £22-50 / 30-45mins

Rodney Quixley, BA NutCert

Archway House, 39 Sunbury Lane, Battersea,
London SW11 3NP ☎0171-228 2564
Iridology, Kinesiology, Nutrition.
Rodney also treats cardiovascular problems,
weight loss and skin restoration.
Mon-Sat 10am-6pm, most days.
Initial Consultation: £40-00 / 1½ hrs
Subsequent visits: £25-00 / ½-1 hr

Nicola Griffin, DiplON

Ultimate Health Clinic, 24 Queens Road, East
Sheen, London SW14 8PJ ☎0181-392 2777
*Nutrition, Vega Tests, Supplements,
Bach Flower Remedies.*
Mrs Griffin uses Vega Tests as means of
diagnosis for candida, gut dysbiosis and food
intolerance. She also runs a weight loss clinic.
Her therapy includes a highly effective bio-
energetic treatment programme from Switzerland.
Mrs Griffin also treats ME.
Mon-Fri 10am-6pm.
Initial Consultation: £45-00 / 1½ hrs
Subsequent visits: £30-00 / 1 hr

Karen Lamb, DiplON

Putney Leisure Centre, The Alternative Treatment
Room, Dryburgh Road, Putney, London
SW15 1BL ☎0181-871 7093
Nutrition, Supplements.
Ms Lamb qualified in 1992 and has successfully
treated cases of candidiasis and gut dysbiosis.
She is about to open a multi-disciplinary clinic in
Kingston. For more information or a free 15
minute consultation contact Karen Lamb on 0181-
332 0514. Wed 10am-6.30 pm.
Initial Consultation: £28-00 / 1 hr
Subsequent visits: £22-00 / 40 mins

Sonja Vanderpool, DiplON

Putney Natural Health Clinic, 11 Montserrat Road,
Putney, London SW15 2LD
☎0181-789 2548
*Nutrition, Aromatherapy, Allergy
Testing.*
At the second session clients receive a comprehensive type-written report, including conclusions drawn from consultation and results from
allergy/food sensitivity tests; dietary and other
recommendations. Supplements offered at a discount. Variable availability.
Initial Consultation: £40-00 / 1½ hrs
Subsequent visits: £30-00 / 1½ hrs

Patrick Holford, BSc DiplON

Institute of Optimum Nutrition, 13 Blades Court
Deodar Road, Putney, London SW15 2NV
☎0181-877 9993
Nutrition, Supplements.
Patrick is the Director of the ION and has writen,
lectured and researched widely. By appointment.
Initial Consultation: £50-00 / 1 hr
Subsequent visits: £30-00 / ½ hr

Rita Nielsen, DiplSPA DipFDZ DiplFR

DiplIR RMT FDZ
127 Moyser Road, Streatham, London
SW16 6SJ ☎0181-769 5652
*Nutrition, Aromatherapy, Reflexology,
Naturopathy, Vega Tests.*
Rita also uses acupuncture to help clients stop
smoking and lose weight. All day, every day.
Initial Consultation: £25-00 / 1 hr
Subsequent visits: £30-00 / 1 hr

T Marshall-Manifold, LicAc BM

Wimbledon Clinic of Natural Medicine, 1 Evelyn
Road, Wimbledon, London SW19 8NU
☎0181-543 5477/540 3389
*Acupuncture, Biological Medicine,
Medigen.*
The clinic's approach to GD and candida is to
restore harmony to the gastric tract. Diagnosis is
helped by means of the analysis of saliva and
urine, measuring the Redox potential (free radical
activity), and recording deviation from the
accepted norm. Treatment is individual to the
patient and may include homoeopathic, herbal,

enzymes, colonic irrigaton, ozone therapy and nutritional support. Mon-Thu 9.30am-6pm.
Initial Consultation: £60-00 / 1 hr
Subsequent visits: £34-00 / ½ hr

Karen Lamb, DipION
The Kingston Clinic, 2 Fife Road, Kingston KT1 1SZ ☎0181-332 0514
Nutrition, Supplements.
Ms Lamb qualified in 1992 and has successfully treated cases of candidiasis and gut dysbiosis. She is about to open a multi-disciplinary clinic in Kingston. For more information or a free 15 minute consultation contact Karen Lamb on 0181-332 0514. Mon-Sat 9am onwards.
Initial Consultation: £30-00 / 1 hr
Subsequent visits: £25-00 / 40 mins

Nina Pearson, BSc (Hons) MD(MA)Hom
ITEC DipSJAc
34 Downside Road, Sutton, Surrey SM2 5HP
☎0181-643 1609
Homoeopathy, Massage, Su Jok Acupuncture, Reflexology.
Nina also treats people with ME. Mon-Fri 9.30am-4pm 7.30-9.30pm.
Initial Consultation: £40-00 / 50 mins
Subsequent visits: £28-00 / 35 mins

Monica Richardson, DipION
101 Malmains Way, Beckenham, Kent BR3 2SF
☎0181-650 3273/289 6546
Nutrition, Supplements.
Monica is curently doing further studying under Erica White. Mon-Tue 10am-noon, 2pm-4pm.
Initial Consultation: £30-00 / 1 hr
Subsequent visits: £20-00 / 40-45 mins

Dr Robert C Kelvinson, PhD RGN
RCT BSc (Hons) DHM ND (USA) DSc (India) IFR
Regent Clinic, 12 Albert Road, Belvedere, Kent DA17 5LJ ☎01322-446 244
Naturopathy, Diet, Herbal Medicine, Homoeopathy.
Second week in every month.
Initial Consultation: £25-00 / 1 hr
Subsequent visits: £18-50 / ½ hr

Colin Nicholls, BA DipPhyt MNIMH
46 High Beeches, Chelsfield, Orpington, Kent BR6 6EF ☎01689-858 068
Herbal Medicine, Essential Oils, Supplements/Probiotics.
Colin treats ME and is also editor of the British Journal of Phytotherapy (Herbalism). Thursdays.
Initial Consultation: £30-00 / 1 hr
Subsequent visits: £18-00 / ½ hr

LONDON WEST

Gaye Annand, MFPhys MISPA MAR
Flat 5, 61 Alderney Street, London SW1V 4HH
☎0171-821 8061
Dowsing, Reflexology, Aromatherapy.
Gaye has success countering the effects of vaccinations and anaesthetics. Mon/Tue/Thu/Fri 9am-5pm; Wed 3-5pm.
Initial Consultation: £32-00 / 1 hr
Subsequent visits: £32-00 / 1 hr

Kim Osborn, DipION
The Harbour Club, Watermeadow Lane, Fulham, London SW6 2RR ☎0171-371 7744
Nutrition, Dietary Therapy, Supplements.
Mon evening; Tue afternoon; Thu evening.
Initial Consultation: £65-00 / 1 hr
Subsequent visits: £40-00 / ½ hr

Dr Duo Gao, MBBS NTCMI (China)
16 Fulham High Street, Fulham, London SW6 3LQ, ☎0171-736 8233
Traditional Chinese Medicine.
Traditional Chinese medicine is an ancient yet sophisticated form of diagnosis and treatment for many physical and emotional problems. Prescriptions are tailored to individual needs - thus two patients with the same Western diagnosis may receive different herbal medicines, depending on condition (Yin/Yang).
Tue-Thu 10am-6pm.
Initial Consultation: £10-00 / 20 mins
Subsequent visits: £10-00 / 20 mins or more.

Tessa Carrs, DipION
25 Hurlingham Gardens, Fulham, London
SW6 3PH ☎0171-736 2043
Dietary Therapy, Nutrition, Supplements.
Tessa has done research in ME and treats this condition. Mon-Fri.
Initial Consultation: £30-00 / 1½ hrs
Subsequent visits: £15-00 / ½ hr

Sonja Vanderpool, DipION
106 Colehill Lane, Fulham, London SW6 5EJ
☎0171-731 4856/0973-314 210
Nutrition, Aromatherapy, Allergy Testing.
At the second session clients receive a comprehensive type-written report, including conclusions drawn from consultation and results from allergy/food sensitivity tests; dietary and other recommendations. Supplements offered at a discount. **Support Group Co-ordinator.**
Mon-Fri 9am-7pm; Sat 10am-1pm.
Initial Consultation: £35-00 / 1½ - 2 hrs
Subsequent visits: £25-00 / 1-1½ hrs

Kim Osborn, DipION
80 Kingwood Road, Fulham, London SW6 6SS
☎0171-381 0205
Nutrition, Dietary Therapy, Supplements. Fri 10am-4pm.
Initial Consultation: £50-00 / 1 hr
Subsequent visits: £40-00 / ½ hr

Dr Charles Innes, MBBS MFHom
The Health Partnership, 12a Thurloe Street, South Kensington, London SW7 2ST
☎0171-589 6414
Dietary Therapy, Homoeopathy, Supplements.
Dr Innes also works at other clinics and takes NHS patients. He also treats ME. Thu 9am-5pm.
Initial Consultation: £65-00 / 1½ hrs
Subsequent visits: £30-00 / ½ hr

Michael Franklin, BSc MA DipNS (USA)
Chelsea Health Centre, 174 Ifield Road, London
SW10 9AF ☎0171-373 8575

Dietary Therapy, Herbal Medicine, Supplements.
Michael specialises in candida, allergies, eating disorders, PMT, migraine, IBS, ME, arthritis, acne, eczema and other chronic conditions. Patients are given a thorough and careful investigation into their problems in order to establish the underlying cause of their symptoms. Wed-Sat.
Initial Consultation: £38-00 / 1 hr 15 mins
Subsequent visits: £38-00 / 1 hr 15 mins

Dr Alan R Hibberd, PhD DCC
FPS(Aust) PhC MRPharmS IAOMT BSAEM
25b Clanricarde Gardens, Bayswater, London
W2 4JL, ☎0171-229 9078 (& Fax)
Vega Tests, Kinesiology, Biochemistry, Pathology.
Dr Hibberd offers natural treatment for gut dysbiosis (including candidiasis and gut protozoal infection), IBS, ME, PMT, allergies, nutritional deficiencies, child hyperactivity and mercury toxicity from amalgam fillings. He carries out ongoing clinical research in the field of nutrition and environmental toxicity and writes broadly on the subject. Mon 9.15am-12.15pm; Tue-Thu 8.30 am-5.30pm; Fri 8.30am-2.30pm.
Initial Consultation: £95-00 p/h / 1 hr 15 mins
Subsequent visits: £95-00 p/h / 45 mins-1hr

Michael Franklin, BSc MA DipNS (USA)
Equilibrium, 150 Chiswick High Road, Chiswick, London W4 1PR ☎0181-742 7701
Dietary Therapy, Herbal Medicine, Supplements.
Michael specialises in candida, allergies, eating disorders, PMT, migraine, IBS, ME, arthritis, acne, eczema and other chronic conditions. Patients are given a thorough and careful investigation into their problems in order to establish the underlying cause of their symp-toms. Wed-Sat.
Initial Consultation: £38-00 / 1hr 15 mins
Subsequent visits: £38-00 / 1 hr 15 mins

Katie Bolland, DThD GNI
Brackenbury Natural Health Centre, 30 Brackenbury Road, Hammersmith, London
W6 0BA ☎0181-741 9264
Nutrition, Iridology, Colonic Hydrotherapy.

A consultation with Katie consists of iris diagnosis and a photo of the eye serving as a record. A detailed case history is taken and the client may be referred for tests to his doctor or an independent laboratory. Advice on diet, supplements and probiotics is individual. Colonic therapy is optional but usually highly recommended. Saturdays.
Initial Consultation: £45 approx / 1½ hrs
Subsequent visits: £40 approx / 1 hr

Suzanne Ross, CNS MAR BAC
15 Holmes Road, Twickenham, Surrey
TW14 RF ☎0181-891 3234
Nutrition, Counselling, Reflexology.
Mon/Fri am & pm; Sat am.
Initial Consultation: £35-00 / 1½ hrs
Subsequent visits: £20-00 / 50 mins

Suzanne Ross, CNS MAR BAC
Maple Leaf Clinic, 20 The Green, Twickenham, Surrey TW2 5AB ☎0181-891 3234
Nutrition, Counselling, Reflexology.
Support Group Initial Contact. Mon evening; Wed morning & eve; Thu eve.
Initial Consultation: £35-00 / 1½ hrs
Subsequent visits: £20-00 / 50 mins

Fiona Robertson, DO MRO ND RGN
Alternatives Complementary Therapy Centre
118 (Old) High Street, Northwood, Middx.
HA6 1BJ ☎01923-828 832
Osteopathy, Naturopathy.
Mon 9am-5pm. (Flexible).
Initial Consultation: £30-00 / 1 hr
Subsequent visits: £25-00 / ½ hr

Anita Christie, MNIMH
14 Munster Road, Teddington, Middx.
TW11 9LL ☎0181-977 8468
Herbal Medicine, Nutrition, Remedial Massage.
Anita also treats ME. Mon/Tue/Wed/Fri am.
Initial Consultation: £28-00 / 1 hr
Subsequent visits: £16-00 / ½ hr

Kate Bridgewater, IAT KF RP OHBD
Kingston Natural Healing Centre, 40 Eastbury Road, Kingston KT2 5AN ☎0181-546 5793
Allergy Testing, Optimum Health Balance, Health Kinesiology.
Mon/Sat 10am-6pm.
Initial Consultation: £30-00 / 1½ hrs
Subsequent visits: £25-00 / 1 hr

GREATER MANCHESTER

Dr Keith Scott-Mumby, MBChB
BSANM
23 Edge Lane, Chorlton, Manchester M21 9HJ
☎0161-881 0448
Allergy Testing, Nutrition, Psycho-therapy.
Dr Mumby may integrate his "Applied Philosophics" and "Life Repair" into his treatment if appropriate. He recommends about 75% of candida patients use drugs and sees many people with ME. He has written several books including the Allergy Handbook (Thorsons). Mon-Thu.
Initial Consultation: £65-00 / 40-50 mins
Subsequent visits: £45-00 / 40-50 mins

Clifford Lomas, DO ND MRN MRO
316B Buxton Road, Stockport SK2 7DD
☎0161-456 2087
Osteopathy, Naturopathy, Diet, Herbs, Hydrotherapy.
Mon 9.30-1.30pm Tue/Thu 9.30-6pm; Wed 10.30-5pm; Fri 3-6.30pm Sat am.
Initial Consultation: £24-00 / 1 hr
Subsequent visits: £20-00 / ½ hr

Margaret Moss, MA (Cantab) UCTD
DiplON
15e Mauldeth Close, Heaton Mersey, Stockport
SK4 3NP ☎0161-432 0964
Nutrition, Dietary Therapy, Anti-Toxic Counselling.
Margaret is a nutritionist who specialises in helping people whose ability to detoxify is inadequate. This includes people with ME, gut dysbiosis, candida albicans or chemical sensitivity. She emphasises the nutrients that are needed for detoxification and reduces dietary and

environmental toxins. **Support Group Initial Contact.** Flexible; can arrange weekends or evenings.
Initial Consultation: £30-00 / 1½ hrs
Subsequent visits: £20-00 p/h / ½-1½ hrs

MERSEYSIDE

Paul Traynor, BSc DipION DipAppSS
37 Hope Street, Liverpool L1 9DZ
☎0151-707 1311
Nutrition, Supplements. Mon-Fri.
Initial Consultation: £35-00 / 1 hr
Subsequent visits: £20-00 / ½ hr

Audrey N Barbasch, ND DO BNA LIA
7 Rutland Road, Southport, Merseyside PR8 6PB
☎01704-530 574
Naturopathy, Osteopathy/Chiropractic, Colonic Hydrotherapy, (S.O.T.), Electro-Crystal Therapy.
Colonic Hydrotherapy charged at £26-00 per hour. Mon/Tue/Wed/Fri 12.30-6pm.
Initial Consultation: £35-00 / 1½-2 hrs
Subsequent visits: £20-00 / 1 hr+

Maria Knowles, MRPharmS MNIMH
22 Wyken Grove, St Helens, Merseyside
WA11 9JA ☎01744-23322
Herbal Medicine, Dietary Therapy.
Mon-Fri 9am-6pm. Answerphone.
Initial Consultation: £20-00 / 1 hr
Subsequent visits: £10-00 / ½ hr

NORFOLK

Dr A N Hill, LMSSA
'County Health', 15 High Street, Holt, Norfolk
NR25 6BN ☎01263-713 974
Homoeopathy, Dietary Therapy, Supplements.
Dr Hill is soon to publish a book on the subject. He sees over 80 patients with ME every year. Wed /Thu; All day.
Initial Consultation: £25-00 / ½ hr
Subsequent visits: £20-00 / ½ hr

Dr A N Hill, LMSSA
'City Health', 21A St. Stevens Road, Norwich
NR1 3SP ☎01603-630 226
Homoeopathy, Dietary Therapy, Supplements.
Dr Hill is soon to publish a book on the subject. He sees over 80 aptients with ME every year. Mon all day.
Initial Consultation: £25-00 / ½ hr
Subsequent visits: £20-00 / ½ hr

NORTHAMPTONSHIRE

Mrs Ann Knott, DTD RCT MCIA
44 Ellesmere Avenue, Brackley, Northants.
NN13 6BX ☎01280-705 951 Fax: 702 853
Dietary Healing, Colonic Hydrotherapy.
The treatment is holistic and based around diet with colonics as necessary. The aim is to source the original cause of the imbalance in the body that caused the illness in the first place. Mrs Knott is herself an ex-candida sufferer for six years who also treats M.E. Variable - by appointment only.
Initial Consultation: £37-50 / 1¼ - 2 hrs
Subsequent visits: £37-50 / Variable

NORTH YORKSHIRE

Rex E Newnham, PhD ND DO DHom
Cracoe House Cottage, Cracoe, N Yorks.
DN37 9QX ☎01756-730 240
Mineral Nutrition, Homoeopathy, Herbal Medicine. By arrangement.
Initial Consultation: £25-00 / 1 hr
Subsequent visits: £5-£30 / Varies

Mrs V J Kearney, MIAT ITEC
2 Ridge Villas, Forest Moor Road, Knaresborough, N Yorks. HG5 8JP ☎01423-864 358
Allergy Testing, Kinesiology, Homoeo-pathy.
Subsequent consultations can usually be managed by phone. Mon-Fri 9.30am-7.30pm.
Initial Consultation: £40-00 / 2 hrs
Subsequent visits: Variable / Variable.

Ms Pauline Andrle, MA (Oxon) MNIMH
NFSH
20 Aldreth Grove, Bishopthorpe Road, York, N
Yorks. YO2 1LB ☎01904-613 644
Herbal Medicine, Spiritual Healing, Supplements. Wed-Fri.
Initial Consultation: £17-50 / 1 hr
Subsequent visits: £7-50 / ½ hr

NOTTINGHAMSHIRE

Maureen Murphy, MNIMH
425 Nottingham Road, Mansfield, Notts.
NG18 4SO ☎01623-20128
*Herbal Medicine, Nutritional Therapy,
Homoeopathy.*
Answerphone at all times.
Initial Consultation: £33-00
Subsequent visits: £14-00

Ann Wilkinson, SCM LicAc DO MRNT
MGO MTAcS
Natural Health Care, 'Appletree', 13 Lincoln Road,
Newark, Notts. NG24 2BU
☎01636-707 156
Osteopathy, Acupuncture, Supplements. Ann also treats ME. Mon-Sat.
**Initial Consultation: 1 hr; fees are discussed
privately.**

Mrs Jackie Hodges, SRN DiplON
6 Church Lane, Plungar, Nottingham NG13 0JD
☎01949-860 697
Nutrition, Supplements.
Jackie, who was a sufferer herself runs a successful support group in Nottingham. Phone
0115-982 353. She also treats children and
people with ME and is currently training in
Kinesiology. **Sup-port Group Co-ordinator.**
Mon/Tue/Fri Mornings. After 6pm most days.
Initial Consultation: £32-00 / Up to 1½ hrs
**Subsequent visits: £22-00 / 1 hr and £15-00 /
½ hr**

Heather Lyons, DiplON MNCA
The Well Being Centre, 11 Musters Road
West Bridgford, Nottingham NG2 7PP

☎0115-982 5353
Nutrition, Supplements.
Diagnosis includes evaluation of Dr Crook's
Candida Questionnaire. Heather's advice includes
measures for intestinal cleansing, de-toxification,
anti-fungal therapy, food intolerance testing,
reflorestation with probiotics and healing of the gut
wall. This is done through a careful food
programme, pulse challenge test, stress
management and a supportive on-going dialogue.
Fridays.
Initial Consultation: £35-00 / 1hr
Subsequent visits: £30-00 / 1 hr

Judy Patterson, MNIMH MSR MIAT
Wellbeing Centre, 11 Musters Road, West
Bridgeford, Nottingham NG2 7PP
☎0115-982 5353
*Herbal Medicine, Supplements,
Reflexology, Diet.* Thu 1pm-5pm.
Initial Consultation: £25-00 / 20 mins
Subsequent visits: £12-00 / 1½ hrs

Mrs Jackie Hodges, SRN DipNut
The Wellbeing Centre, 11 Musters Road
West Bridgeford, Nottingham NG2 7PP
☎0115-982 5353
Nutrition, Supplements.
Jackie, who was a sufferer herself runs a successful support group in Nottingham. Phone
0115-982 353. She also treats children and
people with ME and is currently training in
Kinesiology.
Mon/Tue/Fri 12.45pm-4.45pm.
Initial Consultation: £32-00 / Up to 1½ hrs
Subsequent visits: £22-00 / 1 hr

OXFORDSHIRE

Mrs Clare De Freitas, BA MSc CHM
NIMH
The Abingdon Surgery, 65 Stert Street, Abingdon,
Oxon. OX14 3LB ☎01235-523 126
Herbal Medicine, Nutrition, Massage.
Wed 12-6pm.
Initial Consultation: £25-00 / 1 hr
Subsequent visits: £15-00 / ½ hr

Patricia Ward, ITEC KFRP

The Health Barn, 10 Alvescot Road, Carterton,
Oxon. OX18 3JH ☎01993-843 832
Health Kinesiology, Reflexology, Bach Flower Remedies.
Pat has been a health food shop owner since 1987. She is now applying Health Kinesiology to de-allergise patients to candida and food additives etc, and get the body's energy into balance. She finds aloe vera very effective. **Support Group Initial Contact.**
Mon/Tue/Thu/Fri/Sat 10am-4pm.
Initial Consultation: £28-00 / 1 hr
Subsequent visits: £23-00 / 1 hr

Stan J Harding, MC AMC

40 North Hinksey Lane, Botley, Oxford, Oxon.
OX2 0LY ☎01865-200 489,
Fax: 01865-200 838
McTimoney Chiropractic, Healing, Counselling.
Stan finds raw foods and cleansing important. He also treats people with ME. Five days a week.
Initial Consultation: £40-00 / 1 hr
Subsequent visits: £20-00 / ½ hr

Michael Franklin, BSc MA DipNS (USA)

28 Aysearth Road, Yarnton, Oxford, Oxon.
OX5 1ND ☎01865-375 923
Dietary Therapy, Herbal Medicine, Supplements.
Michael specialises in candida, allergies, eating disorders, PMT, migraine, IBS, ME, arthritis, acne, eczema and other chronic conditions. Patients are given a thorough and careful investigation into their problems in order to establish the underlying cause of their symptoms. Mon-Tue.
Initial Consultation: £38-00 / 1hr 15 mins
Subsequent visits: £38-00 / 1 hr 15 mins

Noëlle Scott, BA MAR DiplON

6 Rupert Way, Thame, Oxon. OX9 3YA
☎01844 212 592
Nutrition, Counselling, Bach Flower Remedies, Reflexology.
Noëlle is an ex-candida sufferer herself who is now healed. She trained as a medical doctor before having to leave on account of her health. She knows from her personal experience how much patients need to be supported. By appointment.
Initial Consultation: £35-00 / Up to 1½ hrs
Subsequent visits: £20-00 / 40 mins

SHROPSHIRE

Carl Ryan, BTech RGN MNIMH

7 West Street, Shrewsbury, Shrops. SY1 2JN
☎01743-351 287
Herbal Medicine.
By appointment. Answerphone 24 hrs.
Initial Consultation: £25-00 / 1 hr
Subsequent visits: £15-00 / ½ hr

Jenny Hargreaves, DThD DNMed DIrid

The Natural Health Centre, 4 The Professional Centre, Bank Farm Road, Radbrook Green, Shrewsbury, Shrops. SY3 6DU
☎01743 248 878
Nutrition, Iridology, Supplements.
Jenny Hargreaves' treatment is holistic and individual to each patient's health problems, past and present. Free initial chat.
Wed morning, evenings by arrangement.
Initial Consultation: £25-00 / 1½ hrs
Subsequent visits: £18-00 / 30-45 mins

Carl Ryan, BTech RGN MNIMH

The Natural Health Centre, 4 The Professional Centre, Bank Farm Road, Redbrook Green, Shrewsbury, Shrops. SY3 6DU
☎01743-248 878
Herbal Medicine.
By appointment. Answerphone 24 hrs.
Initial Consultation: £25-00 / 1 hr
Subsequent visits: £15-00 / ½ hr

Carla Halford, DiplON

Whole Health, Butchers Row, Shrewsbury,
Shrops. SY6 7BJ ☎01694-722 849
Nutrition, Attitudinal Therapy, (Kinesiology).

Carla specialises in treating candida and gut dysbiosis and IBS. She also treats ME. By appointment.
Initial Consultation: £23-00 / 1 hr
Subsequent visits: £23-00 / 1 hr

Carla Halford, DipION
The Creative Health Centre, 52 Hagley Road, Stourbridge, Shrops. DY8 1QD
☎01384-379 141
Nutrition, Attitudinal Therapy, (Kinesiology).
Carla specialises in treating candida, gut dysbiosis and IBS. She also treats ME. Wednesdays.
Initial Consultation: £27-00 / 1 hr
Subsequent visits: £27-00 / 1 hr

SOMERSET

Dr David Dowsen, MB ChB
Cheddar Medical Centre, Roynon Way, Cheddar, Somerset BS27 3NZ
☎01934-744 574
Dietary Therapy, Desensitisation, Complex Homoeopathy, Acupuncture.
Dr Dowsen treats many hundreds of ME patients every year and is currently doing research on gut dysbiosis. Patients can be seen on the NHS under special funding arrangemements. Tue, Fri, Sat.
Initial Consultation: £35-00 / ½ hr
Subsequent visits: £35-00 / 20 mins

Gwynne H Davies, ND DO MNTOS
MBEOA BDA RNT
'Nirvana', 4 Calway Road, Taunton, Somerset TA1 3EQ ☎01823-335 610
Allergy Testing, Nutrition, Osteopathy.
Gwynne also treats people with ME. (See books)
Mon-Wed 9am-1pm & 2-4.30pm.
Initial Consultation: £75-00 / 45 mins
Subsequent visits: £25-00 / ½ hr

Mrs Jill Carter, SRN CIA IFA NFSH
Ringstead, Sutton Montis, Yeovil, Somerset BA22 7HF ☎01963-220 449
Colonic Hydrotherapy, Nutrition, Massage, Shen Tao, Radionics, Spiritual Healing.

Jill also treats ME. Mon-Fri; occasional weekends.
Initial Consultation: £42-00 / 2 hrs+
Subsequent visits: £42-00 / 1½ hrs+

SOUTH YORKSHIRE

Ms Pauline Andrle, MA (Oxon) MNIMH
NFSH
44 Christchurch Road, Doncaster, S Yorks. DN1 2QL, ☎01302-341 514
Herbal Medicine, Spiritual Healing, Supplements. Mon-Tue.
Initial Consultation: £17-50 / 1hr
Subsequent visits: £7-50 / ½ hr

Jan Robertson, SRN SCM MAR
20 Sefton Road, Fulwood, Sheffield S10 3TP
☎0114-230 3298
Chiropody, Reflexology, Nutrition.
Mon-Fri 9am-5pm.
Initial Consultation: £35-00 / 1-1½ hrs
Subsequent visits: £16-00 / 30-45 mins

Brian Hampton, DipION
The Caring Clinic, Barkeds Road, Sheffield S7 1SD ☎0114-255 1345
Nutrition, Colonic Hydrotherapy, Supplements.
Brian also treats ME. colonic irrigation is given by one of his colleagues. **Support Group Initial Contact.**
Weekdays 8.30am-7pm; Sat 9am-1.30pm.
Initial Consultation: £35-25 / 1 hr 15 mins
Subsequent visits: £35-25 / 1 hr or pro rata.
Fees include VAT.

Margaret D'Souza, MEd DipION
239 Abbey Lane, Sheffield S8 0BT
☎0114-236 2428
Nutrition, Kinesiology, (Counselling).
A candida sufferer herself, Margaret's approach includes a) analysis of questionnaire showing symptoms, health history, diet and yeast-related factors; b) muscle testing for food intolerance and candida overgrowth and supplement suitability; c) personal programme to supply essential nutrients to rebalance the gut flora and promote healing of

the gut wall. **Support Group Initial Contact.**
Mon-Fri; days and evenings.
Initial Consultation: £40-00 / 2 hrs
Subsequent visits: £20-00 / 1 hr

STAFFORDSHIRE

Lorna Power, BSc LCPH MHMA (UK)
"Grasshoppers", 1 Anglesey Close, Chasetown,
Staffs. WS7 8XA ☎01543-675 027
Homoeopathy, Nutrition.
By mutually convenient appointment.
Initial Consultation: £40-00 / 1½ hrs
Subsequent visits: £15-00 / ½ hr

Christopher Menzies-Trull, MNIMH
37 Liverpool Road, Stoke-on-Trent, Staffs.
ST4 1AW ☎01782-49789
*Herbal Medicine, (Naturopathy),
Iridology.*
Availability variable - answerphone.
Initial Consultation: £25-00 / 1hr
Subsequent visits: £8-00 / ½ hr

SUFFOLK

Lyn Barnes, DiplON
'Daydreams', 10 Langton Place, Bury St
Edmunds, Suffolk IP33 1RW ☎01284-702
045
Nutrition, Supplements.
Free 20 minute appointment offered (with no
obligation) so that you can find out what nutritional
therapy involves and whether you feel it is the right
therapy for you. First two treatments will take 1½
hrs each. Lyn also treats ME. Wed 1.30-4.30pm.
Initial Consultation: £20-00 / 1½ hrs
Subsequent visits: £18-00 / 1 hr

SURREY

Sue Smith, BSc (Hons) SRN DiplON
HVCert MBRA
2 Broad Walk, Caterham, Surrey CR3 5EP
☎01883-348 046
Reflexology, Nutrition, Supplements.
Mon 2-8pm; Tue 2-6pm; Thu 2-8pm.

Initial Consultation: £23-50 / 1 hr
Subsequent visits: £23-50 / 1 hr

Kate Bridgewater, IAT KF RP OHBD +
6 Queens Reach, Creek Road, East Moseley,
Surrey KT8 9DE ☎0181-979 6888
*Allergy Testing, Optimum Health
Balance, Health Kinesiology.*
Thu/Fri 10am-6pm.
Initial Consultation: £30-00 / 1½ hrs
Subsequent visits: £25-00 / 1 hr

Ian Miller, MC AMC MISP
12 Kingswood Close, Merrow, Guildford, Surrey
GU1 2SD ☎01483-304 744
*McTimoney Chiropractic, Polarity
Therapy, Celloid Minerals, Herbs.*
Mon-Fri 8.30am-7pm.
Initial Consultation: £36-00 / 1 hr
Subsequent visits: £27-00 / 45 mins

Marion Kirkham, DiplON HPA
19 Hodgson Gardens, Weylea Farm, Burpham,
Guildford, Surrey GU4 7YS ☎01483-36429
*Supplements, Dietary Therapy, (Celloid
Mineral Therapy).* Wed 8am-7pm.
Initial Consultation: Free / ½ hr
Subsequent visits: £59-00 / Up to 1½ hrs

Jennie Davis, ITEC RAWDip
17 Sycamore Close, Fetcham, Leatherhead,
Surrey KT22 9EX ☎01372-373 876
*Nutrition, Massage, Reflexology,
Iridology, Kinesiology.*
Ms Davis' massage therapy involves the use of
Hopi candles. She also uses iridology. 9.30am-
2.30pm; Sat 10am-5pm.
Initial Consultation: £35-00 / 1½ hrs
Subsequent visits: £25-00 / 1 hr

Gaynor Greber, DipNut DiplON MNCA
'Ingledale' Natural Health Centre, Tanhouse Farm,
1 Tanhouse Road, Old Oxted, Surrey RH8 9PE
☎01883-717 277

Candida Questionnaire, Nutrition, Supplements.
Tue 10am-2pm.
Initial Consultation: £30-00 / 1 hr
Subsequent visits: £22-00 / ½ hr

Jennifer A Harper, DipDTh DipNatMed
MBRCP MRNT, Manor Cottage, High Street, Ripley, Surrey GU23 6AF ☎01483-224 064
Nutrition, Kinesiology, Bach Flower Remedies.
Jennifer Harper is qualified in nutrition and natural therapies. She has developed her own system, combining holistic therapies and healing in a unique way to help re-balance the body and achieve high levels of health and well-being. Ms Harper has lectured and written articles for a number of well-known magazines and has a BBC radio phone-in programme. Mondays.
Initial Consultation: £40-00 / 1 hr
Subsequent visits: £25-00 / ½ hr

Anita Christie, MNIMH
Pear Tree House, 52 Richmond Road, Staines, Surrey TW18 2AB ☎0181-977 8468
Herbal Medicine, Nutrition, Remedial Massage. Anita also treats ME. Available Thursdays.
Initial Consultation: £30-00 / 1 hr
Subsequent visits: £20-00 / ½ hr

Dr Duo Gao, MBBS NTCMI (China)
1A Cheam Road, Sutton, Surrey SM1 1NT
☎0181-643 4222
Traditional Chinese Medicine.
Traditional Chinese medicine is an ancient yet sophisticated form of diagnosis and treatment for many physical and emotional problems. Prescriptions are tailored to individual needs - thus two patients with the same Western diagnosis may receive different herbal medicines, depending on condition (Yin/Yang). Fri-Sat.
Initial Consultation: £10-00 / 20 mins
Subsequent visits: £10-00 / 20 mins or more.

Michael Burt, DO MRO ND MRN BAc
MBAAR AMIPH
Brabant House, Portsmouth Road, Thames Ditton, Surrey KT7 0EY ☎0181-398 7592

Homoeopathy, Acupuncture, Osteopathy, Radionics.
Mr Burt's format for treatment involves 1) Identification of food allergies, sensitivities and intolerances. 2) Identification of food deficiencies, e.g physiological dysfunction and vitamin/mineral deficiencies. 3) Desensitization, tonification, elimination, detoxification, antidoting, sedation, supply and replacement by means of radionics and homoeopathy. Tue 9am-7pm; Fri 3-7pm.
Initial Consultation: £66-00 / 1½ hr
Subsequent visits: £66-00 / 1½ hr

Sue Smith, BSc (Hons) SRN DipION
HVCert MBRA
Wellbrook Clinic, 21 Stafford Road, Wallington, Surrey SM6 9AN ☎0181-401 0011
Reflexology, Nutrition, Supplements.
Fri 2-8pm.
Initial Consultation: £25-00 / 1hr
Subsequent visits: £25-00 / 1 hr

Dr Keith Scott-Mumby, MBChB
BSANM
60 Berkeley Court, Oatlands Drive, Weybridge, Surrey KT13 9HY ☎01932-231 540
Allergy Testing, Nutrition, Psychotherapy.
Dr Mumby may integrate his "Applied Philosophics" and "Life Repair" into his treatment if appropriate. He recommends about 75% of candida patients use drugs and sees many people with ME. He has written several books including the Allergy Handbook, Thorsons. Thu-Sat.
Initial Consultation: £85-00 / 40-50 mins
Subsequent visits: £50-00 / 40-50 mins

Pauline Varney, MCSP
Redcroft Clinic, 12 Barham Close, Weybridge, Surrey KT13 9PR ☎01932-851 372
Physiotherapy, Vega Machine Tests, Acupuncture, Homoeopathic Nosodes.
Mon/Wed/Thu/Fri 8.20am-1pm; Mon/Wed 6.30pm-8.30pm.
Initial Consultation: £30-00 / 1 hr
Subsequent visits: £25-00 / 40 mins

Lynda Vaughan, RAWNutDip ITEC

'Lauriston', Wych Hill, Woking, Surrey GU22 0HA
☎01483-761 312
Nutrition, Iridology, Kinesiology.
Mon-Fri 10am-6pm.
Initial Consultation: £30-00 / 1-1½ hrs
Subsequent visits: £15-00 / ½ hr

Jennie Davis, ITEC RAWDip
Limetree Centre, Fitsroy House, Lynwood Drive,
Worcester Park, Surrey KT4 7AD
☎0181-330 0100
Nutrition, Massage, Reflexology, Iridology, Kinesiology.
Ms Davis' massage therapy involves the use of
Hopi candles. She also uses iridology. Mon/Tue/
Wed 10am-2.30pm; Sat 10am-5pm.
Initial Consultation: £35-00 / 1½ hrs
Subsequent visits: £25-00 / 1 hr

TYNE & WEAR

Miss Gwenneth Brown, MRN MRO
MIAT
23 High Street, Gosforth, Newcastle NE3 4AD
☎0191-285 1656
Naturopathy, Osteopathy, Homoeopathy. Mon-Fri 7.30am-4pm.
Initial Consultation: £26-50 / 1 hr
Subsequent visits: £21-00 / ½ hr or more

WARWICKSHIRE

Pam Penlington, BEd DipION MRNT
MIAT
The Emporium, 44 The Square, Kenilworth,
Warks. CV8 1EB ☎01926-50 115
Nutrition, Dowsing, Counselling, Healing.
Availability varies
Initial Consultation: £30-00 / 1½ hrs
Subsequent visits: £20-00 / 1 hr

Vivienne Brown, LicAc DipAc
38 Russell Terrace, Leamington Spa, Warks.
CV31 1HE ☎01926-422 388

Acupuncture, Counselling, Supplements.
Vivienne has over twenty years' experience in
acupuncture, including training in China. She also
treats ME. Mon-Fri 9am-5pm.
Initial Consultation: £42-00 / 1½ hrs
Subsequent visits: £25-00 / 1 hr

Jan Trinder, RGN OHN RCT KFRP
The Creative Health Centre, 50A Warwick Street,
Leamington Spa, Warks. CV32 5JS
☎01926-316 500
Kinesiology, Colonic Hydrotherapy, Supplements.
Jan treats people with ME and is a herself a
previous sufferer of candidiasis and ME. Mon
11am-7pm; Tue -Wed 9am-5.30.
Initial Consultation: £45-00 / 1½ hrs
Subsequent visits: £28-00 / 1 hr

Pam Penlington, BEd DipION MRNT
MIAT
The Creative Health Centre, 50A Warwick Street,
Leamington Spa, Warks. CV32 5JS
☎01926-316 500
Nutrition, Dowsing, Counselling, Healing. Thu afternoons.
Initial Consultation: £30-00 / 1½ hrs
Subsequent visits: £20-00 / 1 hr

Jenny Jones, MNIMH
50a Warwick Street, Leamington Spa, Warks.
CV32 5JS
☎01926-317 500
Herbal Medicine, Nutrition.
Support Group Co-ordinator. Wednesdays
Initial Consultation: £35-00 / 1 hr
Subsequent visits: £20-00 / ½ hr

Mrs Jan Hagues, LCSP (Phys) ITEC
6 Bracken Close, Highlands, Rugby, Warks.
CV22 6AL ☎01788-569 528
Remedial Massage, Manipulative Therapy, Celloid Mineral Therapy, Supplements.
Mrs Hagues offers dietary monitoring (£10 to
cover cost for candida patients only); help and
encouragement. She works with a local herbalist

and health shop whose owner also offers advice and a personal service. Treatment includes deep soft tissue massage. Mon/Wed/Fri 9am-5.30pm; Tue 2pm-5.30pm; Sat 9am-1pm.
Initial Consultation: £30-00 / 2 hrs
Subsequent visits: £18-00 / 1 hr

WEST MIDLANDS

Janet E Spence, RCT RIr DipMLD
BRCP CIA GNI SI RNT
The Well Natural Health Centre, 89 Institute Road, King's Heath, Birmingham B14 7EU
☎0121-443 1580
Colonic Hydrotherapy, Iridology, Nutrition, Manual Lymph Drainage, Massage.
Janet treats numerous patients with ME. Fri 3.30-7pm
Initial Consultation: £40-00
Subsequent visits: £25-00

Anne Chiotis, BSc (Hons) ARCS MNIMH
67 Orchard Road, Erdington, Birmingham B24 9JB ☎0121-373 0412
Herbal Medicine, Flower Essences, Yoga/Meditation.
Herbal medicines are extra and cost £6-00 per month. Anne also treats ME. Mon-Sat 10.30-3.30; usually.
Initial Consultation: £39-00 / 1½ hrs
Subsequent visits: £22-00 / 1 hr

Helen Elroy, ITEC IHBCPTE MCIA IAC (USA)
515 Hagley Road, Warley, Birmingham B66 4AX
☎0121-429 9191
Colonic Hydrotherapy.
Mon/Tue/Thu/Fri 10am-8pm; Wed 10am-6pm; Sat 10am-4pm.
Initial Consultation: Free / 15 mins
Subsequent visits: £38-00 / 1 hr 15 mins

Carla Halford, DipION
The Natural World Health Clinic, 596 Bearwood Road, Warley, Birmingham B66 4BW
☎0121-420 2145

Nutrition, Attitudinal Therapy, (Kinesiology).
Carla specialises in treating candida, gut dysbiosis and IBS. She also treats ME.
Wed/Sat.
Initial Consultation: £27-00 / 1 hr
Subsequent visits: £27-00 / 1 hr; up to 50% discount for the unemployed.

Jenny Jones, MNIMH
Hill Cottage, Coventry Road, Berkswell, Coventry, W Midl. CV7 7AZ
☎01676-532 320
Herbal Medicine, Nutrition.
Support Group Initial Contact. Mon-Fri; days and eves.
Initial Consultation: £35-00 / 1 hr
Subsequent visits: £20-00 / ½ hr

Janet E Spence, RCT RIr DipMLD
BRCP CIA GNI SI RNT
Complementary Medicine Centre, 20 Coppice Walk, Cheswick Green, Shirley, Solihull, W Midl. B90 4HY ☎01564-750 140
Colonic Hydrotherapy, Iridology, Nutrition, Manual Lymph Drainage, Massage.
Janet treats numerous patients with ME. Tue-Thu 10am-7pm; occasional Sat 10am-4pm.
Initial Consultation: £40-00
Subsequent visits: £25-00

Christopher Bennetto, DO ND MRO MRN MNIMH
Pendene Complementary Medical Centre, 1 Woodfield Avenue, Wolverhampton, W Midl. WV4 4AG ☎01902-338 332
Naturopathy, Herbal Medicine, Osteopathy.
Christopher also treats ME. Mon-Fri 9am-5.30pm.
Initial Consultation: £40-00 / 40 mins
Subsequent visits: £28-00 / 20 mins

WEST SUSSEX

Ann Rowland, DipION MNCA
Chichester Natural Health Centre, 5 City Business Centre, Basin Road, Chichester, W Sussex

PO19 2DU ☎01243-786 946
Nutrition, Bach Flower Remedies.
Anne also treats ME. Wednesdays.
Initial Consultation: £30-00 / 1hr
Subsequent visits: £18-00 / ½ hr

Mary Halliday, DipION
Kentrigg, St John's Park, Menston, Ilkley, W
Yorks. LS29 6ES ☎01943-874 769
Nutrition, Supplements.
Initial fee covers three months' monitoring, plus 20

Mrs A Warren-Davis, FNIMH
Nortfields Farm Herbary, Fontwell Avenue
Eastergate, Chichester, W Sussex PO20 6RX
☎01243-542 349
Medical Herbalism, Diet, Counselling.
Mrs Davis is a Fellow of NIMH. Mon-Thu 11am-
5pm.
Initial Consultation: £30-00 / 1 hr or more (pro
rata).
Subsequent visits: £15-00 / ½ hr

John Tunnicliff, BSc (Hons) NCA
39 Thakeham Drive, Goring-by-Sea, W Sussex
BN12 5BB ☎01903-243 969
John is due to qualify at the I.O.N in 1996. He was
once a candida sufferer himself and is now a
Support Group Co-ordinator.

Christopher Pick, DCN DLI (Inst) DHH
Stringers Studio, East Street, Petworth, W
Sussex GU28 0AB ☎01798-343 600
Nutrition, Lymphatic Irrigation.
Mon-Fri 9.30am-5.30pm.
Initial Consultation: £40-00 / 1 hr
Subsequent visits: £20-00 / ½ hr

WEST YORKSHIRE

Sarah Goodwin, MNIMH MBRI
The Hebden Bridge Centre of Natural Medicine
33 West End, Hebden Bridge, W Yorks.
HX7 8UQ ☎01422-843 517
*Herbal Medicine, Diet, Iridology, Bach
Flower Remedies.*
Sarah also treats ME. Concessionary fees av-
ailable for those on benefit: Initial consultation,
£15-00; subsequent visits: £7-50. Mon-Tue 10am-
3.30pm; Wed-Thu 10am-7pm.
Initial Consultation: £27-00 / 1½ hrs
Subsequent visits: £13-50 / 45 mins

mins back-up telephone support. **Support Group Co-ordinator.** Flexible, by arrangement.
Initial Consultation: £30-00 / 1½ hrs
Subsequent visits: £25-00 / 1 hr

Rhona J Smith, ITEC Mlat
Complementary Medicine Centre, 20 Cavendish Street, Keighley, W Yorks. BD21 3RG
☎**01535-606 859 (Fri) 644 162**
Nutrition, Aromatherapy, Acupressure, Allergy Testing, Kinesiology, Bach Flower Remedies.
Rhona also offers remedial massage, stress release and relaxation tecniques as well as food and chemical allergy diagnosis and treatment. She is also involved with the Health Education Council in promotion of good nutrition and group work. Friday - all day.
Initial Consultation: £25-00 / 2 hrs
Subsequent visits: £10-00 / 1 hr

Rhona J Smith, ITEC Mlat
Manor House, 15 Yate Lane, Oxenhope, Keighley, W Yorks. BD22 9HL
☎**01535-644 162**
Nutrition, Aromatherapy, Acupressure, Allergy Testing, Kinesiology, Bach Flower Remedies.
Rhona also offers remedial massage, stress release and relaxation tecniques as well as food and chemical allergy diagnosis and treatment. She is also involved with the Health Education Council in promotion of good nutrition and group work. Available evenings.
Initial Consultation: £25-00 / 2 hrs
Subsequent visits: £10-00 / 1 hr

M F Chen, MA Oxon DCHM LicAc
Acupressure Clinic, 249a Otley Road, Leeds LS16 5LQ ☎**0113-278 1267**
Acupressure, Acupuncture, Chinese Herbal Medicine, Supplements.
Ms Chen also treats ME. **Support Group Initial Contact.** Every Month 1st to 14th, by appointment only.
Initial Consultation: £15-00 / 1 hr
Subsequent visits: £15-00 / 1 hr

Alison Denham, MNIMH
Clinic of Alternative Medicine, 46 Chapeltown Pudsey, Leeds LS28 8BS ☎**0113-239 3396**
Herbal Medicine, Dietary Advice, Essential Oils.
The diagnosis of gut dysbiosis is often reached by default when no other diagnosis has been made. Alison takes a full medical history and makes a physical examination before making a diagnosis. Herbs are used in combination to treat the infection and symptoms and are of particular use in viral infections, eg ME. She uses American, Chinese and European and her own plants. Tue/Fri.
Initial Consultation: £19-50 / ½ hr
Subsequent visits: £18-00 / ½ hr

WILTSHIRE

Dr Anthony Dunstan Fox, BSc
MBBS DCH DRCOG RCGP
5 Wyndham Road, Salisbury, Wilts. SP1 3AA
☎**01425-618 801**
Homoeopathy, Diet, Herbs, Vega Tests, Bach Flower Remedies.
Dr Fox treats a large number of patients with ME. Available Thursdays.
Initial Consultation: £46-00 / 40 mins
Subsequent visits: £30-00 / 20 mins

Valerie Bullen, BSc (Hons) MSc
29 Tithe Barn Crescent, Swindon, Wilts. SN1 4JX
☎ **01743-538 893**
Kinesiology, Minerals and Vitamin Therapy, Homoeopathy.
Kinesiologists regard candidiasis as being due to the immune system's inability to clear the organism from the body. This may be because the system is weakened through 'malnutrition' or has failed to recognise the organism and needs to be re-educated. Kinesiology allows the correct cause to be detremined. Valerie also treats ME. Variable - by appointment.
Initial Consultation: £30-00 / ½ hr

Helen Auburn, DiplON
55 Akers Way, Swindon, Wilts. SN2 2NF
☎**01793-495 475**

Nutrition, Supplements. Mon-Fri 6pm 8pm.
Initial Consultation: £25-00 / 1 hr
Subsequent visits: £25-00 / ½ hr

SCOTLAND

Lincoln Coutts, ASK
Riverside Physiotherapy, 585 Holburn Street,
Aberdeen, AB1 7LH ☎01224-211 517
*Kinesiology, (Nutrition), Bach Flower
Remedies.*
The practitioner follows specific correction pro-
cedures indicated by the results of muscle tests,
thus not having to guess a diagnosis or form an
opinion as to the treatment needed. With kin-
esiology the patient receives a specific and hol-
istic treatment, individual to his needs. **Support
Group Co-ordinator.** Tue-Fri 8.30am-5.30pm;
Saturdays by arrangement.
Initial Consultation: £30-00 / 1½ hrs
Subsequent visits: £15-£30 / ½-1 hr

Mrs E McGregor, ITEC Bio-MA IAHP
Cairn Holistic Centre, 'Broombush', Dunscore,
Dumfries, DG2 0UL ☎01387-820 378
*Bio-Magnetic Therapy, Cranio-Sacral
Therapy, Nutrition, Massage, Crystal
Therapy* Mon-Fri 9am-5pm.
Initial Consultation: £20-00 / 1½ hrs
Subsequent visits: £15-00 / 1 hr

Dee Atkinson, BA (Hons) MNIMH
Napiers Clinic and Dispensary, 18 Bristo Place,
Edinburgh, EH1 1EZ ☎0131-225 5542
*Herbal Medicine, Supplements,
Essential Oils.* Mon-Sat 9am-5.30pm.
Initial Consultation: £18-00 / 45 mins
Subsequent visits: £10-00 / ½ hr

Dr Cornelia Fellner
Featherstone, MD RCGP
Centre Director, 'Health Works', 5 Bank Lane,
Forres, IV36 0NU ☎01309-676 691
*Psychosomatic Medicine, Nutrition,
Complex Homoeopathy, Herbalism.*
The reassurance of Dr Featherstone's medical
background and her open-mindedness to any

complementary approach allow the patient to
choose the health care they want. She works
under the NHS in cooperation with other medical
and complementary practitioners who are all
dedicated to 'health care' rather than 'disease
cure'. Vega Tests at £35-00. She finds it appropriate to prescribe antifungal drugs to about
25% of candida patients. Mon-Fri 9am-5pm.
Initial Consultation: £25-00 / ½ hr
Subsequent visits: £25-00 / ½ hr

Dr Sheila Lilian Gibson, MBChB MD
MFHom BSMDH McC.Soc
Glasgow Homoeopathic Hospital, 1000 Great
Western Road, Glasgow, G12 0NR
☎0141-334 9800
*Nutrition, Homoeopathy, Psycho-
therapy.*
Mrs Gibson works at an NHS hospital, hence no
fees are payable. She is also co-author of 'The
complete Wheat-Free Diet' and 'Homoeopathy for
Everyone'. She sees 50-100 ME patients per year.
Tue/Thu/Fri Mornings.
Initial Consultation: Free / Up to 2 hrs
Subsequent visits: Free / ½ hr/Variable.

Dr Robin G. Gibson, MB FRCP DCH
BSNM BSAEN MIATh BSMDH McC.Soc
354 Albert Drive, Glasgow, G41 5PJ
☎0141-427 1505
*Nutrition, Homoeopathy, Psycho-
therapy, Allergy Testing.*
Dr Gibson, a consultant physician, is co-author of
the book 'Homoeopathy for Everyone' and 'The
Complete Wheat-Free Diet'. He also treats ME.
Tue/Thu 9am-7pm.
Initial Consultation: Varies / 1 hr
Subsequent visits: Varies / ½ hr

Jane Ridder-Patrick, BSc MRPharmS
MNIMH
41 Balcastle Gardens, Kilsyth, Glasgow,
G65 9PE ☎01236-824 813
Counselling, Naturopathy, Reflexology.
Mon-Fri 9am-6pm.
Initial Consultation: £25-00 / 1 hr
Subsequent visits: £25-00 / 1 hr

David Mellin, DiplION

80 Hamilton Road, Rutherglen, Glasgow,
G73 3DQ ☎0141-647 6210
Dietary Therapy, Allergy Testing, Supplements. David also treats people with ME.
Mon-Fri 9am-6pm.
Initial Consultation: £20-00 / 1 hr
Subsequent visits: £15-00 / ½ hr

Lincoln Coutts, ASK

Chelsea House Clinic, Chelsea Lane, Inverurie,
AB5 3QQ ☎01467-624 888
Kinesiology, (Nutrition), Bach Flower Remedies.
The practitioner follows specific correction procedures indicated by the results of muscle tests, thus not having to guess a diagnosis or form an opinion as to the treatment needed. With kinesiology the patient receives a specific and holistic treatment, individual to his needs. Mon 10am-8pm.
Initial Consultation: £30-00 / 1 hr
Subsequent visits: £15-£30 / ½-1hr

A Cameron Cunningham, BA (Hons)

DEP C Psychol AFBPsS ND MRN
Falkirk Natural Therapy Centre, 198 Stirling Road,
Larbert, FK5 4SQ ☎01324-557 628 (& Fax)
Nutrition, Naturopathy, Counselling.
Cameron Cunningham qualified as a Naturopath in 1959 and later worked as a Chartered Psychologist. In 1988 he returned to private practice, combining his psychological and naturopathic skills. As well as treating candida and ME, he offers help for stress related problems, back and muscular pain, childhood and family problems. Mon-Fri 9am-5pm.
Initial Consultation: £30-00 / 1 hr
Subsequent visits: £25-00 / 45 mins

WALES

Jenny Hargreaves, DThD DNMed DIrid

Holistic Healing Centre, Regent Street, Llangollen,
Clwyd LL20 8HS ☎01978-861 457
Nutrition, Iridology, Supplements.
Jenny Hargreaves' treatment is holistic and individual to each patient's health problems, past and present. Free initial chat. **Support Group**
Initial Contact. Most Days.
Initial Consultation: £25-00 / 1½ hrs
Subsequent visits: £18-00 / 30-45 mins

Jenny Hargreaves, DThD DNMed DIrid

Hillside House, Bronwylfa, Wrexham, Clwyd
LL14 4LD ☎01978 841 626
Nutrition, Iridology, Supplements.
Jenny Hargreaves' treatment is holistic and individual to each patient's health problems, past and present. Free initial chat. By arrangement only.
Initial Consultation: £25-00 / 1½ hrs
Subsequent visits: £18-00 / 30-45 mins

Mrs Anna V Noon, MNIMH

Baker Street Natural Healing Centre, 1st Floor,
4 Baker Street, Aberystwyth, Dyfed SY23 2BJ
☎01970-615 232
Herbal Medicine, Diet, Lifestyle Advice.
Herbal medicines are extra. Mon 9am-2pm.
Initial Consultation: £20-00 / 1 hr
Subsequent visits: £10-00 / ½ hr

Mrs Anna V Noon, MNIMH

Rhoscellan Fach, Clarach, Aberystwyth, Dyfed
SY23 3DR ☎01970-828 219
Herbal Medicine, Diet, Lifestyle Advice.
Herbal medicines are extra. Tue-Fri daytime, some eves. **Initial Consultation:** £20-00 / 1 hr
Subsequent visits: £10-00 / ½ hr

Kerry J Caldock, RGN BA PhD MNIMH

12 College Road, Upper Bangor, Bangor,
Gwynedd LL57 2AN ☎01248-714 244
Herbal Medicine, Dietary Therapy, Supplements.
Mon/Tue/Fri; answering service.
Initial Consultation: £18-00 / 1hr
Subsequent visits: £12-00 / ½ hr

J Elizabeth Oliver, MSc MIAT LCST

LGSM
3 Fairfield Close, Penrhyn Bay, Llandudno,
Gwynedd LL30 3HU ☎01492-549 805

Dowsing, Nutrition, Kinesiology, (Homoeopathy), Bach Flower Remedies.
Ms Oliver is clinician to the Hyperactive Children's Support Group and 'Foresight.' She also treats ME. By appointment.
Initial Consultation: £25-00 / 1½ hrs
Subsequent visits: £10-00 / ½ hr min

Richard Burden, ND MRN DO MRO
78 Mansel Street, Swansea SA1 5TW
☎01792-654 751
Osteopathy, Naturopathy, Supplements.
Richard also treats ME.
Mon/Tue/Thu/Fri 8.30am-5.30pm.
Initial Consultation: £30-00 / 1hr
Subsequent visits: £18-00 / ½ hr

IRELAND

Dr John Clements, MB BCh
70 Ranelagh Village, Dublin 6 ☎01-660 4810
Allopathy, Acupuncture, Homoeopathy, Eclosion.
Mon/Tue/Thu/Fri 3-7pm
Initial Consultation: IR£20-00 / ½ hr min
Subsequent visits: IR£20-00 / ½ hr

Bridget A Heavey, DipAc LicAc SRN
SCM
Lr Eyre Street, Newbridge, Co Kildare
☎045-431 033/432 317
Acupuncture, Vega Tests, Kinesiology, EAV Testing.
Support Group Initial Contact. Mon-Fri 9 -5
Initial Consultation: IR£35-00 / 1 hr min
Subsequent visits: IR£25-00 / 50 mins-1 hr

Linden M E Moore, RGN CSK LicAc
Ashview Clinic, Lisbarnett Road, Comber,
Co Down BT23 6AW ☎01238-541 669
Kinesiology, Acupuncture, Nutrition.
Tue-Fri, plus 2 eves; Sat am.
Initial Consultation: £25-00 / 1 hr 15 mins
Subsequent visits: £20-00 / 50-60 mins

PRACTITIONERS WHO CONSULT BY POST

If you do not live near a practitioner, or cannot get to one, a postal consultation is a very good option.

ION Nutritionists
Nutritionists trained at the Institute for Optimum Nutrition usually use a standard questionnaire which you fill out before your appointment, and this also works well for postal consultations. Most practitoners charge the same as for face to dace consultations as the written report they send you and telephone calls involve at least the same amount of time.

Radionics practitioners
(See chapter 11 for how radionics works). For a consultation you will usually be asked to send the practitioner a lock of hair, a photo or a signature. Most practitioners give a written report and a telephone conversation with the opportunity to follow up as appropriate. Phone the Radionics Society for a contact.

Erica White, DipION
22 Leigh Hall Road, Leigh-on-Sea, Essex
SS9 1RN ☎01702-720 85
Nutrition, Supplements.
Erica has a very busy practice; she uses detailed questionnaire for postal and personal consul-tations with careful analysis of answers. Fees in clude professional report plus audiotape and three months' support, followed by re-assessment and advice. An ex-sufferer herself, Erica is author of "Beat Candida Cookbook", lecturer and tutor at the Institute for Optimum Nutrition and a committed Christian. She also has many ME patients. Ring for a questionnaire and postal appointment date when Erica will get back to you. Then you will be sent a two-page letter including personal suggestions, fact sheets, her tape or booklet on candida or ME and the price list for the supplements she recommends. Erica has her own range of products (White's Food Supplies) as well as offering proprietary brands such as BioCare, Health plus and Lamberts. **Fee: £45-00**

The Nutrition Line
(Higher Nature's helpline service.)

Penny Davenport, RNT
Sharon Kaye Dip ION
Christine Monson Dip ION
Jannette Swayne Dip ION
Mandy Cohen Dip ION
Burwash Common, E Sussex
TN19 7LX ☎ 0891-615 522
Nutrition, Supplements, Herbal
Medicine.
All five nutritionists offer unbiased personal
advice. (See also entries under East Sussex)
**Fee: 39p per minute cheap rate and 49p at
other times.**
Weekdays 11am-7pm

Keith Mason, PhD BRCP
The Mill House, Breamore, Fordingbridge, Hants.
SP6 2AF ☎01725-513 018
Radionics, Metaphysical Assessment,
Element Therapy, Celloid Minerals, Diet,
Homoeopathy.
Keith investigates the underlying biochemical and
metaphysical (ie energetic or pre-physical)
influences on your character. These may include
electromagnetic fields. Suggestions for treatment
will often be at an energetic level. Assessment via
hair sample. Ring for package and guidelines.
You will receive a written, personal biochemical
and metaphysical assessment detailing the
underlying causes, and be asked to report back
afer a month.
Initial Assessment Fee: £65-00.
Further Check-up, if needed, averages £17-50.

Ann Rowland, DipION MNCA
Old Bell Cottage, Rogate, Petersfield, Hants.
GU31 5EF ☎01730-821 725 (& Fax)
Nutrition, Bach Flower Remedies.
Anne also treats ME. Includes two telephone
follow-ups. **Fee: £40-00**

Noëlle Scott, BA MAR DiplON
6 Rupert Way, Thame, Oxon. OX9 3YA
☎01844 212 592
Nutrition, Counselling, Bach Flower
Remedies, Reflexology.
Noëlle is an ex-candida sufferer herself who is
now healed. She trained as a medical doctor
before having to leave on account of her health.
She knows from her personal experience how
much patients need to be supported.
Initial Consultation: £35-00
Subsequent Fee: £20-00

Mary Halliday, DiplON
Kentrigg, St John's Park, Menston, Ilkley, W
Yorks. LS29 6ES ☎01943-874 769
Nutrition, Supplements.
Initial fee covers 3 months monitoring, plus 20
minutes back-up telephone support.
Fee: £30-00
Follow-up: £15-00

WHAT THEIR LETTERS STAND FOR

AIPTI	Association of Independent Therapists International
ANM	Association of Natural Medicine
AOC	Aromatherapy Organisations Council
AR	Association of Reflexology
ASK	Association of Systematic Kinesiology
BA	Bachelor of Arts
BA (Hons)	Bachelor of Arts, Honours
BAAR	British Acupuncture Association and Register
BAC	British Association for Counselling
BAc.	Bachelor of Acupuncture
BAFATT	British Association for Autogenic Training
BAMA	British Alternative Medicine Association
BANMA	British Alternative Nutritional Medicine Association
BAWA	British Association of Western Acupuncture
BCA	British Chiropractic Association
BCh	Bachelor of Surgery
BCMA	British Complementary Medicine Association
BDA	British Dietetic Association
BEd	Bachelor of Education
BIAT	British Institute of Allergy Therapists
Bio-MA	Bio-Magnetic Association
BM	Bachelor of Medicine
BMA	British Medical Association
BMAS	British Medical Acupuncture Society
BNA	British Naturopathic Association
BRA	British Reflexology Association
BRCP	British Register of Complementary Practitioners
BS	Bachelor of Surgery
BSAEM	British Society for Allergy and Environmental Medicine
BSANM	British Society for Allergy and Nutritional Medicine
BSc	Bachelor of Science
BSc (Hons)	Bachelor of Science, Honours
BSENM	British Society of Environmental and Nutritional Medicine
BSI	British Society of Iridologists
BSMDH	British Society for Medical and Dental Hypnosis
BSNM	British Society for Nutritional Medicine
BTech	Bachelor of Technology
CBiol	Chartered Biologist

CCAM	Council for Complementary and Alternative Medicine
CertEd	Certificate of Education
CertHealthEd	Certificate of Health Education
ChB	Bachelor of Surgery
CHM	Certificate in Herbal Medicine
CHNH	College of Herbs and Natural Healing
CIA	Colonic International Association
CSK	Certificate in Systematic Kinesiology
DA	Diploma in Aromatherapy
DAc	Doctor of Acupuncture
DC	Doctor of Chiropractic (British Chiropractic Association)
DCH	Diploma in Chinese Herbalism
DCHM	Diploma in Chinese Herbal Medecine
DCM	Diploma in Chinese Medicine
DCN	Diploma in Clinical Nutrition
DHD	Diploma in Dietary Healing
DHH	Diploma in Holistic Health
DHom	Diploma in Homoeopathy
DipAc	Diploma in Acupuncture
DipCNS	Diploma from Centre for Nutritional Studies
DipDTh	Diploma in Dietary Therapy
DipFDZ	Diploma from the Federation of Danish Reflexologists
DipIFR	Diploma in International Federation of Reflexologists
DipION	Diploma from Institute for Optimum Nutrition
DipISM	Diploma Institute of Stress Management
DipISPA	Diploma from the International Society of Professional Aromatherapists
DipNatMed	Diploma in Natural Medicine
DipNut	Diploma in Nutrition
DipNutCouns	Diploma in Nutritional Counselling
DipPhyt	Diploma in Phytotherapy
DipPsych	Diploma in Hypnosis and Psychotherapy
DIrid	Diploma in Iridology
DLI	Diploma in Lymphatic Irrigation
DNMed	Diploma in Nutritional Medicine
DO	Doctor of Osteopathy
DSc	Doctor of Science
DTD	Dietary Healing Diploma
DThD	Dietary Therapy Diploma
FBM	Foundation of Biological Medicine
FICGT	Fellow of the Institute of Crystal and Gem Therapists
FNIMH	Fellow of the National Institute of Medical Herbalists

FRCP	Fellow of the Royal College of Physicians
FRCS	Fellow of the Royal College of Surgeons
GCRN	General Council and Register of Naturopaths
GCRO	General Council and Register of Osteopaths
GNI	Guild of Naturopathic Iridologists
GP	General Practitioner
HAR	Holistic Association of Reflexologists
HPA	Health Practitioners Association
IACT	International Association of Colour Therapists
IAHP	Inter-Association of Healthcare Practitioners
IAPM	International Academy of Preventative Medicine
IAT	Institute of Allergy Therapists
ICAK	Institute of Complementary Applied Kinesiology
ICM	Institute of Complementary Medicine
IFA	International Federation of Aromatherapists
IFADip	Diploma from the International Federation of Aromatherapists
IFR	International Federation of Reflexologists
IOB	Institute of Biology
ISPA	International Society of Professional Aromatherapists
ITEC	International Therapy Examination Council
KF	Kinesiology Federation
KFRP	Kinesiology Federation Registered Professional
LCH	Licentiate in Homoeopathy
LCPH	College of Practical Homoeopathy (Midlands)
LCSP	London & Counties Society of Psychotherapists
LDS	Licentiate in Dental Surgery
LicAc	Licentiate in Acupuncture
LMSSA	Licensed in Medicine by the Society of Apothacaries
MA	Master of Arts
MAc	Master of Acupuncture
MAR	Member of the Association of Reflexologists
MAVR	Member of the Association of Vacuflex Reflexologists
MB	Bachelor of Medicine
MBRA	Member of the British Reflexology Association
MBRI	Member of the British Register of Iridologists
MBSR	Member of the British Society of Reflexologists
MC	McTimoney Chiropractor
McC. Soc	McCarrison Society
MCHNH	Member of the College of Herbs and Natural Healing
MCIA	Member of the Colonic International Association
MCO	Member of the College of Osteopaths

MCrOA	Member of the Cranial Osteopathic Association
MCSP	Member of the Chartered Society of Physiotherapists
MD	Doctor of Medicine
MEd	Master of Education
MFDZ	Member of the Federation of Danish Reflexologists
MFHom	Member of the Faculty of Homoeopathy
MH	Master Herbalist
MHMA	Member of the Herbal Medicine Association
MHMA (UK)	Member of the Homoeopathic Medical Association (UK)
MHPA	Member of the Health Practitioners Association
MIAT	Member of the Institute of Allergy Therapists
MIBiol	Member of the Institute of Biology
MICRA	Registered Member of College of Iris Ananlysis
MIFA	Member of the International Federation of Aromatherapists
MIFR	Member of the Interantional Federation of Reflexologists
MIIR	Member of the International Institute of Reflexology
MIPC	Member of the Institute of pure Chiropractic
MIr	Master Iridologist
MISPA	Member of International Society of Professional Aromatherapists
MMCA	Member of the McTimoney Chiropractic Association
MNCA	Member of the Nutrition Consultants Association
MNIMH	Member of the National Insitiute of Medical Herbalists
MNS	Member of the Nutrition Society
MPhil	Master of Phliosophy
MRCGP	Member of the Royal College of General Practitioners
MRCP	Member of the Royal College of Physicians
MRCS	Member of the Royal College of Surgeons
MRN	Member of the Register of Naturopaths
MRO	Member of the Register of Osteopaths
MRPharmS	Member of the Royal Pharmaceutical Society of Great Britain
MRS	Member of Reflexologist Society
MSc	Master of Science
MTAcS	Member of the Traditional Acupuncture Society
NCA	Nutrition Consultants Association
NCP	National Council of Psychotherapists
ND	Doctor of Naturopathy
NFSH	Natitonal Federation od Spiritual Healers
NHN	Natural Health Network
NHP	Natural Health Practitioner
NIMH	National Institute of Medical Herbalists
NMS	Natural Medicines Society

NutCert	Certificate of Nutrition
OHN	Occupational Health Nurse
PhD	Doctor of Philosophy
RCGP	Royal College of General Practitioners
RCHM	Register of Chinese Herbal Medicine
RCT	Registered Colonic Therapist
RCTh	Registered Celloid Therapist
RGN	Registered General Nurse
RIr	Registered Iridologist
RNT	Register of Nutritional Therapies
RS	Reflexologists' Society
SCM	State Certified Midwife
SHL	Society of Homoeopaths Licenciate
SMDH	Society of Medical and Dental Hypnosis
SNC	Society for Nutritional Councillors
SRN	State Registered Nurse
TAS	Traditional Acupuncture Society

INDEX OF PRACTITIONERS